2-WEEK
TOTAL
BODY WITHDRAWN
TURNAROUND

The 14-Day Plan That Jumpstarts
Weight Loss, Maximizes Fat Burn, and
Makes Over Your Fitness Mindset Forever

CHRIS FREYTAG
With Alyssa Shaffer

AND THE EDITORS OF
Prevention.

RODALE

PHOTOGRAPHS ON PAGES
96, 97, 134, 176, 202, 246, 276, 318
© Shay Peretz

PHOTOGRAPHS ON PAGES
xiv, 17, 27, 32, 40, 97, 135, 177, 203, 247, 277, 319, 338, 341, 348, 351, 374, 379
© Tim Pearson

PHOTOGRAPHS ON PAGES
42–47, 63–73, 80–91, 100–111, 118–129, 137–147, 154–165,
182–195, 206–218, 226–239, 256–269, 280–293, 300–313, 359–365
© Karen Pearson

BOOK DESIGN BY Donna Agajanian

Library of Congress Cataloging-in-Publication Data
Freytag, Chris.
    2-week total body turnaround : the 14-day plan that jumpstarts weight loss, maximizes fat burn, and makes over your fitness mindset forever / Chris Freytag.
        p.   cm.
    Includes bibliographical references and index.
    ISBN-13 978–1–60529–862–7 direct hardcover
    ISBN-10 1–60529–862–X direct hardcover
    ISBN-13 978–1–60529–863–4 trade paperback
    ISBN-10 1–60529–863–8 trade paperback
    1. Reducing exercises—Popular works.   2. Reducing diets—Recipes—Popular works.   I. Title.   II. Title: Two week total body turnaround.
RA781.6.F72   2009
613.7'12—dc22   2008047535

Distributed to the trade by Macmillan

    4   6   8   10   9   7   5   3   hardcover
2   4   6   8   10   9   7   5   3   1   paperback

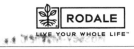

We inspire and enable people to improve their lives and the world around them
For more of our products visit **rodalestore.com** or call 800-848-4735

FOR MY FAMILY,
WHO LIVE AND BREATHE IT
WITH ME EVERY DAY ☺

—CHRIS FREYTAG

FOR MY MOTHER, BONNIE,
WHO TAUGHT ME EVERY STEP FORWARD
IS A STEP TOWARD SUCCESS

—ALYSSA SHAFFER

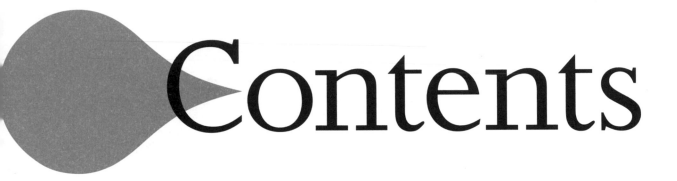

Contents

PART I: **PREPARE**
Get Ready for Success

PART II: **ACHIEVE**
Make It Happen Day-by-Day

PART III: **MAINTAIN**
Make It Last for Life

A big thank-you goes to the 2-Week Total Body Turnaround Test Panel: Linda Agnes, Terrie Allen, Laurie Champ, Donna Crotteau, Julie Frothingham, Nancy Haley, Shelley Jacobs, Michele Kerlin, Michelle Knapek, Kelly Liddle, Linda Madden, Dene Maloney, Roxanne McCain, Teresa McDonald, Tami McKibben, Colleen O'Neil, Cindy Pariseau, Sue Purkat, Joann Quackenbush, Anne Randall, Seleta Randle, Dee Rasmusson, Kim Regenhard, Barb Rustad, Jane Starman, Roxanne Sinkie, Michelle Skrypec, Maria Slavens, Stephanie Teig, Diane Von Bank. You proved to me and yourselves

ACKNOWLEDGMENTS

that this program is for real. Each and every one of you has inspired me to share this jumpstart with everyone willing to try! Your continued success makes me proud.

A big thank-you to my husband and kids, who support and participate in my quest to share the knowledge of health and fitness with others. I know my kids will always remember that a glass half full is better than a glass half empty. Of course, a thank-you to my parents, who taught me that success is the sum of hard work and passion.

To Alyssa Shaffer, my coauthor and friend, who was a rock star partner in this project. Your talent as a journalist, dedication to the project, and friendship are much appreciated.

To my editor, Andrea Au Levitt, who got behind the project with excitement. Your guidance and advice have been valuable.

I am grateful to Leah McLaughlin and Liz Vaccariello for being so supportive of this project. A big thank-you to the rest of the fabulous *Prevention* team— Donna, Rosalie, and Rebecca—you amaze me with your creativity and hard work! And big hugs to Kim, Kate, and Shelby, who keep me organized and on task in the office.

And finally, thank you to everyone else who has touched this book—photographers, stylists, friends, and *Prevention* family—you are wonderful.

Stay Healthy,

Chris Freytag

WELCOME!

"Every accomplishment starts with the decision to try."

—*Anonymous*

Let's Get Started

Sometimes all you need to light a fire is a little spark. Consider this book your own personal ember—the firestarter you need to get back on track to a sleeker, healthier body and a happier you. The 2-Week Total Body Turnaround will help you rev up your metabolism, blast calories, and drop inches everywhere (especially in your belly) in just 14 days. But more importantly, it will provide a jumpstart to help get you back on the path to a lifetime of healthy habits that will last.

Two weeks certainly doesn't sound like a lot of time. But in just 14 days, this exclusive program—tried and tested with women just like you—will help you regain your energy, increase your endurance, and feel stronger and more confident than ever.

This program is based on my 17-plus years in the health and fitness industry as a personal trainer and coach, group fitness instructor, weight management consultant, and motivational speaker. I've worked with hundreds of women of all ages and shapes, and over the years I've come to learn that women need a program that is realistic to follow with a busy schedule, will yield results quickly, and will motivate them to stay with it for the long haul.

Do You Need a Turnaround?

We've all had times when we need a little push in the right direction. Maybe you're someone who had always been active, but got sick or injured and had to take a break. Perhaps you took a vacation and couldn't get motivated to start moving again, or became so swamped at work or busy with family obligations that even the idea of lacing up your shoes and squeezing in a workout seemed impossible. Or maybe you've just succumbed to one of any other dozens of distractions that have kept you from exercising regularly or eating right, and fell naturally into inertia.

What if you've never been very active? Former exercisers aren't the only ones who will benefit from this program. If you have been planted on the couch for so long that just getting off it seems like way too big a barrier to get past, you've come to the right place. You won't stay sedentary for long after reading through this book, which is loaded with dozens of stay-motivated tips designed to get you moving and keep you moving.

And even frequent exercise enthusiasts need help: If you're stuck in a rut that you can't climb out of or are just plain bored with your current program, consider this your prescription for a mind/body makeover. Over the course of the next 2 weeks, you'll revitalize your routine, break through a plateau, and jumpstart your way to real, measurable results.

2 Weeks for Lasting Change

No matter what your situation, the 2-Week Total Body Turnaround is designed to help you feel revitalized, confident, and stronger than ever. We all know the myriad benefits of working out, from combating diabetes, heart disease, and cancer to building strong healthy bones, fighting stress, and boosting your mood. I'm here to help you get started in achieving all of these benefits and more.

Of course, it also helps when the changes you see are a lot more immediate. And there's nothing more gratifying than having your pants feel a little looser, or the needle on the scale slip down a few numbers. When I first came up with this program, I knew it was going to be successful,

"Tell me and I'll forget.
Show me and I'll remember.
Involve me and I'll understand."—Confucius

because it puts together everything I've known to be true about losing weight and making a change for a healthy lifestyle—targeted strength moves, fat-blasting cardio exercise, smart eating tips. But I was eager to put it into action to see how it worked on "real people," just like you. So I recruited a test panel of 30 women who were at a stage of their lives when, for various reasons, they felt they really needed to make a change. Some stories may sound familiar: A few never lost the baby weight from nearly a decade ago; others started new, stressful jobs and hadn't had time to fit in exercise or were simply balancing the demands of family and everyday life. Others said they'd just been slowly accumulating pounds each year, and hadn't realized how heavy or out of shape they had become.

Some had moving stories from the start: widows who had gained weight since losing their spouses, breast-cancer survivors who put on extra pounds with each chemotherapy treatment, a mother who used food for comfort when coping with a sick child, a patient who went into early menopause following a hysterectomy. Some were motivated by upcoming vacations, others by the thought that they just wanted to be in shape for themselves and their families.

Their results were more than just awesome—they were awe-inspiring. In just 2 weeks, they lost an *average* of nearly 6 pounds and 10½ inches, with some losing as much as 12 pounds and more than 22 inches! They unanimously reported that their energy levels soared, they slept better, and they simply felt stronger and healthier. And they even continued to burn more calories all day long, even at rest. But perhaps even more importantly, they discovered newfound confidence in themselves and in what they could achieve when they set out to make a difference in their lives and their health.

What to Expect

So what exactly will you be doing over the next 14 days? I promise you won't be spending hours a day in a boot-camp-like program pounding out hundreds of situps and pushups or going into a starvation-mode diet where bread and pasta are your enemies. Instead, what you'll find is a realistic, research-based program that builds muscle, burns fat, and boosts your metabolism in just 1 hour a day.

Each day you'll follow a clearly laid-out plan to help you tone up and lose weight. You'll do an hour of exercise each day, with a combination of strength and cardio. My signature strength-training exercises—tried-and-tested to be among the most effective ever—will firm up all of your major muscle groups in just 30 minutes a day. You'll alternate your focus between upper body plus core, lower body plus core, and total body moves with each workout. In addition, you'll spend 30 minutes each day with my do-anywhere walking program, which will rev up your daily calorie burn. You'll also have a full day of active rest and recovery each week. If weight loss is a primary goal, I recommend you follow the no-deprivation, customized diet, which will have you sampling a wide range of delicious foods that will fit into everyone's taste and budget. This diet features a sensible mix of carbohydrates, protein, and fat, with three healthy meals and two snacks built into your day so you never go too long without eating or allow yourself to get too hungry. Plus, the program was designed to mesh perfectly with the exercises you'll be doing, so your body will be ideally fueled for activity each and every day. You'll learn what to choose, what to avoid, and how to make smart choices when it comes to getting results that last.

The third, and equally important, part of the plan has to do with mental fitness. I tell my clients: Motivation gets you started; habit keeps you going. Fifty percent of getting into shape is mental. It's about connecting the brain with the program, and melding together willpower, motivation, and focus. I'll give you all the tips and strategies you need over the next 2 weeks to get you started and feeling energized with my "Turnaround Tips" and secrets of positive self-talk, plus fail-proof ways to keep feeling strong and form a habit of healthy living. Keep this book with you and refer to it whenever you need a little reminder of all that you can accomplish if you just set your mind to it!

For a sneak peek at your total program, take a look at the chart on page 320. You can also use the chart as a handy reference once you've mastered all the exercises.

The Tao of 2 Weeks

Why did I choose 2 weeks as the focal point for this plan? I wanted to pick a length of time that was short enough to be completely doable, yet long enough to provide measurable results. Two weeks is enough time to see real changes in your body and your outlook—the kind that will keep you coming back for more. I'm not going to tell you that you won't be working here: Real success does entail real work. But along the way you'll have plenty of fun and find results you never dreamed were possible in such a short amount of time.

For 2 weeks—14 days—I'm going to tell you exactly what exercises to do, what to eat, and how to stay motivated from the time you wake up until you get some much-deserved rest. I'll start with a quick fitness assessment so you can find the exercises most appropriate for your level. Then I'll get into the plan specifics and how to make it work into your schedule, no matter how busy it may be. Finally, I'll tell you exactly what to expect from the program, from how to handle slight muscle soreness (don't worry . . . it's a good thing!) to the best foods to eat before and after exercise. After just a few days, you'll already start to feel more confident and energized. By the end of Week 1, you'll feel stronger and more powerful. After Week 2, you'll see noticeable weight loss—your clothes will feel looser and you'll feel lighter, healthier, and totally recharged!

2 Weeks to Commit, a Lifetime to Be Fit!

Every person coming into this plan may have a different goal in mind. You might have a special event such as a wedding or a beach vacation and feel you need to fast-track your results with a dedicated exercise and diet program. That's one way to find big success in a short time. After the 2 weeks are up, you may want to repeat the program to continue your weight-loss

REAL TURNAROUND SUCCESS STORY
"I see real changes everywhere in my body."
DIANE VON BANK

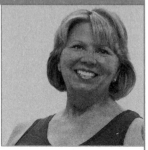

HALFWAY INTO HER 2-WEEK Total Body Turnaround, Diane noticed something different about the way her pants were fitting. "Because there was less fat on my butt and thighs, the hem of my favorite dress slacks was dragging on the floor!" A day or so later, she noticed that her cheekbones were looking much more pronounced. By the end of her 2-week plan, her arms grew more defined. After 14 days, she'd lost more than 5 pounds and 9 inches. "My husband tells me he can feel the difference every time he hugs me!" she exclaims.

When she started the program, Diane had slowly been accumulating extra pounds over the years. Shoulder surgery in the summer turned her into a couch potato by the time fall came around, and she worried about what the next 10 years would bring. Seeking something that would give her both structure and accountability, she signed up to try the Turnaround plan.

She immediately liked the balanced nature of the plan, with its emphasis on both clean eating and exercise, and in its easy way of splitting half of the workout into cardio and half into strength. Despite a busy work and travel schedule, she made exercise her priority. "I preplanned easy dinners so I could fit in my workout and still have time to wind down before bed, and made my lunch the same time I prepared dinner so it wouldn't get forgotten in the next day's morning rush." Sunday evenings were spent cleaning and chopping vegetables and fruits for the work week, so she could easily prepare salads and lunch boxes. And she relished the bite-size nature of the plan itself. "You can do almost anything for 2 weeks—it doesn't feel like such a mountainous task, and you get rewarded with results for your efforts. I like the idea of doing 2 weeks, then 2 weeks again and again. Life is really full of special events. This 2-week jumpstart was the perfect way to start down that path."

and fitness success, perhaps with a slightly more modified version (for details on entering a maintenance phase, see page 379). Or you can keep coming back to the 2-Week Total Body Turnaround as a way to jumpstart your weight loss every 6 weeks or so. You can also continue to pull some of your favorite elements from the book—my body-changing strength moves, my endorphin-boosting interval plans—into your now-regular fitness routine. But I hope you will see the 2-Week Total Body Turnaround as the key to establishing long-term healthy habits. Think of it as a guidebook for fitness, healthy eating, and motivational success for the rest of your life!

How Do I Know It Works?

I'm confident that if you follow this plan, you will have a jumpstart on your health and fitness and get results you never thought possible in such a short amount of time, without resorting to extreme measures of diet or exercise. But don't just take my word for it: Throughout this book, you'll "listen in" to what our test panel had to say through each and every day of the plan. You'll hear what they loved and what they felt was a struggle, albeit a worthwhile one that helped them complete every step of the program. Their stories will inspire you along the way. Remember, you are not alone!

Just the Beginning

What about after the 2 weeks are up? As I mentioned earlier, there are many ways to use this program to get the results you want. If you liked the challenge and want to continue seeing amazing results, repeat! This plan is so packed with innovative exercises and sensible, effective eating tips that you could do it consistently for months on end.

But if you don't have the time to devote to the complete program going forward, I'll give you the next steps you need to take to continue making forward progress and propel yourself into a lifestyle that works. Consider this the beginning of a long and happy relationship with your body. It's a 2-week plan that will turn around your attitude, your exercise program, your eating habits, and your life.

Ready to begin?

"To realize your true potential . . . move away from your comfort zone and work in uncharted land."—*Kevin C. Hall*

PREPARE

"Ability is what you're capable of doing.
Motivation determines what you do.
Attitude determines how well you do it."
—Lou Holtz, *legendary football coach*

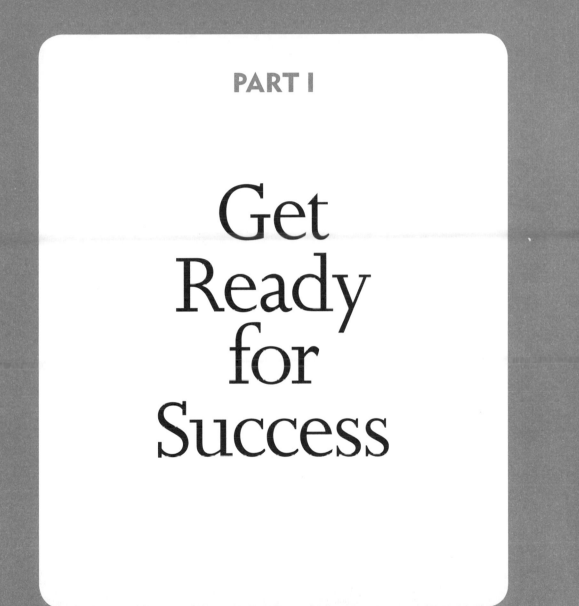

PART I

Get Ready for Success

Time to Turn Things Around

Congratulations! Now that you've decided to make a commitment to yourself, it's time to get started! This chapter will give you all the information you need to get moving in the right direction, so you don't miss a single benefit from completing the 2-Week Total Body Turnaround plan.

I Love Mondays

No, I'm not crazy: I love Monday because it represents a fresh start, and it's the perfect time to get your 2-Week Total Body Turnaround under way! Of course, you can start your 2-Week Total Body Turnaround any day of the week, but I strongly recommend making Monday your first day.

Numerous studies from around the world have shown that health-related issues—strokes, heart attacks, accidents/injuries, etc.—occur more often on Mondays than any other day of the week. So you might think of Monday as a bit of a downer. But hear me out: Monday can also be looked at as an opportunity to make the simple changes you need in order to live a healthier, happier life.

Leaders in the field of public health, including experts at Columbia University Mailman School of Public Health and Johns Hopkins Bloomberg School of Public Health, agree: Together with Syracuse University Newhouse School of Public Communications, they've created a campaign called "Healthy Monday." Its primary purpose is to dedicate each and every Monday as a day of health—a time when we can take action to establish healthier behaviors, whether it's losing weight, beginning an exercise routine, stopping smoking, eating more healthfully, and so on. They've teamed up with some big health organizations such as the American Cancer Society and the American Heart Association, with the idea of promoting Mondays as a day to get people to cut calories, drink less, and get their butts off the couch! Their motto: "Monday is the day all health breaks loose! A great day to do healthy, go healthy, be healthy."[1]

I've been doing a special "Motivation Monday" segment on the local NBC affiliate in Minneapolis for years—it's a tradition for my viewers to get motivated to be their very best on Monday!

I also like Monday as the start day for your plan because it's clean and simple: It's the time when most of us go back to work, our kids go back to school, and mail starts up again. Just like Friday begs the question, "What am I going to do this weekend?" Monday is the natural day to ask yourself: "What's going on this week?" On Monday, we typically take stock of all the things we have in store for the week—upcoming activities, grocery shopping, appointments, ball games . . . you get the idea. It's a fresh start each and every week, a new beginning 52 times a year! I love the idea of Monday as a trigger date for your weekly goals, efforts, and dreams.

And a trigger date like this is important: Studies have shown that when subjects have a regular reminder or cue, they're more likely to take action when it comes to their health, whether it's participating in breast self-exams or cervical-cancer screenings or keeping up with immunization schedules. Sure, you can resolve to be healthier, exercise more, and eat less when New Year's comes around. Unfortunately, nearly half of us will fail to keep those resolutions by the time February 1 rolls around. So if you end up having a burger and fries over the weekend or missed a few workouts during the week because you were way too busy, tired, or sick to fit them in, use the following Monday to get back on track. After all, Monday comes around every 7 days, so you never have to wait too long to get moving again!

Mondays also make sense for another practical reason: You can use the weekend as a time to prepare yourself. Don't worry, you don't have to spend a small fortune equipping your home or devote hours to getting ready. But spending just a little time over the weekend to help prepare yourself mentally and physically will greatly help to make the next 2 weeks go smoothly. Whether it's going to the grocery store and making some smart food choices for your family or planning out your week of workouts, the weekend is a perfect time to get ready for the fantastic changes that lie ahead!

Outfit Yourself for Activity

The beauty of the 2-Week Total Body Turnaround is that you don't need a lot of fancy equipment to get a great workout. All of the moves we give here can be done with simple dumbbells, or, in some cases, even your own body weight. You may also need some common household items, such as a sturdy

GOOD TO KNOW

Optimism not only helps you stay the course, it can also keep you healthier! Researchers from the University of California, Los Angeles, found that healthy first-year law students who were confident they would do well in school were not only happier, they also had a better-functioning immune system than students who were negative about their own performance.[2]

GOOD TO KNOW

Having a clear goal is a great way to keep on track for success. Researchers at the University of Iowa found that men and women who wrote down specific goals about diet or physical activity were more likely to follow through on their plans than those who had a general weight-loss goal or no clear game plan.[3]

chair. If you don't already have them, hit the sporting-goods store or fitness department at your local retailer and invest in at least two sets of dumbbells, one that's a light to medium weight (say, 3 to 5 pounds), and one that's a heavier weight (like 8 to 10 pounds). Use the section "Determine Your Starting Point" (beginning on page 8) to help determine which size weights you should buy.

In addition to the muscle-sculpting strength moves you'll be doing with the dumbbells, you'll also be doing a daily dose of cardio exercise. We recommend walking, which we'll explain a bit more in the next chapter. And while the beauty of walking is that you can do it almost anywhere, without any major equipment, you should invest in a pair of comfortable walking shoes to see you through the length of this program and beyond. Choose a style that fits you best and provides you what you need in terms of comfort and support. Some walkers prefer running shoes, which tend to have a bit more cushioning, but the flip side is that sometimes running shoes are overbuilt, which can make your shins feel stressed and tender. A walking shoe should be flexible enough that it will bend and twist through the middle. As you walk, you'll land on your heel and then push off onto your toes, so you want the shoe to flex with you. You'll also need a style that has a relatively flat heel to give you a smooth stride.

Once you've got your footwear settled, make sure you have appropriate clothes to exercise in. Cotton is great, but for comfort, there's no beating moisture-wicking fabrics like Coolmax or Dri-Fit, which help keep sweat away from your skin so you don't get all cold and clammy. You'll also avoid chafing. If you choose to walk outdoors, eliminate any excuses (rain clouds, anyone?) by dressing for unexpected weather, which means wearing a moisture-wicking inner layer, an insulated middle layer (for cooler weather), and a water-resistant outer layer. No matter where you walk, make sure you have a supportive sports bra and sweat-wicking socks to keep you comfortable with every step.

Get Your Mind On Board

It can also be helpful to use the weekend before your 2-Week Total Body Turnaround kickoff to organize your thoughts, as well as your cupboards and gear. Take a few moments to write down exactly what it is that you want to accomplish over the next 2 weeks. What has brought you to this point? What do you see yourself doing when the 2 weeks are over? Commit to yourself now that you are going to see the next 2 weeks through to completion. On the next page, write down any obstacles that you think might thwart you, then determine how you will best sidestep them.

I really consider this one of the most important parts of your 2-Week

My Commitment Contract

I am starting this program on this day _____

Because _____

_____

_____

_____

At the end of 2 weeks I want to feel _____

_____

_____

_____

When the 2 weeks are over, I will _____

_____

_____

_____

In the past, _____

_____

_____ has typically stood in the way of my accomplishing similar goals.

I will sidestep these obstacles this time by _____

_____

_____

_____

CHECKLIST

I have shared my needs with my family and friends so they can support me. ☐

I have gone to the grocery store and stocked up on healthy foods. ☐

I have checked my calendar to make sure I have 14 days blocked off to commit to this plan. ☐

I have at least one light and one moderately heavy set of dumbbells. ☐

I have a good pair of athletic shoes. ☐

Total Body Turnaround. Look at this time as a chance to "flip the switch," mentally. This is your chance to launch your body and mind into a brand-new place. Everything you do over the next 14 days is important, and your mind needs to be as fully involved as your body. I want you to have this book on your bedside table when you wake up, then bring it with you to the office or carry it around your home, every day. Whenever you need some motivation, open it up and reboot! I'm here to connect with you whenever you need me.

Remember, this program is only 14 days—that's just 2 weeks out of your life. It's all about being specific: small steps, in a set amount of time. Yes, this program is intense—but it's supposed to be. It won't work if you're bored or slightly disengaged. I need your complete attention! Mark 14 days off your calendar, and be accountable to each one. Yes, you will work harder than you ever thought you could, but you'll also feel more powerful than you ever thought you could. Focus on your goals, and you'll be ready to take this to the next stage—the next 2 weeks after the first 2. The finish line of any program is just the beginning of a whole new race, and I'm here to help you prove it.

Women today lead incredibly full lives—we balance work, family, and home. So, things may occur that make everything you set out to do less than perfect. My advice: Strive for progress, not perfection. When you set realistic goals like having more energy, getting a better night's sleep, being in a happier mood, or having a better temperament, then you, just like our test panel, will surely lose inches and pounds. Take the steps you need to live a cleaner life, and weight loss will happen. The bottom line is this: Success is all about how much you care. Do you care? Are you ready? If so, you can become a success story with the 2-Week Total Body Turnaround. I'm proud of you already!

Determine Your Starting Point

I know you're anxious to get these next 2 weeks under way, but before you dive into the program, take some time (maybe this weekend!) to determine your fitness level. You might think you already know where you stand (frequent gym-goer, permanent fixture on the couch, or, more likely, somewhere in between), but by taking some basic fitness measurements, you have an objective starting point. Use these results to track your progress over the next 2 weeks and beyond. You can also use this assessment to help you determine if you should do the challenging (harder) version of the exercise portion of the plan, or whether you should stick with the basic program.

I also like fitness tests because they paint the picture of where you are now—not where you were 10 years ago. You may have been an athlete in high school or ran a marathon in your twenties, but a lot can change over the years, and your body usually doesn't keep up with your mind. I recommend checking yourself again after the 2 weeks are up and then again after 2 weeks, at least until you reach your better-body goals.

These tests were designed to measure some fitness fundamentals, whether aerobic endurance, strength, or flexibility. Fitness, after all, covers a lot of ground. You can be very strong, but still not able to run more than a few blocks. Or you might be able to walk for miles, but be unable to lean over to tie your shoes. There are dozens of different tests out there, but the simplest ones can be the best at helping to establish your baseline fitness level. Take the time to complete each of these before you begin your 2-Week Total Body Turnaround, and then again at the end of the 2 weeks. Check back in with yourself every 2 weeks or so. (We've provided a blank test log for you on page 14 that you can photocopy and reuse as often as you'd like.) I'm counting on you to keep up with your exercise routine. You'll be surprised at how much the numbers change if you stick with your commitment to live healthier!

WHAT YOU'LL NEED: A watch with a second hand or stopwatch, comfortable walking shoes, stairs, a yardstick or tape measure, and some tape.

WALKING TEST

Exercise physiologists often use something called the Rockport Walking Test (named after the footwear company) as a way to help measure aerobic endurance. Basically, it measures how long it takes you to walk a mile at as quick a pace as possible. It's a pretty straightforward routine, and involves one of my favorite activities—walking!

1. Measure out a distance of 1 mile (if you're doing this outside, use the walking maps on Prevention.com, or go to a local track and figure out how many loops you need to do in order to complete 1 mile).

2. Figure out your pre-walk heart rate. Do this after you've rested or sat for awhile. Press your middle and index fingers on the main artery along the middle of either side of your neck and count the number of beats you feel for 10 seconds. Then multiply by 6 to determine the right number of beats per minute.

> **Heart rate before walk:** _____ beats per minute

3. Walk 1 mile as fast as you can. Pace yourself so that you can complete the entire distance. Of course, if you need to rest or stop along the way, that's okay—but remember that the clock needs to keep on ticking!

4. Once you've walked the full mile distance, stop your watch and take note of your complete time. Then immediately take your heart rate a second time.

Time to walk 1 mile: _____ minutes _____ seconds

Heart rate after walk: _____ beats per minute

STAIR CLIMB

This test is a measurement of your maximum aerobic capacity, or VO_2 max. Although it's a little more intense than the 1-mile walking test, it's a good way to help determine just how far you can push yourself.

Climb four flights of stairs (12 to 14 steps each) as fast as you can. If you only have 1 set, run up and then walk quickly down; repeat for a total of 6 times. Record your time and heart rate below.

Time to climb 4 flights of stairs: _____ minutes _____ seconds

Heart rate after climbing: _____ beats per minute

PUSHUPS

The classic pushup is a great way to measure both upper-body strength and muscular endurance, or how long you can do the exercise without getting tired. You'll also be doing pushups in the 2-Week Total Body Turnaround plan, but with a bit of a twist! In the meantime, this will be a good way to "practice" for the 2 weeks ahead!

Begin on the floor on all fours, palms under shoulders, with your head in line with your spine. Bring your knees together and drop your hips so your body is 45 degrees to the floor and a straight line from head to knees. Slowly lower your upper body toward the floor, bending your elbows 90 degrees. Straighten your arms and repeat. Do as many pushups as you can in 1 minute.

Pushups in 1 minute: _____

(Note: For a challenge, try doing this test as a full pushup, with your legs extended behind you and the tips of your toes touching the floor. Just be sure to use the same measurement—full or modified pushup—each time you retest!)

PLANK

Just as pushups measure upper-body endurance, the plank is a good way to determine your core-strength endurance—those all-important abdominal muscles that are so key to everything you do! Yup, you'll be seeing planks on the 2-Week Total Body Turnaround plan as well, but with a fun variation!

Lie face down on the floor, and get into a plank position. Place your forearms on the floor, elbows under shoulders, and keep your legs extended behind you. Lift up, balancing on the balls of your feet and your forearms. Keep your abdominals tight to help support your body weight. Hold here for as long as possible, then record your time.

Time in plank position: _____ minutes _____ seconds

CHAIR SQUATS

Use this test to help evaluate the strength and endurance of your lower-body muscles, especially your quadriceps and glutes. By using a chair, you're able to keep the right form, and also determine just how low you need to squat down (it makes it a lot harder to cheat!). Just use a standard-size chair like a kitchen or desk chair (no wheels!).

Stand a little in front of the chair, feet about hip-distance apart with arms at sides. Bend your knees, sitting back as if you're about to sit in the chair. Let your butt just lightly touch the seat (don't sit all the way down). Keep your weight over your heels, and don't allow your knees to move past your toes. Stand up and repeat. Do as many squats as you can in 1 minute. If you have to stop and rest, that's okay—but keep that watch running.

Squats in 1 minute: _____

SIT AND REACH

This is a classic test to help measure flexibility in the all-too-tight hamstrings and lower back. It looks at how far you can bring your upper body forward while you're seated. Try to do this test after you've warmed up a little (so after the previous aerobic and strength tests, or even after you've just walked in place for a few minutes). As you probably know, it's never a good idea to stretch a cold muscle, because you can injure yourself. It's also helpful if you can have a friend or family member measure your results.

Place the yardstick or tape measure with the zero mark closest to you, and tape it in place at about the 15-inch mark. Sit over the yardstick so it's between your legs, and keep your feet about 12 inches apart, legs straight. Bring your heels even with the tape at the 15-inch mark. Stack your hands, one over the other, middle fingers aligned and pointing forward. Slowly bend forward, being careful not to jerk or bounce your upper body. Slide your fingers along the yardstick as far as possible. Measure how many inches you've moved forward at the farthest point. Repeat the test a total of 3 times and record your best results.

Forward flexibility (best of 3 tries): _____ inches

BALANCE DRILLS

Balance is sometimes called the fourth pillar of fitness, after strength, cardio exercise, and flexibility. It's important in everything you do, especially as you get older. The better balance you have, the less likely you are to fall and get injured—even if it's while doing something as simple as stepping off a curb. Best of all, you'll see changes in your balance very quickly. Just a few minutes a day of exercises that work your balance go a long way toward improving your performance!

Stand tall, feet together, and arms at your sides. Lift your right foot a few inches off the floor, either to the side or behind you. Hold here as long as you possibly can. Record your time and repeat with your left leg.

Next, do this same exercise with your eyes closed. (You'll be surprised at how much more difficult this becomes!) This is a great way to measure your progress as you move forward in the plan.

Single-leg balance, eyes open (right foot): _____ minutes _____ seconds
Single-leg balance, eyes open (left foot): _____ minutes _____ seconds

Single-leg balance, eyes closed (right foot): _____ minutes _____ seconds
Single-leg balance, eyes closed (left foot): _____ minutes _____ seconds

BODY MEASUREMENTS

Numbers on the scale aren't everything when it comes to measuring progress. Another good indicator of how well you're doing when it comes to shedding body fat is to look at how many inches you're losing. It's not hard to determine your starting point: Take a tape measure and measure the circumference of some key points of your body. (To make it more accurate, it's helpful to have a friend or your spouse do this for you; if you go to the gym, you can ask one of the trainers to help, as well.) The women on our test panel were amazed at how quickly their measurements shrank—often 2 or more inches each from their waist, hips, and thighs in 14 days! Often measurements are one of the first things to change on your body, even more quickly than pounds, simply because you may be bloated or dealing with inflammation. You'll be surprised to see how small changes really do add up to big results.

Here are the key areas to measure:

1. Natural waistline (right at your belly button)
Start of 2 weeks_____ end of 2 weeks_____

2. Hips (at the fullest part of butt)
Start of 2 weeks_____ end of 2 weeks_____

3. Right thigh (at the fullest part)
Start of 2 weeks_____ end of 2 weeks_____

4. Left thigh (at the fullest part)
Start of 2 weeks_____ end of 2 weeks_____

5. Chest (around the middle of the bust)
Start of 2 weeks_____ end of 2 weeks_____

6. Calves (at the fullest part)
Start of 2 weeks_____ end of 2 weeks_____

7. Right biceps (at the fullest part)
Start of 2 weeks_____ end of 2 weeks_____

8. Left biceps (at the fullest part)
Start of 2 weeks_____ end of 2 weeks _____

Prepare Yourself: At the Grocery Store

You don't need to make a big investment before starting the 2-Week Total Body Turnaround, but it does help to start the plan on the right foot—which means having what you need in place so there are fewer obstacles in your path. Having plenty of fruits, vegetables, low-fat dairy, and lean meat in your refrigerator and whole grains plus other smart snacks in your cupboard can go a long way toward making sure you don't veer off course once the 2 weeks begin. I'll give you more details about what to eat in Your 2-Week Total Body Turnaround Eating Plan, starting on page 49. But take this weekend as an opportunity to "junk-food proof" your house. If you've ever had to childproof your home, you'll know what this means—think about all those temptations as imminent dangers for your diet, and get rid of them. Clear out the ice cream, chips, and cookies—don't just hide them in your freezer or somewhere in the cupboard where you won't see them.

My 2-Week Success Log

Photocopy this page and fill it out at the end of your 2-Week Total Body Turnaround (and every 2 weeks or so after that) to track your progress.

WALKING TEST

Heart rate before walk: _____ beats per minute

Time to walk 1 mile: ____ minutes ____ seconds

Heart rate after walk: _____ beats per minute

STAIR CLIMB

Time to climb 4 flights of stairs: ____ minutes ____ seconds

Heart rate after climbing: _____ beats per minute

PUSHUPS

Pushups in 1 minute: _____

PLANK

Time in plank position: ____ minutes ____ seconds

CHAIR SQUATS

Squats in 1 minute: ____

SIT AND REACH

Forward flexibility (best of 3 tries): ____ inches

BALANCE DRILLS

Single-leg balance, eyes open: _____ minutes _____ seconds

Single-leg balance, eyes closed: _____ minutes _____ seconds

BODY MEASUREMENTS

1. Natural waistline: _____ inches
2. Hips: _____ inches
3. Right thigh: _____ inches
4. Left thigh: _____ inches
5. Chest: _____ inches
6. Calves: _____ inches
7. Right biceps: _____ inches
8. Left biceps: _____ inches

If your family simply can't live without some treats, try to buy foods they like but that won't tempt you. For example, I, for one, am not at all tempted by Lucky Charms or Chex Mix, but I can eat a whole box of Wheat Thins when stressed. Be sure to avoid your trigger foods, and tell your family about your intentions to begin (and complete!) this program and make a commitment to exercise regularly and eat healthier. Then ask them for their support—many a well-meaning diet has been sabotaged by a spouse or family member who can't help but snack on chips or sweets in front of someone who is trying to lose weight.

Next, make up a list of what you want to eat for the next week or so (you're probably best off making at least two trips to the store to buy fruits and vegetables over the next 14 days so you can ensure that everything is fresh and tasty). You'll read more about what makes a healthy food choice in your 2-Week Total Body Turnaround eating plan, but take some time now to see what makes sense for you.

WHOLE GRAINS: You'll want plenty of healthy whole grains like oatmeal; whole-wheat bread, pasta, or wraps; brown rice; or grains like quinoa or bulgur. Grocery store aisles are teeming with smart grain choices, many of which have a hearty, satisfying taste, are a good source of fiber, and are very filling.

FRUITS AND VEGETABLES: I always try to buy the freshest produce, which often means whatever is in season: root vegetables and citrus fruits like oranges or grapefruit in the winter months, or summer-fresh choices like strawberries, blueberries, peaches, or crisp salad greens. Whatever you pick, try to eat the colors of the rainbow every day: red, like tomatoes or red peppers; green, like broccoli or spinach; purple, like beets or eggplant; orange, like carrots or butternut squash; yellow, like summer squash . . . you get the idea. Most vegetables are rich in vitamins and other important antioxidants; the more variety you have, the more widespread the sources of disease-fighting phytochemicals.

DAIRY: Low-fat dairy is not only tasty and satisfying (hello, who doesn't like creamy yogurt or some yummy cheese?), but it may also be very important if you're looking to lose weight. Studies have found that adults who eat a high-dairy diet have lost significantly more weight and fat than those who consume a low-dairy diet containing the same number of calories.[4] Other research has shown that eating three to four servings of dairy a day is more effective when it comes to dropping pounds than taking calcium supplements or eating calcium-fortified foods.[5] Plus, as you well know, dairy is good for building strong bones. Smart options include low-fat or fat-free milk, yogurt, or cheese, plus other low-fat items like cottage cheese, ricotta, and certain spreads.

PROTEIN: Head for the meat section and stock up on lean meats like sirloin or pork tenderloin, as well as fresh chicken breast or turkey. Go to the seafood aisle for smart choices like tuna, salmon, or shrimp. Not a meat eater? Get your protein fill with tofu, edamame, or other beans. I buy flank steak—a very lean cut—and use a special tool that pokes holes in the meat, so you only have to marinate it for about 15 minutes. It's so easy and fast, and very yummy!

ADDITIONAL CHOICES: To help your body stay satisfied, you'll also need to include some healthy fats in your diet, such as avocados, olive oil, and nuts. Even some peanut butter (opt for the natural kind) can be a great snack in moderation, especially when served with some fruit like an apple or banana or on a slice of whole-wheat bread. Finally, don't forget the water: If you're not a fan of the bottled kind, get a simple filter and use it now, so you have a chilled, full container of water in your refrigerator come Monday morning. I really like flavored water, but you don't have to buy the artificially flavored kind. Add something simple, like cucumbers, strawberries, mint leaves, orange or lime slices, or even pear! Let it sit for a while so the water becomes infused with the flavor. It's incredibly refreshing and a great way to hydrate and feel satisfied with zero calories.

Think Positive

Studies of successful weight loss have shown that in order to achieve long-term success, you need to upend negative thinking patterns. In other words, you need to act healthy to be healthy. So how do you change your behavior to get there? One of the most widely accepted models of behavioral change, known as the scientific-sounding transtheoretical model of behavioral change, says, quite simply, that if you want to establish long-term change, you need to go through five key steps: precontemplation, contemplation, preparation, action, and maintenance.[6]

In the precontemplation stage, most people probably aren't planning on taking any action for the foreseeable future (usually the next 6 months). So just by picking up this book and showing a willingness to establish a change, you've already passed through Stage 1! That means you've entered Stage 2: contemplation. You have an intention to live a healthier lifestyle and plan on jumpstarting it with the 2-Week Total Body Turnaround. But you haven't started yet. What's been holding you back? Maybe you just need that kick in the butt—that's where I come in! I'm here to be both your coach and cheerleader, firm but understanding. I may push you, but you'll also find strength and encouragement, plus the tools to be empowered to push through, stay with it, and prove to yourself that you can do it. Stay tuned for Stage 3: preparation, which is what this chapter is all about. You're about to take action, which means it's time to get ready for the plan to begin by getting the foods you need, the clothes or sneakers, and so on.

I get really excited about Stage 4: action! It all begins on Day 1, when you'll start the exercise program and healthy food plan. Days 1 to 14 are all

REAL TURNAROUND SUCCESS STORY
"I've learned not to use food as a crutch."
SHELLEY JACOBS, 42

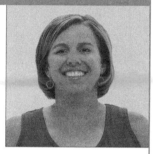

WHEN HER SON COLE was born, Shelley and her husband thought he just had a bad case of jaundice. But doctors soon discovered that her infant had a serious liver disease that caused his bile ducts to become blocked, so his body was slowly poisoning itself. Emergency surgery unblocked the ducts, but Cole was placed on a transplant list and will eventually need a new liver.

"There was a moment in the hospital where my mom said to me, 'You need to eat to take care of yourself and be strong,' and I think something in my brain clicked. Suddenly food became a stress relief."

Although Cole did miraculously well after his diagnosis, Shelley, 42, says she'd gotten to the point where she was no longer taking care of herself. Over the past few years, other stresses—struggling with secondary infertility leading up to the birth of her daughter, Courtney, now 4; coping with a single income when she quit her job to stay at home with her children; taking Cole, now 8 and still awaiting a liver transplant, to various doctors—meant more poor eating choices and less time to exercise, until she realized that at 5 feet 3 inches and about 165 pounds, she needed to lose at least 30 pounds to get back into good health.

The structure of the plan, she says, has helped her get excited again about exercise and her choices. "I feel so much better about myself. For the first time in a long time, I feel like I'm in control again." In the 2 weeks on the program, she dropped almost 5 pounds and 9 inches, including more than 2 inches off her waist. "These little changes have made me want to work harder to see larger ones," she notes.

Perhaps even more importantly, she says, being on the plan has greatly helped to reduce her stress levels. "The other day I was really impatient with my children, and I realized later that I hadn't exercised that day. It made me appreciate that exercising regularly really does have an effect on my mood. I think as a mom I get hung up on not exercising because it takes time away from my kids, but it's also not good for my kids to see me unhealthy."

Although she modified the program slightly after the 2 weeks were up, she still tries to work out at least every other day and has kept up her healthy eating choices, serving more fruit to her family and making easy switches like having brown rice instead of white. She says she's still taking things 2 weeks at a time. "This has been a great springboard to help me find a new way of thinking about things. It's all about making the right choices."

about taking action to turn around your lifestyle and institute a lifetime of healthy living. I think you'll find Stage 4 to be one of the most gratifying things you can do for yourself. And then there's Stage 5: maintenance. This stage may not come for some time—you may wish to repeat the 2-Week Total Body Turnaround again and again or modify it based on your needs or schedule. But once you have achieved your goals, this is the phase you'll want to stay in for the long haul—a healthy, happy place that will make you feel good about yourself.

Step Forward

As you will see in the next chapter, the 2-Week Total Body Turnaround takes an integrated approach to helping you take a healthier approach to living. I've been a trainer for almost 20 years, helping people just like you take the steps they need to succeed, and I can tell you that sometimes the hardest thing to do is just to take that first baby step forward and remember that you are going to be making a positive change for life.

On the very first day of the program, Linda Agnes e-mailed me to say, "I'm psyched. I need this!" Linda, age 40, had gained more than 40 pounds over a 2-year period. She told me she was sick of living an unhealthy life and wanted to make a change. On a scale of 1 to 10, she put her motivation level as a 10+ for desire, but a 6 when it came to actually committing to exercising and watching her diet. Her report on Day 2: "This is hard!" But I knew that she could do it, because she was ready to. And she did. In her own words: "I sucked it up, wiped my tears, and powered through to become a new woman!" After the 2 weeks were up, Linda lost an amazing 12 pounds and 16 inches off her body, including 4½ inches from her waist. (Read more about her inspiring story on page 176.)

I'd like to give you a little more detail about what you can expect over the next 14 days before diving into the program. Begin with the understanding that this is something that will not only change your body, but also your entire attitude. You're making a commitment to yourself, and to your family, that you want to think, live, and be healthier. With that in mind, consider this plan not only a physical turnaround, but also a psychological one. What you do and think over the next 2 weeks will have a profound impact on your success both in the near term and in the distant future. Two weeks, when compared to your entire life, is nothing—a mere blip. But when you consider these 2 weeks being the launching point toward eating more healthfully and exercising regularly, the shift is monumental.

Of course, you'll be getting plenty of the physical, as well. In the next

2 weeks you will work every major muscle group (and some not-so major ones!) to the fullest extent, sculpting muscle mass and creating a strong, lean foundation on which you can continue to build in just a half-hour a day. Each day, you'll also be undertaking an energizing 30-minute cardio program that will challenge you to push yourself out of your comfort zone, while at the same time blasting fat and boosting your metabolism. It's not all hard work: I've also built in 2 full rest days where I'll encourage you to be as active as possible, whether it's playing vigorously with your kids or getting up from behind your desk whenever possible.

In addition, for results that are as remarkable as those achieved by our test panel, I recommend following the 2-Week Total Body Turnaround food plan. This simple plan, based on a 1,600-calorie diet, makes it very easy to track exactly what you should be eating, from grains and vegetables to dairy products and healthy fats. Even if you don't follow the food plan to the letter, remember to be aware of your basic diet. If you do every last rep of each exercise and every second of cardio, then go out and eat a half a pepperoni pizza or a pint of premium ice cream, you'll be negating all of your hard efforts. Think of the start of this program as a time to clean up your diet—it's a fresh slate for you and your body, which means everything you put into it and everything you do with it.

Remember, too, that this is not an all-or-nothing approach to life—or even to the next 2 weeks. Two weeks is not a huge commitment, timewise, but you might still have the occasional hiccup—a meeting that runs late and upends your plan to exercise after work, last-minute dinner plans that happen to involve a less-than-healthy eatery, a sick child, or even a case of the sniffles for yourself. (On our test panel, the women had plenty of distractions—graduation parties, birthdays, a daughter who was getting married, business trips, even a cold—but they made it happen!)

If you think you'll need to miss a day of the plan because life throws up a big roadblock, look at our FAST routine in Part III. This 15-minute plan is designed to work every major muscle in your body while also getting your heart rate up so you start to work up a sweat and burn about 135 calories. It's not ideal, especially when you have such a short time to commit to making a difference. But it's better than doing nothing, and it will help you commit to seeing the program through to the end without getting lost or discouraged! Also remember that, while I've tried to provide everything you need to see you through the next 2 weeks, you might need some flexibility. So switch days if you need to: If you have to take a business trip on Day 8, flip it with Day 6. You are in charge here, and I know you can do it!

Get Set to Work It Out!

By now, I hope you're psyched up and ready to go. I know I am! But first, I want to take some time to explain why this program is truly different from other types of exercise plans you may have tried in the past, and why it is scientifically proven to get the results you want.

As a trainer, I see the value of exercise every single day with my clients. It really is a fountain of youth in so many ways. Exercise helps to fight heart disease, cut cancer risk, prevent diabetes, reduce high blood pressure, ward off osteoporosis—the list goes on and on.

Scientists who study these things have shown that if you exercise on a regular basis, you can live a longer, healthier, happier life. One recent study from Finland found that over a 20-year period, men and women who were physically active were up to 21 percent less likely to develop cardiovascular disease or die of any other natural causes.[7] And researchers from the well-respected Framingham Heart Study of more than 5,000 men and women found that active subjects lived almost 4 years longer than inactive ones.[8]

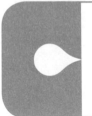

"You can't cross the sea merely by standing and staring at the water."
—Rabindranath Tagore, Bengali poet

So what makes up a good exercise plan? The American Council on Exercise says there are two primary areas you need to focus on in order to live a healthier life: cardio and strength training.

Strength in Numbers

Let's look at the strength part of the equation first. Resistance training is basically strengthening your muscles by moving them against any type of resistance, whether it's with a piece of equipment like a dumbbell or weight stack or even just against your own body weight. Most of us have tried strength training at some point, cranking out some crunches or pushups or even going to a body-sculpting class at the gym. So you likely know that feeling of muscle fatigue you get after repeating an exercise a bunch of times. That's the sign that you're working the muscle to the point that it's getting stronger. And stronger muscles do more than just help you lug a heavy bag of groceries in from the car or carry your child across the room (although that's a key benefit!). Resistance training will increase the amount of lean muscle on your body while helping to decrease the percentage of body fat.

Lifting weights is the fastest way to build muscle. That's important for many reasons, not the least of which is the role muscle plays in metabolism. Muscles are a lot more metabolically active than fat, which basically means that muscle burns more calories at rest than fat. So the more muscle you have on your body, the more calories you'll burn all day long—even when you're just sitting around. It's the golden ticket for weight loss. In one 8-week study, women and men who did only cardio exercise lost 4 pounds but gained no muscle, while those who did half the amount of cardio and an equal amount of strength training shed 10 pounds of fat and added 2 pounds of muscle.[9]

If you add 3 extra pounds of muscle to your body, you'll increase your metabolism by about 7 percent, which means about 100 extra calories burned each day![10] On the other hand, if you're on a diet, you often will lose muscle along with fat, which decreases your resting metabolic rate (RMR), or the minimum amount of calories your body needs to function. Drop your RMR by 20 percent, and that's 300 less calories your body naturally burns a day.

It's also crucial to protect your body against natural muscle loss: Starting in your thirties, women begin to lose about ½ pound of muscle a year. Do the math and you'll see that if you aren't proactive about maintaining your muscle mass, you will be facing some pretty dim statistics. That's one reason the weight starts to sneak on with each decade: Our bodies become less metabolically active, so we are burning fewer calories each year. Since it's the rare person who also cuts back on the amount of calories consumed, that imbalance leads to weight gain—about 3½ pounds a decade. The good news is you don't have to just sit by and let your strength dwindle. If you are consistent, you can achieve noticeable results in as little as 2 weeks!

THE TURNAROUND DIFFERENCE, PART 1: Building Strength

When I set out to design this program, I combed through the research to find the very best way to get maximum results in minimum time through resistance training. Here's what I discovered: It's all in the timing when it comes to "pumping iron." Slowing down to a 6-second repetition (usually 2 counts to lift, 4 counts to lower) has been shown to be among the most effective ways to build muscle strength. There are a couple of key reasons why.

The first one has to do with something called concentric and eccentric training. Simply put, the concentric part of an exercise is when the muscle shortens in length, usually the lifting phase. If you think about a very basic move like a biceps curl, the concentric part of the move is when you curl that weight toward your shoulder. The eccentric part is the lengthening phase—when you lower the weight and straighten your elbow back to the starting position.

Your muscles need to work in both of these phases for optimal growth. But researchers have long known that your muscles are significantly stronger in the eccentric part of an exercise. This has to do with the way the muscle fibers work against resistance as they lengthen. During the eccentric phase, nerve impulses signal motor units to fire, even though there are fewer motor units involved than during the concentric phase. Because fewer fibers are involved, there's more stress on each one. And stress leads to muscle breakdown; the more breakdown you have, the more the muscle has to rebuild, and it's this rebuilding of muscle that gets you stronger. With this program, you're taking more time in the eccentric phase (4 counts) than the concentric one (2 counts) in order to build muscle where you are strongest.

The bottom line is this: Putting an emphasis on the eccentric part of an

"Walking is man's best medicine."
—Hippocrates

exercise is one of the quickest ways to get results. In the eccentric phase of exercise, internal muscle friction increases effective force output by about 20 percent. Numerous studies have found that training with an emphasis on eccentric contractions yields greater strength adaptations than an emphasis on the concentric training. Many experts have pronounced eccentric training as superior to concentric for inducing muscle hypertrophy (the ability to build lean muscle tissue).

Now that your head is probably spinning, what does all this science boil down to? When you put more emphasis on the lowering phase of activity, your muscles are able to work harder, and when they work harder, you get faster results. (You're also preventing gravity from doing some of the work for you, another bonus.)

Want proof this workout works? Let me count the ways:

- In a study from the University of Texas Medical Branch at Galveston, subjects who trained for 5 weeks following a program with a similar concentric/eccentric training emphasis to the 2-Week Total Body Turnaround had nearly twice the strength gains as those who only placed an emphasis on the concentric phase of exercise.[12]

- A study from East Carolina University found that placing an emphasis on the eccentric overload resulted in a 46 percent increase in strength in just 1 week![13]

- A 2007 study published in the *Journal of Strength and Conditioning Research* found women were up to 160 percent stronger in the eccentric phase of an exercise than in the concentric phase over the course of a 2-week testing period.[14]

- A 2007 study from Penn State University found that eccentric training not only significantly increased lean muscle, it also helped improve bone density and bone mineral content among women.[15]

Take Your Time

The second key way the 2-Week Total Body Turnaround strength plan works is the amount of time it takes to do each repetition. No more flying through the workout, whipping the weights around: Slowing the movement down for each repetition of the exercise helps eliminate one of the biggest "cheats" that many of us make during resistance training. When you swing a weight through the air, you're relying heavily on momentum, which will compromise your results. By slowing down the exercise to a 6-second count, you'll eliminate this momentum, so your muscles work harder through the full range of motion.

The longer repetition has another big advantage: You're increasing the amount of time your muscles work under tension. And research has shown that more time under tension equals better results. One study from the *Journal of Sports Medicine and Physical Fitness* found men and women who slowed down the amount of time it took to perform one repetition had about a 50 percent increase in strength after about 8 weeks of training.[17]

One point I'd like to make has nothing to do with research studies or important scientific journals: When you take the time to really slow down and think about every aspect of an exercise, whether you're lifting and lowering a weight or just doing a simple pushup, you're helping to cement the relationship between your mind and your body. Taking your time and counting out each beat of an exercise means you're not just going through the movements: You're getting your brain as involved in the exercises as your muscles, and that will help ensure your success over the course of the next 2 weeks and well beyond.

The "Afterburn" Effect

I have more great news: The strength exercises you do on the 2-Week Total Body Turnaround keep on working for you even after you've finished each workout. You can thank what's known as excess post-exercise oxygen consumption, or EPOC—otherwise known as afterburn. Simply put, this is the amount of extra calories your body continues to burn after a workout is over. Research has shown that a workout that challenges your muscles like the ones you'll do almost every day on the 2-Week Total Body Turnaround *can boost your resting metabolism for up to 36 to 48 hours post exercise.*[18, 19] That means your body continues to burn more calories each and every day of this 2-week period beyond what you're already burning through exercise and daily activity, whether you're taking a shower, reading the paper, or walking the dog. The longer and more intense your exercise plan, the greater and longer the afterburn will be. Research shows that the greatest boost comes in the 2 hours immediately following your workout, and the type of intensity makes a big difference in the level of afterburn. I'll also talk about afterburn as it relates to your cardio exercise in a little bit.

THE TURNAROUND DIFFERENCE, PART 2: Burn Fat with Cardio

Now that we've covered all of the fabulous benefits that you'll get from doing the strength exercises on the 2-Week Total Body Turnaround, let's talk about cardio, a.k.a. aerobic exercise. Cardio is crucial when it comes to burning body fat and excess calories and taking care of your heart. According to the guidelines issued by the American Council on Exercise, both moderate- and vigorous-intensity physical activity will help you reap the benefits; you just have to spend more time if you exercise at a moderate pace than you would at a vigorous one.

Moderate-intensity activity means you're working hard enough to raise your heart rate and break a sweat, but not so hard that you can't carry on a conversation (think: brisk walking). With vigorous intensity, you're working at a rate of near breathlessness, which basically means it's hard to say more than a few words at a time (think: a steady-paced run). If you're short on time, the secret is to work harder, not longer, because you'll burn more calories at a higher intensity. But even being active throughout the day can help add up to more calories burned! (I'll cover that idea a little more in Part II.)

REAL TURNAROUND SUCCESS STORY
"I found my motivation again."
CINDY PARISEAU, 52

SIX YEARS AGO, CINDY considered herself a relatively fit and active person. She was a regular at her local Y's aerobics classes, so much so that at one point she was even asked to become an instructor. But when her son Bill, then 21, was critically injured in a tragic accident, her whole world was turned upside down. "He broke his neck diving off a dock and was left a quadriplegic. For the next 5 years, we devoted our lives to helping him get back on track," she says.

Thanks in large part to the support of his family, Bill finished his degree from the University of Minnesota in a few years and now works in medical technology. But Cindy suddenly found herself without her regular role as a caregiver. "I realized that I had completely lost my fitness routine. I knew I needed to do something but wasn't sure what. When I heard about the 2-week plan, it sounded like the perfect way to get myself started again."

Adding strength training and intervals—two workout components she had never really focused on—made a big difference to Cindy's results. After 2 weeks on the plan, she had shed an amazing 22 inches, including several inches from her hips, waist, and thighs. She also found she had a lot more energy to cope with her job as a construction supervisor for a power company, as well as taking care of Bill's needs.

Even a full year after the plan, Cindy continues to exercise 6 days a week and follow a healthy eating program. "I don't feel deprived or under the gun—I eat what I want but in moderation." She's down about 10 pounds and a full clothing size and remains e-mail buddies with another test panel member for support. But most importantly, she adds, she's found her motivation again. "I'm back to being faithful to my routine. I think I'm even more into it! And I don't see myself going off it again."

Walk This Way

Hands down, my favorite choice of aerobic exercise is walking. Reason #1: It's so ridiculously easy. There's not a lot of equipment to buy, and you've mastered it since you were a toddler. You just lace up your shoes and go. In addition, walking is a low-impact activity, which means it won't hurt your joints or leave you feeling achy or injured. And, best of all, it's backed by dozens upon dozens of studies as being one of the most effective, proven methods of improving fitness and aiding weight loss, in addition to its myriad health benefits. One of the largest of these is the National Weight Control Registry, a group of more than 5,000 individuals who have lost at least 30 pounds and kept the weight off for at least 1 year. Almost 95 percent of the participants reported that, in addition to dietary changes, they lost the weight and kept it off in large part by increasing their physical activity—most frequently by walking.[23]

Blast Away Belly Fat

If you're in the early stages of menopause, or perhaps even fully immersed in "the change," you may have noticed a gradual increase in abdominal pooch—an area health expert Dr. Pamela Peeke has cleverly termed the "menopot." This abdominal fat is largely due to the hormonal changes that occur during the throes of menopause, especially an increase in the levels of a stress-related hormone called cortisol.

Your body releases cortisol whenever you face a stressful situation—heavy traffic, a crazy work deadline, an inconsolable child. Together with adrenaline, it figures into the ancient "fight-or-flight" response, which floods your bloodstream with glucose, fatty acids, and triglycerides. Over time, prolonged exposure to life's daily stresses and all of the chemical reactions they bring about can cause weight gain and fatigue—not to mention numerous other health complaints.

Several studies have linked cortisol with fat storage and weight gain, especially visceral, or deep, fat. All of us have some visceral fat; it helps protect our organs and maintain a core body temperature, and it even acts as a deep energy reserve. But too much visceral fat is associated with high blood sugar, high triglycerides, high cholesterol, and high blood pressure—all of which can lead to cardiovascular disease, diabetes, and stroke.

Now here's the good news: Studies have shown that cardiovascular exercise, like the kind you'll be doing in the 2-Week Total Body Turnaround, can greatly help reduce cortisol levels and the amount of both visceral and abdominal fat.

Walking seems to be especially effective at targeting belly fat. A recent

Japanese analysis of 16 different studies regarding exercise and belly fat found that brisk walking or jogging a minimum of 2½ hours a week (about 20 minutes a day) was enough to reduce belly fat by 1 inch. The greater the amount of aerobic exercise, the better the results![24]

Intervals: The Long and Short of It

Just going out for a leisurely stroll may be fine if you're doing some window shopping, but to really reap all of the benefits of aerobic exercise, you have to focus on the intensity of your walk. And there's no better way to do this than by doing intervals. You may already be familiar with the idea of interval training—it's gotten quite a bit of attention over the past few years from researchers, trainers, and coaches because it's one of the best ways to maximize your results and improve your fitness level in a minimum amount of time.

Intervals are basically periodic bursts of intensity followed by a recovery period. For example, after warming up for a few minutes, you might walk as fast as you can for 30 seconds to 1 minute, then bring it back down to a moderate pace for another minute. Then repeat! There are many kinds of intervals: Some use speed bursts; some will have you walking up a steep incline, like a hill; some last just a half-minute or so; others can have you huffing and puffing for up to 5 minutes. But what all of these workouts have in common is that they push you out of your comfort zone, then give you a chance to catch your breath before doing it again.

Numerous studies back intervals as being a fantastic way to not only improve your fitness (so you can go longer and stronger), but also to burn more calories and fat than you would if you just headed out for a walk at a steady pace for the same amount of time. One recent study found subjects who practiced interval training burned 36 percent more fat post exercise and improved cardiovascular fitness by 13 percent.[25] And a recent Australian study found that women who exercised at a high intensity for 8 seconds, then recovered for 12 seconds, for a total of 20 minutes, 3 times a week, *lost five times as much weight* as those who exercised 3 days a week for 40 minutes at a steady speed—without making any significant changes in their diets.[26]

Because you're moving out of your comfort zone, intervals will also help you become more aerobically fit, which means you'll be able to burn more calories with each and every workout. One study found that after just 2 weeks of interval training, subjects doubled their endurance levels.[27]

Just like with your strength workouts, doing intervals is also a great way to pump up your afterburn, or your ability to burn fat even after you're done exercising. Although this number is largely dependent on the time and

Walk away from . . . breast cancer.
Women who performed the equivalent of 1¾ to 2½ hours per week of brisk walking had an 18 percent lower risk of breast cancer than inactive women.[28]

Walk away from . . . heart disease.
A landmark study of more than 70,000 nurses ages 40–65 found the more a woman walked, the lower her chances of having a coronary event. Those who walked 3 or more hours a week had a 35 percent less risk compared to those who walked infrequently. Plus, it's never too late to start: Sedentary women who became active when they reached middle age or later had a lower risk of coronary events than their couch-potato counterparts.[29]

intensity of your workout (the longer and harder you go, the higher the afterburn), over time the extra calories do add up. Research has shown that you can burn an extra 65 to 150 calories post workout due to EPOC.[31]

What's that mean in the long run? Say you're burning an average of 100 additional calories, mostly from fat, post workout. According to Dr. Len Kravitz from the University of New Mexico, if you were to exercise 5 days a week, over the course of a year you would burn up to 26,000 calories (5 workouts a week x 52 weeks x 100 EPOC calories), which equals about 7 pounds of fat—and we're not even counting the calories you burn during the exercise itself.

There's another important reason that I love intervals. It brings us back again to the importance of thinking about what your body is doing. So often my clients will tell me they're just going through the motions, doing the same-old 3-mile jog or power walk on the treadmill or outside. They never really push themselves hard enough outside of their comfort zones. When you practice hard/moderate intervals, you'll challenge yourself in a way you might never have thought possible. After all, you might not be able to go out and run hard for a half hour, but if you incorporate small speed bursts into your walk, you're getting your body used to working at a higher intensity. And after a while, your overall effort level is going to feel easier. The only way you are going to see lasting results is to challenge yourself! That's when you are going to experience the addictive endorphin rush that comes with exercise.

Power It Up

So now you know . . . intervals rule! But that doesn't mean interval training is the only type of exercise you should do. I'm also still a big believer in the good old-fashioned steady-paced workout, also known as tempo training. These types of workouts—where you exercise at as challenging a level (about 75 percent of your maximum heart rate) as you can maintain for at least 30 minutes—are also important in helping to build your body's fat-burning engines.

Tempo training improves your aerobic fitness by increasing your lactate threshold, or the point where lactic acid begins to build up in the muscle. This is important for runners, but it also figures in for walkers because it makes you more aerobically efficient. Steady-paced power walks are also important as part of an overall training program because they can provide a bit of a relief from the challenges of an interval workout, so there's less wear and tear on your muscles and joints. That said, I still recommend doing some "mini-bursts" during your power walk to boost results and ensure that you are not just going through the motions.

Turn Your Body into a Fat-Burning Machine

Yes, it's good for your heart, your lungs, and your mind. But if you're interested in losing weight, aerobic exercise is crucial. A 2000 review from Washington University School of Medicine later summarized by Dr. Kravitz found that with regular cardiovascular exercise come a number of changes that help enhance fat metabolism, or your body's ability to use fat for fuel. Dr. Kravitz notes that aerobic exercise:

● Increases the amount of oxygen brought to your muscles through the bloodstream and takes oxygen out of cells through capillaries, helping the cells themselves burn fat more efficiently

● Makes muscle and fat cells more sensitive to the hormone epinephrine, which in turn improves the release of fatty acids into the blood

● Improves circulation, which means fatty acids will get to the muscles for fuel more quickly

● Helps the protein transporters move fatty acids into the muscle cells themselves and increases the amount of fatty acids allowed to enter into the muscle so the fat is more readily available for fuel

● Increases the number and size of cellular mitochondria, which act as the "fat-burning furnace" within cells themselves

● Speeds up the breakdown of fatty acid molecules used during aerobic exercise[32]

Details, Details

Now that you know all about the *why* of the 2-Week Total Body Turnaround, it's time to talk about the *how*. I'm asking you to take the next 14 days and use them as a way to jumpstart your whole system into getting results. You will work hard over the next 14 days—my plan calls for a half hour of cardio and a half hour of strength every day, with a couple of active "off" days. Commit right here and now to shifting your body into "drive," and get ready to go on a journey that will change your life. Everything you need is right here.

Let's start with the strength part of our program. Except for two "off" days (and we'll get into what those are all about a little later), you will be doing some form of strength training each day for the next 2 weeks. I've created a strength program that will challenge every muscle for maximum results in minimum time. How? Through a method called circuit training.

Circuit training has been studied and practiced for decades, but it's only recently come into its own as an extremely time-efficient and effective way

GOOD TO KNOW

You'll get the same aerobic benefits splitting your workout into smaller chunks as one longer, continuous plan. Studies have shown three 10-minute workouts offer the same fitness and health benefits as one 30-minute one.[33]

to build muscle while keeping your heart rate elevated. Unlike traditional strength training, where you'll do each exercise in an extremely precise fashion, say, 2 sets of 12 to 15 reps with a 30- to 60-second rest between each set, circuit training has you moving nonstop. The more you move, the more calories you burn—and the more you can pack into each and every workout! After you finish the given number of reps for each exercise, move onto the next. Ideally, you'll do each strength workout twice through (they're six moves each), which will take about a half hour. However, since

REAL TURNAROUND SUCCESS STORY
"I'm getting healthy again after a heart attack."
COLLEEN O'NEIL, 46

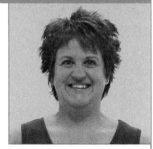

A FEW YEARS AGO, at age 42, Colleen—who exercised regularly, never smoked, drank only occasionally, and had no known history of heart disease—began to feel "funny" while waiting in line at the grocery store. "I just started to feel this odd pressure in my chest, then I felt nauseous, and my arms felt weighted down. I ignored it for a while, but by the time I got home, it had gotten more intense. Finally, my husband and some friends convinced me to go to the emergency room, and, sure enough, they told me I had a heart attack."

Colleen had battled her weight for much of her life, but she felt angry that the heart attack had come when she was actually working out several days a week and watching her diet—and was only about 10 or 15 pounds overweight at the time. "I'm not sure if it was intentional or not, but I quit exercising entirely and started eating more." Her weight crept up little by little until she realized she'd gained nearly 30 pounds. "I just couldn't stay committed to going out and exercising."

Finally, she realized that if she was going to stay healthy, she needed to make a change for the better. "I needed a challenge: Something with a little oomph that would get me going again. I wanted to focus on getting back to where I needed to be, and on making good choices."

After wading through many diet plans in her life, a key difference for her with the 2-Week Total Body Turnaround was the time frame involved. "Knowing I only had to take this 2 weeks at a time meant I wasn't bogged down with the idea of losing a ton of weight. I just focused on the 2 weeks at hand, and then when they were up, the next 2, and so on, and so on."

By the end of her first 2 weeks, her legs looked more toned, her pants felt baggier, and she'd packed up her size 14s. "I refuse to wear them again!" she says. "Packing them up was great motivation to keep going." Although the scale was down only a little more than 3 pounds, she'd dropped nearly 14 inches, including 2 from her waist and 3 from her hips. She's continued to take things 2 weeks at a time, walking every day with a new puppy, taking Spinning classes at the gym, and lifting weights. "I've gotten myself back to a healthy place again. I'm still struggling sometimes to find a balance, but I know I can't give up."

the moves themselves might be new to you, it may take a little longer to learn them, especially during the first few days of the plan. And that's okay. Just try to keep moving throughout the whole strength workout so you're never just sitting around. By Week 2, you'll be doing many of the exercises with balance factors thrown in, so while some of the exercises may be familiar, they will also be more challenging.

You'll certainly feel your heart rate going higher when you go through these strength moves. Recent studies have confirmed that a circuit workout can give an aerobic boost even if you're not doing cardio bursts between sets. Spanish researchers tested a heavy-resistance circuit-training program with minimal rest between sets against a traditional one where subjects rested up to 3 minutes between sets: They found those who did the circuit had a significantly higher average heart rate (about 70 percent of their max; equivalent to a brisk walk or jog) compared with the traditional weight-training group.[34]

Your Strength Plan, Explained

Almost each day for the next 2 weeks, you'll be doing my unique "burn and firm" strength exercises in a circuit that focuses on different areas of the body. I call them this because not only will you feel your muscles burning (think: working!), but you'll also be burning body fat with each workout. One day you might be doing an upper-body circuit, the next day a lower-body one, and the following a total-body workout. This way, one group of muscles will have some time to rest and recover, which we know is the key to getting stronger, while you strengthen other target areas. Each of these workouts will also target the core, so your abs will be getting plenty of exercise! That's because your core is so integral to everything that you do. If your abs and lower back are weak, you won't be able to power through the exercises as effectively, and it can even compromise your aerobic workouts.

Each circuit consists of six exercises. Do them in the order I've given you, moving from one to the next and taking as little rest as possible. Try to do the circuit twice through. If you're learning the moves and it feels like

GOOD TO KNOW

A review of studies by researchers in the Netherlands found that the better your cardiovascular fitness, the more bloodflow goes to the brain. This increases the number of new neural connections, as well as the production of chemicals that carry messages to the nerves—all of which makes you mentally sharper.[35]

"Luck doesn't just happen—luck is preparation meeting opportunity!"

—*Seneca, 1st-century Roman philosopher*

GOOD TO KNOW

To get more out of virtually every resistance exercise, engage your core muscles, especially your deep abdominals (the ones that contract when you're trying to zip up a tight pair of pants). A recent Canadian study found even in basic strength moves like deadlifts and squats, the abdominal and lower back muscles play a significant role. The stronger your core, the better results you'll get all over—not to mention flatter-looking abs![36]

you can only get it done once through, that's okay, at least in the beginning. However, for best results, try to repeat. It should take about 30 minutes.

Start with a weight that feels challenging enough to lift that by the end of the last rep, your muscles really feel like they have been working hard—not so hard that you're experiencing real pain, but also not so easy that you think you could do another 20 reps. For many of the exercises, that might mean a lighter weight for some of the shoulder and arm exercises and a heavier one for those moves that work bigger muscle groups, like the chest and back. Note that if you have lifted weights in the past, you may discover that because the exercises are slowed down, you may have to go with a slightly lighter weight than you are used to (for example, 5 pounds instead of 8).

As you'll see when you go through the plan each day, each exercise is designed with a 6-count rep: 2 counts in the concentric (lifting) phase, and 4 counts in the eccentric (lowering) phase. Remember, with some exercises (like squats and lunges), you might be lowering before you lift. You may not be used to lifting weights this slowly, so take some time to get used to it! Slowing down each exercise with an emphasis on the eccentric phase is crucial to maximizing your results.

The second week of the program offers a more challenging variation of the first, either by adding some balancing element or increasing the amount of weight you're lifting. It's a great way to maximize your results so you get more out of each and every minute of your workout—and beyond! I'm counting on you to challenge your body through each day of the next 2 weeks, and one great way to do this is to shift the emphasis on the exercises that you are doing to those that help with your balance. They place a greater focus on your core, burn more calories, and simply work you harder than you might have thought possible!

Ideally, you'll take on the challenge and do the more intense exercise, but if you simply can't do the move or can't maintain your form properly to complete the slow rep count, I'd rather see you revert to the exercises from the first week. (And hey, do the variation on a third or fourth week!) Without proper form, you not only won't get the full benefits, you also could risk injury, and that's not something anyone wants.

Your Cardio Plan, Explained

Over the next 14 days, you'll also be doing several types of cardio workouts that I've put together. These are some of my favorite routines, based on both the latest research for the most effective exercise plans and also workouts that I have given to my clients with awesome results. I realize you're also doing the strength routine each day, and few of us can spare hours upon hours exercising each day. That's why I've designed each of these workouts to take no more than 30 minutes.

To keep you motivated, I've tried to offer a variety of workouts. Some gradually build in intensity, some use mini speed bursts, and some even incorporate hills or incline. I've suggested a different walking workout to do each day, but keep in mind that you can mix and match them as you wish. If, for example, you don't live in a hilly area, simply substitute another workout for the incline day. You can also do any of these on a treadmill or outside. And if walking is just not your thing, feel free to substitute a different type of aerobic activity that you enjoy more—cycling, using the elliptical machine, stair climber, or rower, even swimming. The most successful exercisers are those who do what they love. So if you would much rather go for a bike ride than lace up your sneakers and walk, hop on! Or if the weather doesn't seem like it's going to cooperate and you have access to a treadmill, keep your workout indoors. That said, if the skies are gray and you don't have a gym or treadmill, don't let that stop you. This is a 14-day plan and every day counts: So put on that rain gear and go outside! A little rain won't hurt you, especially if you dress the part. If the elements really won't cooperate, try walking indoors at the local mall.

The most important part of your cardio workouts is to make sure you are exercising at the right intensity level. There are a few ways to keep tabs on how hard you are working during exercise. I like three: rate of perceived exertion (RPE), talk test, and zone training with a heart-rate monitor. Use them separately or, for best results, all together.

RPE and Talk Test: A Perfect Match

RPE is a well-established training method that researchers have used for decades as a way to help subjects monitor just how hard they are working during exercise. It's pretty straightforward: You are responsible for determining how difficult an exercise feels, on a scale of 1 to 10. Level 1 is the easiest (think: lying with your feet up on the sofa) and 10 the hardest (sprinting to catch the plane before it leaves).

I also really like the "talk test" method. It's pretty much as easy as it sounds: You determine how easy or difficult it is to speak while you're exercising. The more breathless you are, the harder you're working. At a low range of intensity, you can easily chat with a friend; if you're going all out, you might barely be able to grunt a word. Numerous studies have shown this surprisingly simple test is also one of the most effective at validating intensity levels.

The beauty of both RPE and the talk test is that they're super easy to

GOOD TO KNOW

Adding a balance challenge to a strength exercise not only is more practical (the better balance you have, the lower your risk of injury, especially as you get older), it also equals a better workout. When you wobble, you're engaging your abdominal muscles, as well as those on the standing leg (especially your glutes). Result: A better workout for your abs and butt. The good news is that improvements in balance come quickly! In one study, 11 healthy women in their seventies improved their balance by 25 percent over the course of a 5-week training program.[37]

follow and highly individualized—after all, one person's sprint can be another's warmup. But for best results, I recommend using both of these methods together. As you read through each day's cardio workout, you'll see a chart with a corresponding RPE and talk test, but in general, here's how the workout should generally feel during each phase:

RPE	PACE	TALK TEST	FEELS LIKE
1–3	Warmup/cooldown	Chat with ease	You're comfortable
4–5	Brisk	Can speak in full sentences but with some effort	You're running a little late to meet a friend
6–7	Very brisk	Speak mostly in short phrases with some huffing and puffing	You're late for a doctor's appointment
8–9	Power push	Hard to say more than a couple of short words	You're late to meet your boss or pick up your kids
10	Sprint	Can't speak at all	Your plane is about to leave; you can't sustain for more than a minute or so

Have a Heart (Rate)

The third method of determining your exercise intensity is zone, or heart-rate, training. The method is a bit more involved, but it's also among the most personalized and accurate ways to determine your exercise intensity. So if you like gadgets, read on! Heart-rate monitors (which cost about $70 and up) help you keep close tabs on your effort level by monitoring the number of times your heart beats per minute. It acts like a little window into your body's mechanics and helps you determine if you are exercising hard enough, too hard, or at just the right level. One of the best ways to get the most out of this device is to use your heart rate along with your rate of perceived exertion and the talk test—the three together can go a long way toward making sure you're working at the right intensity for results.

Heart-Rate Training 101

Your heart-rate monitor tells you exactly how fast your heart is beating (in beats per minute). But in order for this number to make sense, you need to determine your training zones. There's a little math involved here, but don't worry: I'll make it easy for you.

First off, you need to determine your maximum heart rate—approximately the highest number of times your heart can beat per minute. There are several formulas out there to compute this, but perhaps the easiest one is simply to subtract your age from 220. We'll use a 40-year-old woman as an example: 220 - 40 = 180, so in our example, the maximum heart rate is 180 BPM.

Next up is to determine the training zones, based on a percentage of maximum heart rate. Each of these zones can also correspond to your rate of perceived exertion.

ZONE	INTENSITY	% OF MAX HEART RATE
1	Light (warmup/cooldown)	50 to 60
2	Moderate (brisk)	60 to 70
3	Moderate to high (very brisk)	70 to 80
4	High (power)	80 to 90
5	Very high (sprint)	90 to 100

HOW TO DETERMINE YOUR ZONES

To calculate your training zones, simply calculate the lower and upper percentages of your maximum heart rate. For Zone 1, you'd multiply .50 (or 50 percent) times max heart rate and .60 (60 percent) times max heart rate.

In our example, remember the maximum heart rate for our 40-year-old woman is 180. So her Zone 1 would be:

.50 × 180 = 90

.60 × 180 = 108

In Zone 1, she would want to maintain a heart rate of 90 to 108 beats per minute (BPM).

Here's a worksheet to help you try this for yourself.

Step 1: Compute your maximum heart rate.

220 - your age = _____ (MHR)

Step 2: Multiply your maximum heart rate (MHR) by the given percentage for each training zone.

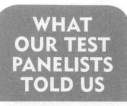

WHAT OUR TEST PANELISTS TOLD US

"When I've worked out before, I would go into autopilot and not really think about what I was doing. You couldn't do that with these workouts—there was always something new to keep you engaged."
—**Barb R., 52**

"I like walking, and doing the intervals really shook things up a bit. There was a time that I just hated the thought of walking a really hilly road near our house, but I did it almost every day over the 2 weeks. It kept me challenged, and when I was finished, I felt so good about myself!"
—**Roxann M., 49**

Zone 1: .50 × MHR = _____

.60 × MHR = _____

(50%)   (%60)
Zone 1 training is between _____ and _____ BPM

Zone 2: .70 × MHR = _____

(you already know .60 × MHR from Zone 1)

(60%)   (70%)
Zone 2 training is between _____ and _____ BPM

Zone 3: .80 × MHR = _____

(you already know .70 × MHR from Zone 2)

(70%)   (80%)
Zone 3 training is between _____ and _____ BPM

Zone 4: .90 × MHR = _____

(you already know .80 × MHR from Zone 3)

(80%)   (90%)
Zone 4 training is between _____ and _____ BPM

Zone 5*

(you already know .90 × MHR from Zone 4)

(90%)   (100%)
Zone 5 training is between _____ and _____ BPM

(*NOTE: *You probably won't hit this zone during training; if you do, it's a sign you need to take the intensity down quickly.*)

Putting It All Together

For each cardio exercise, we've given guidelines for RPE, talk test, and heart-rate zone. Here's how it all breaks down when you're exercising:

INTENSITY	RPE	TALK TEST	ZONE
Easy (warmup/cooldown)	2-3	Easy conversation	1 (50-60%)
Light/moderate (brisk walk)	4-5	Some breathlessness, speak in sentences	2 (60-70%)
Moderate/high	6-7	Mostly breathless, speak in short phrases	3 (70-80%)
High	8-9	Very breathless, speak one or two words	4 (80-90%)
Very high/sprint	10	Out of breath, can't speak	5 (90-100%)

Which Comes First, Cardio or Strength?

My clients often ask me what order they should do their workouts in. I usually like to start with cardio: It gets me going and I feel more energized during my strength workouts. And there's another bonus: You'll get a bigger afterburn if you do your resistance training after your cardio. Researchers who tested four types of training—strength only, cardio only, strength followed by cardio, and cardio followed by strength—found post workout metabolism levels were almost 50 percent higher among subjects in the strength-only and the cardio/strength group than in the strength/cardio group, and almost 90 percent higher than in the cardio-only group.[38] But at the end of the day, do what works for you. Make the workouts fit into your schedule.

How Do I Fit It All In?

You've committed to taking the next 2 weeks to jumpstart your way to a healthier life. But you don't live in a vacuum—I know your responsibilities don't stop just because you need them to. Believe me, I know how hard it is to juggle work, family, and personal time. Over the past 20 years, I personally have met my own roadblocks and detours. I've had some injuries. I've had some family events and work-related things that have interfered with my "perfect" workout plan. But I always say: "Strive for progress, not perfection." Perfection leads to disappointment. Being a mother of three teenagers has lots of surprises. I constantly remind myself of the advice we always hear from flight attendants: "Secure your own oxygen mask before assisting others." I have to take care of myself to be able to adequately take care of my family.

REAL TURNAROUND SUCCESS STORY
"I survived 2 weeks jam-packed with parties!"
KELLY LIDDLE, 46

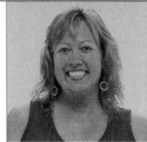

KELLY PROBABLY COULDN'T HAVE picked a worse time to start her 2-Week Total Body Turnaround. During the 14 days she was on the plan, she attended one wedding reception, one bridal shower, one bachelorette party, seven graduation parties, one golf tournament, and a weekend of town celebrations. Yet most of the time, she reports, her willpower won out.

"I exercised right before I had to get into the shower, then had some seltzer to fill me up, and packed a cooler with sugar-free iced tea and carbonated water mixed with Crystal Light. That way I didn't feel too bad when everyone around me was drinking, because I had my own beverages."

Her austerity paid off: After the 2 weeks were up, she'd lost more than 7 pounds and 13 inches, including more than 2 from her waist and $4\frac{1}{2}$ from her hips.

But she wasn't always so dedicated to eating well and exercising. Kelly, 46, says her weight has fluctuated for most of her life. "I'd think I should exercise, then find every excuse not to." Constant snacking on junk food—chips, dips, cookies, and cake—contributed to her weight gain. She recalls, "At one point I was craving sweets, and I lined a baking pan with crackers, then poured on caramel, chocolate, and nuts. When it was finished, I had a corner piece. That tasted so good that I had another, and another. By the end of the day, the whole pan was gone. So I made another pan, ate just one corner piece, and served that to my family so they wouldn't know what I'd done." Eventually, she says, she reached 157 pounds—at 5 feet 4 inches, it was the heaviest she'd ever been.

Soon her 17-year-old daughter was begging her not to buy any more junk food. "She's very slender," says Kelly, "but she was worried about having that in the house, because she didn't want to gain weight."

Kelly said the plan helped her stay energized through all of her many festivities. "I slept better at night and felt more rested in the morning." When her sweet tooth struck, she made smoothies with yogurt and frozen fruit and some protein powder; when she had salty cravings, she reached for pretzel crisps and hot-air popcorn. "I always kept to my calorie count, even with all of the social engagements I was attending."

Since the 2 weeks (and her many parties) have passed, Kelly has kept up her commitment to eating right and exercising more. She brought her weights with her on an 8-day vacation with her family and squeezed in her strength and walking sessions. A year later, she's lost a total of 26 pounds. And while she's relaxed a bit when she does hit the social scene, she's kept some of her healthy eating mantras in mind: "When I go to a party, I really think twice about having things like dips and chips. It's okay once in a while, but then I have to make up for it after and get back on track."

We women have so much to offer to the world. It's something we have to remind ourselves of every day. If you have a family and are constantly balancing work, kids, chores, and life, you're facing what I call the mother load. But nobody cares how much you know until they know how much you care! If you care about yourself, you can take that positive attitude to help others, especially your family. Once you learn to care about yourself, you can be a better parent, friend, co-worker—you name it!

I've packed a lot into one hourlong workout routine. But if you can't find the time to squeeze out 60 minutes in your schedule, it's okay to split things up. The important thing is to find the way to make this work for you. It's only 2 weeks! That may mean doing your cardio in the morning and the strength plan when you come home, or maybe doing one part in the morning and another at lunch. Whatever works for you: But I want you to commit to carving out 1 hour over a day to completing this program. Remember it's just for 2 weeks. You can do it!

Being Flexible: Your 2-Week Stretches

My clients are always asking me, "Is it worth it to stretch?" My answer is a definite: Yes! Stretching helps you stand taller and is good for your posture, which helps you look a few pounds thinner almost instantly! It improves your range of motion and flexibility in your joints, so you can tone your muscles more effectively and do your cardio more efficiently, which means you'll burn more calories. And it makes the little things in life—like turning around to talk to someone or reaching up to change the lightbulb—that much easier to handle.

I've always found that stretching is crucial to relieve daily aches and pains and recover from muscle soreness. While research lately on the benefits of stretching has been mixed, there is evidence it works. In one study, researchers put subjects through a high-intensity exercise, then tested them for soreness: The least flexible subjects felt significantly more muscle tenderness and pain than the most flexible ones. They also had less strength and more indications of muscle damage.[39]

It's important to remember that you should never stretch a cold muscle, or stretch past the point of slight discomfort. You should feel a gentle pull of the muscle toward the end of its range of motion. If you start to cramp or tremble, you're stretching too hard, so ease up. The best time to stretch is really after your cardio workout, while your muscles are still warm. Otherwise, warm up for just a few minutes by walking around, marching in place, or hopping on a stationary bike or elliptical. The American College of Sports Medicine recommends holding each stretch for 10 to 30 seconds. Incorporate the following stretches into your routine for at least 5 minutes every day.

WHAT OUR TEST PANELISTS TOLD US

"At first, I had to force myself to get up and out of bed in the morning to walk, but I grew to love that time—outside, no interruptions, just me and my dog (and sometimes the rain!). Then I did the weight workout at night. It was my sanctuary and my time."
—Maria S., 45

"I liked to do the cardio in the morning, before my kids woke up. It felt good to have it done and not looming over my head. Then I did my strength at night in front of the TV."
—Shelley J., 42

FORWARD BEND

STRETCHES: hamstrings, lower back

Sit tall on floor with legs extended in front of you. Wrap a small towel or resistance band behind the bottom of your feet, holding one end in each hand. Slowly lean forward, rounding your back and looking down at your legs, pulling on the ends of the towel to help deepen the stretch. Stay here for 10 to 30 seconds, sit up, and release.

"L" STRETCH

STRETCHES: hamstrings

Lie face up on the floor, legs extended. Bend left knee toward chest and place towel or resistance band under sole of left foot, holding one end in each hand. Straighten leg forward and slowly pull leg toward you, keeping knee slightly bent. Use the towel to help you move further into the stretch, but stop at the point of discomfort. Hold here for 10 to 30 seconds. Lower, and switch sides.

SHOULDER STRETCH

STRETCHES: tops of shoulders

Stand tall with feet hip-distance apart. Cross right arm in front of chest, placing left hand on right forearm. Gently pull on right arm with left, feeling the stretch in the top of your shoulder. Hold for 10 to 30 seconds; switch sides.

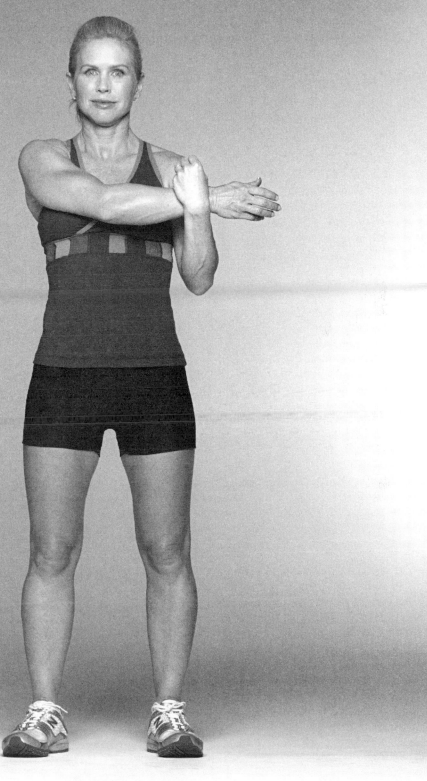

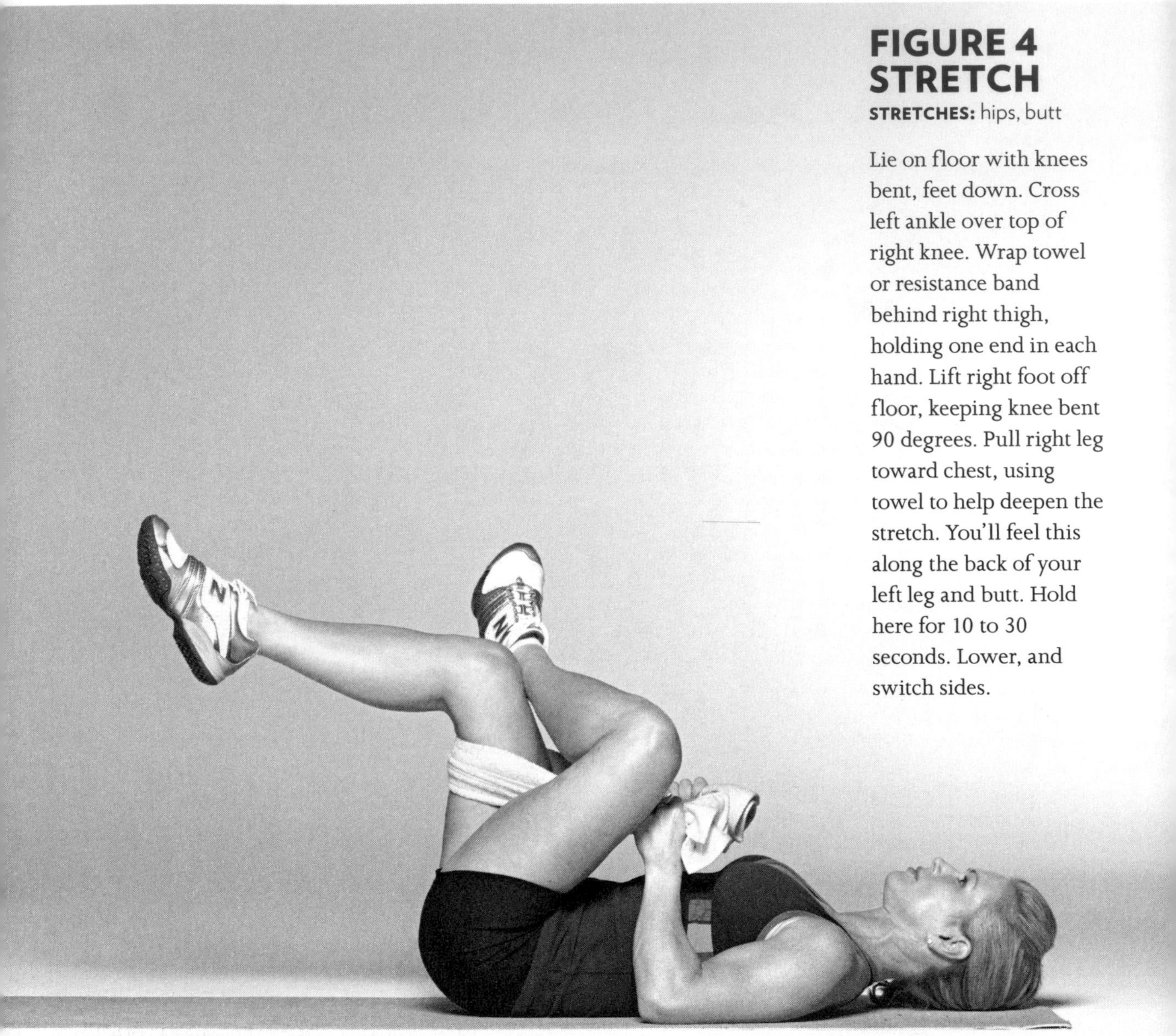

FIGURE 4 STRETCH

STRETCHES: hips, butt

Lie on floor with knees bent, feet down. Cross left ankle over top of right knee. Wrap towel or resistance band behind right thigh, holding one end in each hand. Lift right foot off floor, keeping knee bent 90 degrees. Pull right leg toward chest, using towel to help deepen the stretch. You'll feel this along the back of your left leg and butt. Hold here for 10 to 30 seconds. Lower, and switch sides.

PIGEON STRETCH

STRETCHES: hips, thighs, chest, back

Begin on all fours, knees on floor under hips and palms on floor under shoulders. Bring right knee forward on floor under right shoulder, shin under left shoulder, and extend left leg on floor behind you, keeping leg down. Square your hips to the floor. Push into fingertips, lifting torso away from right thigh as you lengthen your spine and expand your chest. Hold here for 10 to 30 seconds. Switch legs and repeat.

BUTTERFLY STRETCH

STRETCHES: inner thighs, groin

Sit tall with soles of feet pressed together, knees bent out to sides. Place towel under both feet, holding one end in each hand. Lean forward, pulling on the towel to deepen your stretch. Never force your knees down. Instead gently press your elbows into your thighs to release toward the floor. Hold for 10 to 30 seconds.

CHEST STRETCH
STRETCHES: chest

Stand tall with feet hip-distance apart, arms at sides holding towel behind body with one end in each hand. Raise arms behind you, using the towel to help deepen the stretch. Hold for 10 to 30 seconds.

Your 2-Week Total Body Turnaround Eating Plan

Being active is just one very important part of the healthy living equation. Equally important is your diet. For many of you, "diet" has really become a four-letter word. Like many women on our test panel, you've probably tried your fair share of diets over the years, and had some success—at least at first. But the problem with most diets is that they don't offer a long-lasting solution because they don't provide real opportunities to change. Instead, I'm asking you to look at your eating habits and make them better. It's as easy as that.

I'm a big believer in "clean" eating. That's about as easy as it sounds. To make your body healthier, eliminate as many of the preservatives, additives, processed sugars, and general junk from your diet as possible. Clean eating means fresh fruits and vegetables, low-fat or fat-free dairy, and lean meats, poultry, or fish. It means delicious whole grains or grain alternatives like brown rice, quinoa, and oats. It means avoiding most of the interior aisles

"Tell me what you eat,
and I will tell you what you are."
—Jean Anthelme Brillat-Savarin, French gastronome

at the grocery store and hitting up the perimeter, where you find produce, meat, and dairy, not the processed, boxed foods loaded with additives and artificial stuff.

When you're shopping for food or eating at a restaurant, keep three words in mind: plant, tree, animal. Your food should look like it came from something living, and should be easily identifiable—broccoli that looks like broccoli, fish that looks like fish. Fill your grocery cart with colorful choices, so by the time you hit the inner aisles, your cart should already be pretty full. And have a shopping list in hand before you hit the store: Guidelines from the National Heart, Lung, and Blood Institute show you can reduce healthy cooking time by using a shopping list and keeping your kitchen well stocked. Finally, be a label reader: Pay attention to both serving sizes and servings per container, and compare total calories in products, choosing the lower-option ones where you can.

The Calorie Connection

At the end of the day, losing weight boils down to a very simple equation: calories in versus calories out. There are no gimmicks, no fads, no secrets. It all comes down to basic arithmetic. If today you consume 2,000 calories and you burn 2,250, you are losing weight. If you eat 2,000 calories and you only burn 1,500, you are gaining weight. (Burn more than you eat, and you lose weight. Eat more than you burn, and you gain weight.) This is, of course, a broad simplification of how our bodies work. Hormones, genetics, medications, and the many complex biochemical processes that are out of our control all figure in. But calories consumed through what you eat, and calories burned through how much you exercise, is the weight-loss bottom line. Every extra pound on your body represents 3,500 calories you consumed but didn't need. To lose that extra pound, you now have to create a 3,500-calorie deficit. You can't do it in a day or two. The best way to lose weight is to start consuming a little fewer calories and start moving your body a little more. If you cut 500 calories from your typical diet each day, you'd lose approximately 1 pound a week (500 calories × 7 days = 3,500 calories). Think of your cardio as your quick calorie burn—if you overindulge on the weekend, for example, you can make up for it by doing a little extra cardio on Monday. But remember that your strength training is your constant calorie burn—it keeps your body burning more calories all day long.

The Choice Is Yours

I've always found that my clients do better when they get to choose what to eat. If you don't like fish, for example, you're going to be in big trouble if three of your weekly meals are tuna, salmon, and flounder. So, with the help of Cynthia Sass, MPH, RD, and Heather Jones, RD, I've put together a do-it-yourself eating plan that allows you to decide what to eat, based on some simple guidelines. There is a wide range of delicious foods that will fit everyone's taste and budget.

Let's start with a few basic principles. First off, I've given you a sensible mix of carbohydrates, protein, and fat—there are no extreme highs or lows here, just healthy choices that will help you stay satisfied. And you'll be eating at regular intervals—five times a day—so you never go too long without eating or allow yourself to get too hungry. Plus, the program is designed to mesh perfectly with the exercises you'll be doing, so your body will be fueled for activity each and every day.

Here's how it breaks down: Your goal is 1,600 calories a day with a mix of carbohydrates (about 45 percent), fat (about 25 percent), and protein (30 percent). You'll eat three healthy meals (about 400 calories each) and two satisfying snacks (about 200 calories each). (Note that these numbers are for women; a man doing the 2-Week Total Body Turnaround will boost his total calorie count to 2,000.)

Research has shown that following a diet like this, with slight caloric restrictions combined with a moderate carbohydrate and fat and higher protein balance, along with the correct timing, is an ideal mix to help you lose weight without losing energy. So you'll have all the healthy fuel you need to keep you energized through the workouts and recover afterward.

Protein vs. Carbs

Anyone who has attempted weight loss in the past few years has certainly come across the whole "high-protein" versus "low-fat" approach to dieting. I'll talk more about protein and its benefits in Part II, but I designed this meal plan to give you enough protein to reap the benefits without going too far overboard. In addition, we're keeping our carbohydrate levels high enough to make sure you're getting all the energy you need for your workouts, and your fat content high enough that you stay satisfied yet low enough to get results.

When to Eat

I'll leave the exact timing up to you, but at a minimum you should be eating a healthy breakfast, lunch, and dinner, plus snacks. Some people like to have a snack mid-morning and then again after lunch to hold them over to dinner; others prefer a light snack (read: dessert!) at night. But try to eat about every 3 to 4 hours so your blood sugar levels don't dip too low (which can leave you starving and ready to eat everything in your home!). You'll also be fueled for exercise, especially if you decide to split your routine and do part in the morning and part later in the day. But I usually recommend avoiding late-night snacking, which can frequently turn into late-night bingeing.

Portion Control

Portion control is really everything when it comes to making good food choices. Almonds are among the healthiest foods out there, but if you eat the entire tin, you'll consume about 1,500 calories or more! Many of our test panelists found that keeping a set of measuring cups on the counter helped them to figure out the right amount that they should be eating with each meal or snack. Here are some good guidelines to keep in mind:

- Your fist = A medium portion of fruit or 1 cup of rice or pasta
- Your thumb = A 1-ounce serving of cheese
- The tip of your thumb = 1 teaspoon of butter or oil
- The palm of your hand (without fingers and thumb) = One 4-ounce serving of meat, poultry, or fish
- One cupped handful = 1 serving of cereal, pretzels, or chips

The Plan Principles

This is a customized plan, meaning you can mix and match among the food choices to find what you love. If this seems too overwhelming, follow our daily suggested menus in Part II, which lay out some great healthy eating options for one full week. Once you get the idea of how to combine the different food groups, you'll find the possibilities are endless.

TURNAROUND FOOD CHOICES

Each day you should eat:

- 4 servings of vegetables
- 2 servings of fruit
- 4 servings of grains/starchy veggies
- 3 servings of dairy
- 3 servings of protein
- 3 servings of fat

Here are some examples for each food group:

VEGETABLES

Number of Servings per Day: 4; 2 at lunch, 2 at dinner; aim for at least 3 different colors each day

Fresh vegetables— 1 serving equals 1 cup raw or ¹/₂ cup cooked:	Cauliflower	Radishes	Roasted red peppers, jarred in water	Frozen—1 serving equals 1 cup before cooking:
Artichokes	Celery	Spaghetti squash	Salsa	Asparagus
Asparagus	Coleslaw mix	Spinach	Tomato sauce	Broccoli
Broccoli	Cucumbers	Tomatoes	Tomatoes, stewed or diced	French-cut green beans
Brussels sprouts	Eggplant	Zucchini		Spinach
Cabbage	Lettuce, all types			Sugar snap peas
Carrots	Mushrooms	**Canned or jarred— 1 serving equals ¹/₂ cup:**		Yellow wax beans
	Onions	Artichoke hearts, canned in water		
	Peppers			

FRUITS

Number of Servings per Day: 2; 1 at breakfast, 1 as a snack; aim for 2 different colors each day

Fresh—1 serving equals 1 cup or 1 medium piece the size of a tennis ball:	Mangoes	Star fruit	Peaches	100% any variety fruit juice
Apples, all varieties	Melons, all types	Tangerines	Raspberries	
Apricots	Nectarines		Strawberries	**Dried—1 serving equals ¹/₄ cup, unsweetened:**
Bananas, small	Oranges	**Frozen—1 serving equals 1 cup in frozen state:**		Dried blueberries, cherries, apricots, plums, figs, pears, peaches, mangoes, etc.
Cherries	Papayas	Any unsweetened variety, including:	**Canned—1 serving equals ¹/₂ cup:**	
Grapefruits	Passion fruit		Any variety, unsweetened or canned in natural juice (natural applesauce, mandarin oranges, pineapple, etc.)	
Grapes, all varieties	Peaches	Blackberries		Raisins, regular or golden
Kiwifruit	Pears	Blueberries		
	Plums	Cherries		
	Pomegranates	Mangoes		

GRAINS/STARCHY VEGETABLES

Number of Servings per Day: 4; 2 at breakfast, 1 at lunch, 1 at dinner; aim for 3 whole-grain servings and 1 starchy veggie daily

Starchy vegetables— 1 serving equals ¹/₂ cup cooked:	Fresh—1 serving equals:	Frozen—1 serving equals:	Waffles, whole grain, 1	Cream of wheat, ¹/₂ cup cooked
Beans, all varieties (black, pinto, refried, etc.)	English muffins, whole grain, half	Corn, white or yellow, ¹/₂ cup heated	**Grains—1 serving equals:**	Oatmeal, ¹/₂ cup cooked
Plantains	Multigrain bread, 1 slice	Green peas, ¹/₂ cup heated	Cereal, whole grain, ¹/₂ cup dry	Pasta, whole wheat, ¹/₂ cup cooked
Potatoes, red	Pita, 100% oat bran or whole wheat, half	Lima beans, ¹/₂ cup heated	Couscous, ¹/₂ cup cooked	Popcorn, light microwave (no trans fat), 3 cups popped
Potatoes, sweet	Tortillas, corn, 2	Pancakes, whole grain, 1	Crackers, whole grain, ¹/₂ cup	Rice, brown or wild, ¹/₂ cup cooked
	Wraps, 100% whole grain, half			

DAIRY OR DAIRY SUBSTITUTES

Number of Servings per Day: 3; 1 at breakfast, 2 as snacks; use only skim or fat-free milk, yogurt, cottage and ricotta cheese, and reduced-fat cheeses

Crumbled or shredded cheese— 1 serving equals ¼ cup:	Jack	American	**Others—1 serving equals:**	Soymilk, 8 oz or 1 cup
	Parmesan	Gouda	Cottage cheese, nonfat, ½ cup	String cheese, 1 string
	Romano	Mozzarella	Milk, skim, 8 oz or 1 cup	Yogurt, Greek or regular, fat-free, low-fat, or soy, 8 oz or 1 cup
Blue	**Sliced cheese— 1 serving equals 1 slice, about the size of a coaster:**	Provolone	Ricotta, nonfat, ½ cup	
Colby		Swiss		
Feta				
Gorgonzola				

PROTEIN

Number of Servings per Day: 3; 1 at breakfast, lunch, and dinner; choose fish 2 or 3 times a week and a vegetarian source (tofu, veggie burgers) at least twice a week

Unless otherwise stated, 1 serving equals 3 oz or 1 piece about the size of a cassette tape or deck of cards cooked or prepared:	Beef, ground, 98% lean or greater	Egg whites, 1 cup liquid or whites from 5 eggs	Shrimp, frozen or tiny canned	Tuna, chunk light, canned in water
	Canadian bacon	Pork tenderloin	Sirloin, trimmed	Turkey, deli
	Chicken breast	Salmon, wild, fresh or canned	Soy-based vegetarian products (tofu, veggie burgers, dogs, patties, etc.)	Turkey, ground, leanest possible
	Clams, minced, canned			Turkey breast

FAT

Number of Servings per Day: 3; 1 at breakfast, lunch, and dinner; choose plant-based fats as often as possible and aim for variety

1 serving equals:	Mayonnaise, light or reduced fat, 2 Tbsp	Nuts or seeds, chopped or sliced, including walnuts, almonds, pecans, peanuts, cashews, pistachios, pine nuts, sunflower seeds,	pumpkin seeds, 2 Tbsp	Olives, 10 medium black or green
Avocado—⅕ of medium size	Nut butters, including peanut, cashew, almond, soy, or walnut butter, 2 Tbsp		Oil-based salad dressings, 2 Tbsp	Pesto, 1 Tbsp
Cream cheese, light or reduced fat, 2 Tbsp				Vegetable oils, 1 Tbsp

BEVERAGES—WATER

Number of Servings per Day: 2 liters; drink with each meal; don't rely on thirst to guide your intake—carry a water bottle or pour a glass with each of your 5 meals

MEAL GUIDELINES:

Suggested amounts for each meal

BREAKFAST

2 grains/starchy veggies

1 dairy

1 protein

1 fruit

1 fat

A.M. SNACK

1 dairy

1 fruit

LUNCH

1 grain/starchy veggie

1 protein

2 veggies

1 fat

P.M. SNACK

1 dairy

DINNER

1 grain/starchy veggie

1 protein

2 veggies

1 fat

Here's a sample menu so that you can see how these guidelines work on a typical day. We'll give you a menu like this for each of the 14 days of your 2-Week Total Body Turnaround.

SAMPLE MENU DAY 1

BREAKFAST

1 cup whole-grain cereal topped with 1 cup skim milk and 2 tablespoons sliced almonds. Serve with 3 ounces Canadian bacon and ½ grapefruit.

PER SERVING: 450 calories; 13 g total fat; 2 g sat fat; 67 g carbohydrates; 9 g fiber; 24 g protein; 19 mg cholesterol; 620 mg sodium

SNACK

1 cup nonfat/low-fat yogurt

PER SERVING: 140 calories; 0 g total fat; 0 g sat fat; 19 g carbohydrates; 0 g fiber; 14 g protein; 4 mg cholesterol; 190 mg sodium

LUNCH

Turkey Meatball Pocket

PER SERVING: 341 calories; 17 g total fat; 3 g sat fat; 29 g carbohydrates; 5 g fiber; 21 g protein; 67 mg cholesterol; 658 mg sodium

SNACK

1 sliced pear with ¼ cup crumbled blue cheese

PER SERVING: 220 calories; 10 g total fat; 6 g sat fat; 28 g carbohydrates; 6 g fiber; 8 g protein; 25 mg cholesterol; 470 mg sodium

DINNER

Garlic Lemon Shrimp

PER SERVING: 357 calories; 11 g total fat; 2 g sat fat; 32 g carbohydrates; 6 g fiber; 25 g protein; 130 mg cholesterol; 161 mg sodium

TURKEY MEATBALL POCKET

3 ounces ground turkey

$^1/_2$ teaspoon garlic powder

$^1/_4$ teaspoon Italian seasoning

$^1/_8$ teaspoon black pepper

$^1/_2$ whole wheat pita pocket

$^1/_4$ cup marinara sauce

1 cup mixed greens

$^1/_2$ cup thinly sliced cucumbers

$1^1/_2$ teaspoons olive oil

1 teaspoon red wine vinegar

Preheat the oven to 375°F. In a small bowl, combine the turkey, garlic powder, Italian seasoning, and pepper, and mix well. Form into 1″ balls; place on a baking sheet. Bake for 10 to 15 minutes, or until cooked through. Remove from the oven and place the meatballs in an open pita pocket. Place the marinara sauce in a microwaveable bowl, then microwave on high 12 to 15 seconds, or until warm. Spoon the sauce over the meatballs. Toss the mixed greens and cucumber together in a small bowl. Drizzle with olive oil and vinegar before serving.

MAKES 1 SERVING

PER SERVING: 341 calories; 17 g total fat; 3 g sat fat; 29 g carbohydrates; 5 g fiber; 21 g protein; 67 mg cholesterol; 658 mg sodium

NOTE: *This recipe is a little high in sodium (you want to aim for no more than 600 mg per meal), which you should normally avoid, but you'll be sweating a lot throughout the 2-Week Total Body Turnaround, so you can get away with it today.*

GARLIC LEMON SHRIMP

2 teaspoons olive oil

$1^1/_2$ cups broccoli florets

2 cloves garlic, chopped

4 ounces peeled and deveined shrimp

$^1/_4$ cup white wine

1 teaspoon lemon juice

$^1/_8$ teaspoon black pepper

$^1/_2$ cup cooked whole grain pasta (1 ounce dry)

Heat the oil in a medium skillet on medium high; add the broccoli. Cook, stirring frequently, until tender, about 3 minutes. Turn the heat to medium, and add the garlic and shrimp. Cook for 2 minutes, tossing quickly. Stir in the wine and lemon juice, and cook an additional 1 to 2 minutes, tossing to coat. Sprinkle with pepper. Spoon the mixture over the pasta ($1^3/_4$ cups shrimp and broccoli over $^1/_2$ cup pasta).

MAKES 1 SERVING ($1^3/_4$ CUPS SHRIMP AND BROCCOLI OVER $^1/_2$ CUP PASTA)

PER SERVING: 357 calories; 11 g total fat; 2 g sat fat; 32 g carbohydrates; 6 g fiber; 25 g protein; 130 mg cholesterol; 161 mg sodium

NOTE: *If your local grocery store doesn't carry peeled and deveined shrimp, ask the seafood counter to do it for you.*

ACHIEVE

"Excellence can be obtained if you care more than others think is wise, risk more than others think is safe, dream more than others think is practical, and expect more than others think is possible."
—*Anonymous*

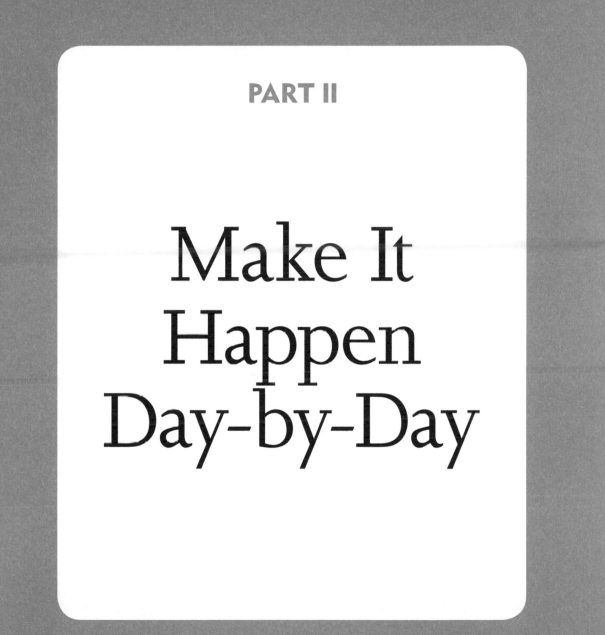

PART II

Make It Happen Day-by-Day

WEEK 1

We're ready to go! I hope you're as excited as I am to dive into your 2-Week Total Body Turnaround. Each day, you'll be doing a 30-minute strength workout and a 30-minute cardio program. The strength routines will focus on a specific area of your body. As I've mentioned, I recommend walking for your cardio, but you can adapt my plan to whatever aerobic activity you like best. At the end of the week, you'll get a day of active rest!

Also, don't forget to stretch for 5 minutes at some point during each day—ideally after your cardio routine.

I'll also give you some suggested daily menu plans. Try these delicious recipes or incorporate your own favorite foods. Each day, we'll also focus on a specific nutrient or food type to help you learn more about ways to establish long-term healthy habits. Finally, I'll give you my favorite daily motivational tips to help keep you on track for success!

Let's get started!

DAY 1

1 ☐ ☐ ☐ ☐ ☐ ☐ ☐ ☐ ☐ ☐ ☐ ☐ ☐

Here we go! We're kicking off your 2-Week Total Body Turnaround with an interval workout that will get you energized for the whole day, followed by a strength routine that focuses on shaping your upper body. Remember, you can do this program all at once (it will take an hour) or do the cardio in the morning and the strength routine in the afternoon or evening (or vice versa)—whatever works for you and your schedule!

For the cardio portion, use both your rate of perceived exertion and the talk test to help you determine whether you are exercising at the right intensity. For those speed bursts, you should be working really hard—they only last a minute each, so make every second count. You can do it! You'll have a full 2 minutes to recover after each one. If you're doing the workout outdoors, simply keep the speed intervals in mind—1 minute fast, 2 minutes recovery.

Also, don't forget to stretch for 5 minutes at some point during the day.

CARDIO: Speed Bursts

INTENSITY	TIME	RPE	TALK TEST
Warm up (heart rate: Zone 2)	4 min.	4–5	You can speak in full sentences (slightly breathless)
Speed burst (heart rate: Zone 4)	1 min.	8–9	You can only say short words (very breathless)
Recover (heart rate: Zone 2)	2 min.	4–5	You can speak in full sentences (slightly breathless)
Repeat speed burst/recovery combo 7 more times for a total of 8 intervals (heart rate: Zone 4/2), going directly from final recovery into cooldown.			
Cool down (heart rate: Zone 1)	2 min.	3	You can speak easily

STRENGTH: Upper Body + Core

This strength workout is designed to target all of the muscles of your upper body, including your arms, back, chest, and shoulders, as well as your core (abs and lower back). Remember that we're focusing on a slower-paced movement than you might be used to. Really take the time to focus on how long it takes to lift and lower the weight for each repetition. Do each exercise in the order given, moving from one to the next after you complete each set. Since you're first learning these, you may only have time to do this once through in a half hour, but as you learn the moves, you should be able to get through the full circuit twice.

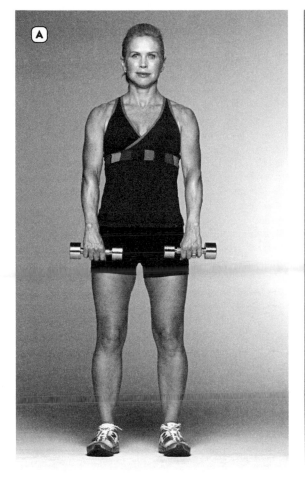

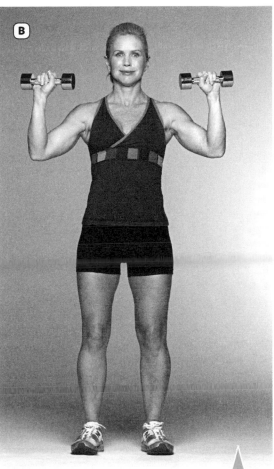

TANK TOP TONER

TARGETS: Arms, back, shoulders

A. Stand holding dumbbells in front of thighs, palms facing legs.

B. Bending elbows, lift weights to chin on count 1 in a reverse curl (palms will now face forward).

C. (not shown) Straighten arms forward on count 2, reaching up and out. Slowly lower straight arms back to start position, taking 4 counts. Repeat from beginning, 8 to 12 times.

GOOD FORM TIP:
Relax your shoulders away from your ears—you'll take the pressure off of your neck and focus more on your shoulders to do the work.

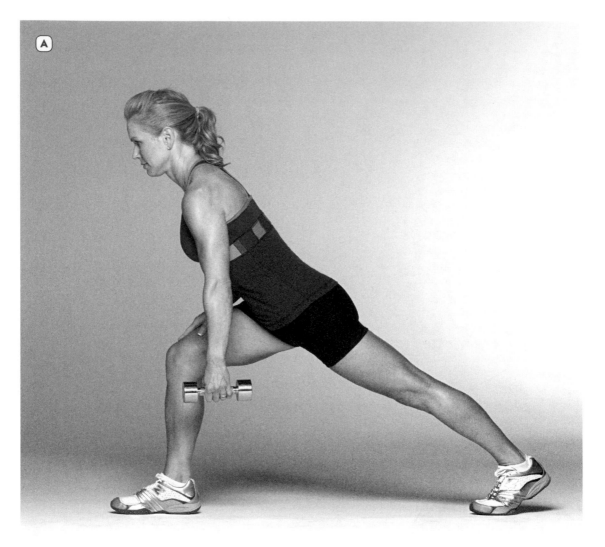

SINGLE-ARM ROW

TARGETS: Back

A. Stand with feet staggered, right foot in front of left, leaning forward slightly with dumbbell in left hand next to inside of right thigh, right hand resting on top of right thigh. Keep your back straight and abs tight, and think about maintaining a long spine.

B. Using the left shoulder blade, draw elbow up toward ceiling for 2 counts (your hand should end up near your hip bone; do not shrug your shoulder). Take 4 full counts to lower to start position. Repeat 8 to 12 times, then switch positions, with left leg in front and weight in right hand.

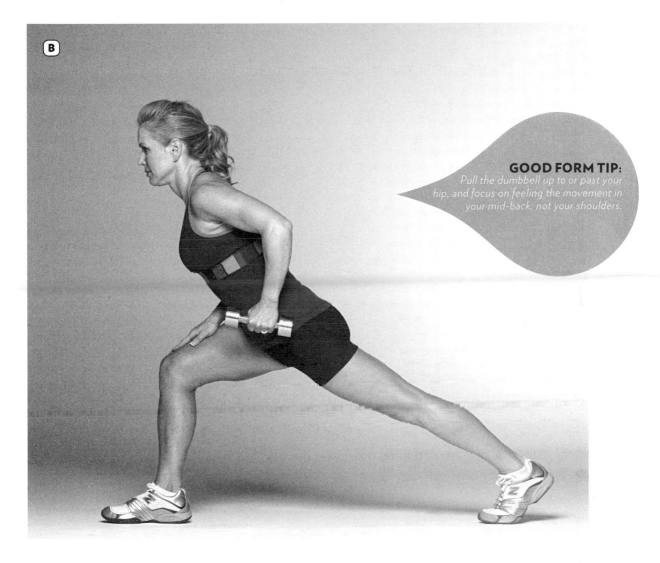

B

GOOD FORM TIP: *Pull the dumbbell up to or past your hip, and focus on feeling the movement in your mid-back, not your shoulders.*

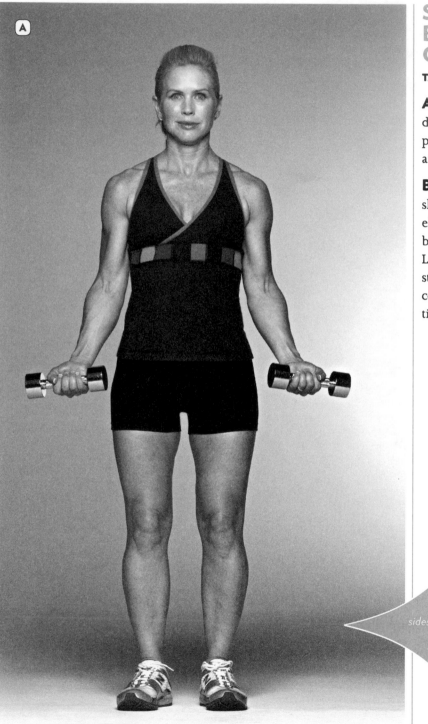

A

STANDING BICEPS CURL

TARGETS: Biceps

A. Stand holding dumbbells at sides, palms facing up and arms straight.

B. Curl weights toward shoulders by bending elbows and contracting biceps for 2 counts. Lower slowly back to start position in 4 counts. Repeat 8 to 12 times.

GOOD FORM TIP:
Keep your elbows close to your sides and your torso upright and still. You'll work more of your biceps and less of your shoulders.

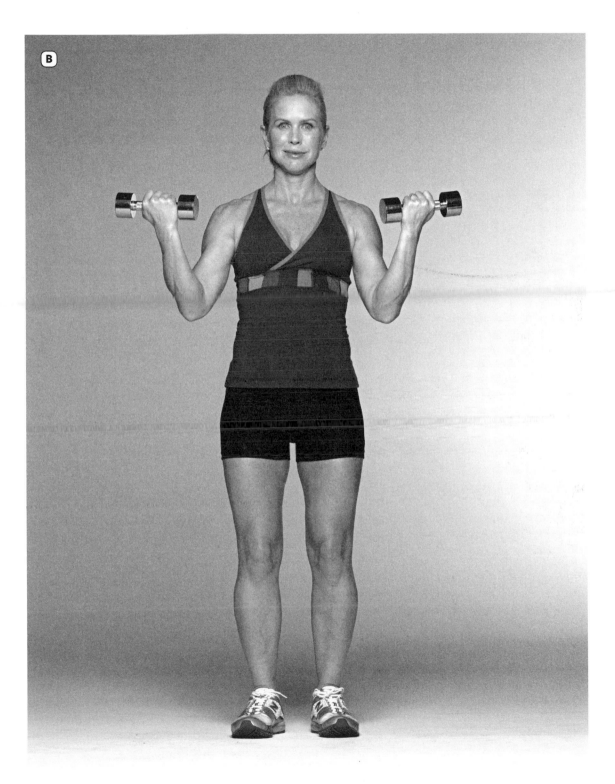

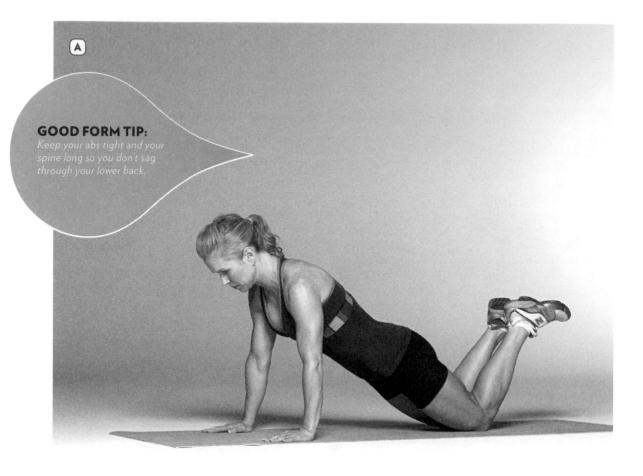

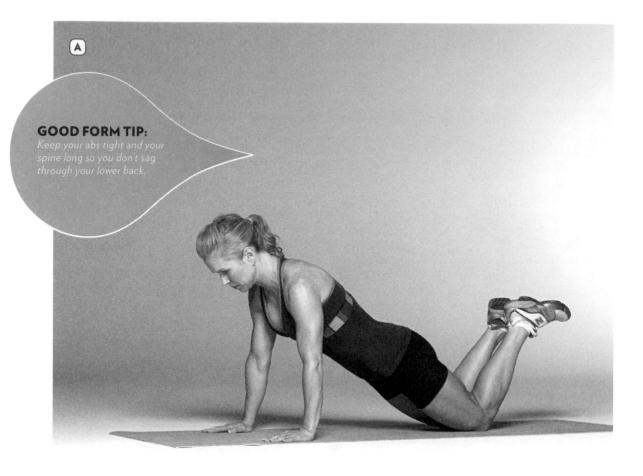

A

GOOD FORM TIP:
*Keep your abs tight and your
spine long so you don't sag
through your lower back.*

PUSHUP SHOULDER TAP

TARGETS: Chest, triceps, shoulders

A. Start in modified pushup position, hands shoulder-width apart on floor and knees down, forming a 45-degree angle while maintaining a straight line through your spine.

B. Lower chest slowly to floor for 4 counts, keeping abs tight and body in a straight line.

C. Push back up to start position for 2 counts, tapping left hand to right shoulder on count 2. Repeat, this time tapping right hand to left shoulder on 2nd count. Do a total of 6 to 8 on each side.

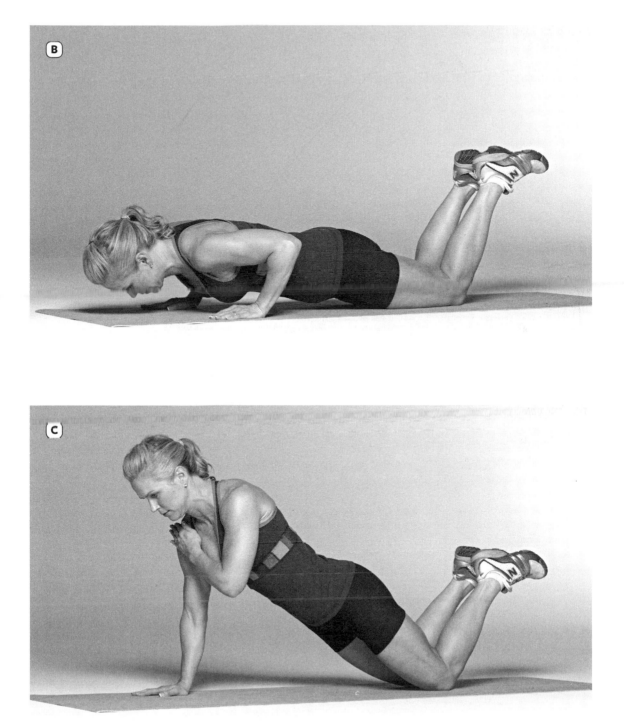

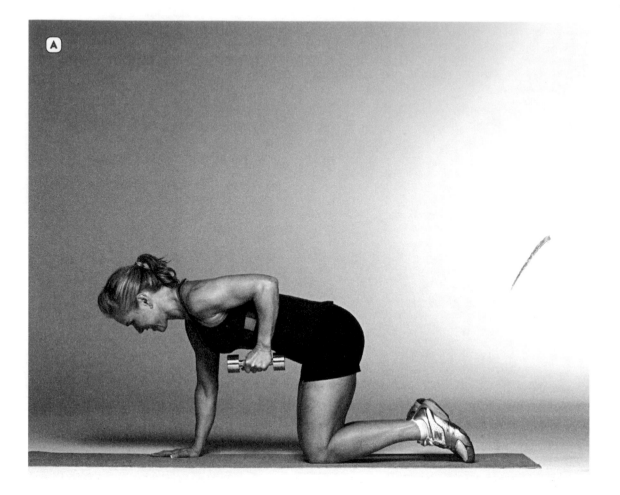

TRICEPS KICKBACK

TARGETS: Triceps

A. Start on all fours, holding dumbbell in left hand and abdominals tight, keeping back flat. Lift elbow next to ribs to begin.

B. Extend arm, pressing dumbbell back for 2 counts until arm is straight. Slowly bend arm to bring weight back toward body in 4 counts. Repeat.

Do not let shoulder move during the exercise; focus on straightening and bending just the elbow joint. Repeat 8 to 12 times. Switch sides and repeat another 8 to 12 times.

GOOD FORM TIP:
Keep your elbow glued to your side and your shoulder steady. Only push the weight back from the elbow joint, not your shoulder.

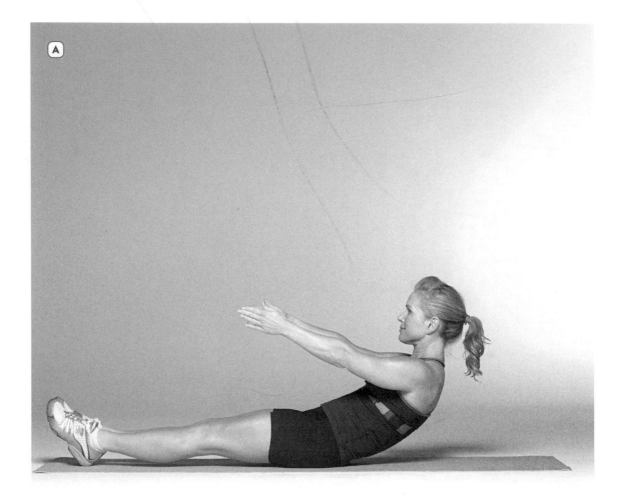

FULL BODY ROLLUP

TARGETS: Abs

A. Lie face up on the floor, legs slightly bent and arms extended next to head, shoulders relaxed, palms facing each other. Pressing your shoulders down, slowly roll up off the floor in 4 counts, keeping abs pulled in and arms extended.

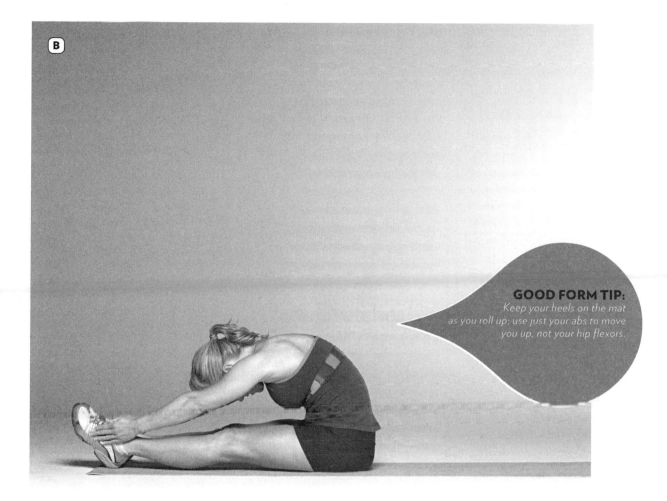

GOOD FORM TIP:
Keep your heels on the mat as you roll up; use just your abs to move you up, not your hip flexors.

B. Finish by reaching forward toward your toes. Slowly roll back down to floor to starting position, taking about 6 to 8 counts to lower. Repeat 6 to 8 times.

DAY 1 TURNAROUND TIP
Learn Your 3 Cs

I want you to write down on a slip of paper or sticky note what I call my 3 Cs: commitment, consistency, and convenience. These C-words are instrumental in helping you begin to make successful changes to your lifestyle. Stick them in a place you will be able to see them over and over these next few days (on the cabinet, the bathroom mirror, the fridge—any place you look at each and every day).

The first step involves making a *commitment* to a healthier lifestyle. Just by picking up this book and getting to this point, you've already done just that. Half of losing weight and getting fit is mental—it's often you against your mind. Stick with this commitment you have made to yourself, and remember, I'll be here with you every step along the way. Keep me with you: I want this book on your nightstand, in your kitchen, or on your desk—wherever you can look at it every day for instruction and for mental strength. It's about having a constant reminder and a constant motivator.

The next thing to consider is *consistency*. We're all busy—I know I am! I have endless lists—making sure the bills are paid, the kids are where they are supposed to be, the laundry is done, the family has dinner, and on and on. There never seems to be enough time in the day to finish everything I need to do. But I know that keeping fit is important to me, and so I look at it like the other things I need to do in the course of a day: get dressed in the morning, load the dishwasher after breakfast, get in a workout, shower. It's a fundamental part of my day, just like brushing teeth. We all need it!

It all comes down to squeezing it in. The best advice I can give is to exercise whenever it fits into your schedule. For most of us, that usually is in the morning. It's my favorite time to exercise. I have a house full of teenagers and a job, and by midday, my list of things "still to do" is incredibly long. If I left my workout till later in the afternoon or evening, I'd probably have to skip it. In fact, I like to start my day early. The sun is just coming up and there's no stress on the horizon at least for the next hour. I love it.

Finally, there is the matter of *convenience*. Let's face it: The more convenient something is, the more often you'll do it. Pick a way to get your workouts in that is convenient. Do you like to walk with co-workers or friends in the evening? Can you put a treadmill in front of the TV and walk during your favorite show? Can you do your strength training right away in the morning before a hundred distractions pop up? Make exercise convenient and the excuses will disappear. (Don't join a health club that's too far away—you'll never go!)

Remember, you've made the *commitment*, and by being *consistent* and thinking about *convenience*, you are on your way to living a healthier life!

PROTEIN IS ONE OF the most important nutrients for your body—without it you simply can't function. There are more than 10,000 different proteins in your body; in your muscles, bones, skin, hair, nails—you get the idea. Protein makes up the enzymes that power all of the chemical reactions in your body, as well as the hemoglobin that carries oxygen in your blood.

There are about 20 basic building blocks of protein, also known as amino acids, which your body then strings together in a wide variety of structures. Unlike fat and carbs (stored as glucose), the body can't hold onto amino acids, so you need a fresh supply of amino acids every day to keep your body humming. Your body can produce or modify about half of the amino acids it needs, but the other half (also known as essential amino acids) must come from your diet. Complete proteins (from animal sources,

LEARN ABOUT: **PROTEIN**

like meat, fish, and dairy products) contain all of the essential amino acids. Incomplete proteins (usually from fruits, vegetables, grains, and nuts) lack one or more of the essential amino acids, which is why vegetarians need a wide variety of protein-containing foods each day.

Protein has the same number of calories per gram as carbs (which has 4 calories per gram), and half that of fat (9 calories per gram). But since your body has to break down each gram of protein that you eat into its individual amino acids, it takes more energy and time to digest, which not only slightly boosts your metabolism, but also keeps you feeling fuller, longer. Plus, its slower digestion won't raise your blood sugar levels as rapidly as a carb-rich food like pasta. One study found those who followed a 6-month diet with at least 25 percent of the calories from protein lost twice as much fat as those who got only 12 percent of their calories from protein.[1] Another found those on a high-protein diet lost 60 percent more weight than those on the low-protein end.[2] Protein is also crucial for building and repairing muscle fibers, and since you're going to be working on toning and sculpting your muscles almost every day during the next 2 weeks, you'll want to make sure you have enough protein to let your muscles do their jobs!

But too much protein can also be problematic. For one, many foods that are high in protein—a juicy porterhouse steak, for example—are also high in fat, especially artery-clogging saturated fat. Eating a lot of red meat has also been linked to an increased risk of colon cancer.

The Institute of Medicine recommends that adults get a minimum of 0.8 grams of protein for every kilogram of body weight (or else the body will break down its own tissue). That translates to 8 grams of protein for every 20 pounds, or 64 grams for a 160-pound woman. With the 2-Week Total Body Turnaround, you'll have 1 serving of protein with each meal, or 3 servings per day (not including 3 servings of dairy). And remember, there are lots of good protein choices beyond the meat department—tofu and other soybean products, beans, nuts, eggs, fish, and even peanut butter are all great options.

MEAL GUIDELINES:
Suggested amounts for each meal

BREAKFAST
2 grains/starchy veggies

1 dairy

1 protein

1 fruit

1 fat

A.M. SNACK
1 dairy

1 fruit

LUNCH
1 grain/starchy veggie

1 protein

2 veggies

1 fat

P.M. SNACK
1 dairy

DINNER
1 grain/starchy veggie

1 protein

2 veggies

1 fat

DAY 1 SUGGESTED MENU

BREAKFAST
1 cup whole-grain cereal topped with 1 cup skim milk and 2 tablespoons sliced almonds. Serve with 3 ounces Canadian bacon and $1/2$ grapefruit.

PER SERVING: 450 calories; 13 g total fat; 2 g sat fat; 67 g carbohydrates; 9 g fiber; 24 g protein; 19 mg cholesterol; 620 mg sodium

SNACK
1 sliced pear with $1/4$ cup crumbled blue cheese

PER SERVING: 220 calories; 10 g total fat; 6 g sat fat; 28 g carbohydrates; 6 g fiber; 8 g protein; 25 mg cholesterol; 470 mg sodium

LUNCH
Turkey Meatball Pocket

PER SERVING: 341 calories; 17 g total fat; 3 g sat fat; 29 g carbohydrates; 5 g fiber; 21 g protein; 67 mg cholesterol; 658 mg sodium

SNACK
1 cup nonfat or low-fat yogurt

PER SERVING: 140 calories; 0 g total fat; 0 g sat fat; 19 g carbohydrates; 0 g fiber; 14 g protein; 4 mg cholesterol; 190 mg sodium

DINNER
Garlic Lemon Shrimp

PER SERVING: 357 calories; 11 g total fat; 2 g sat fat; 32 g carbohydrates; 6 g fiber; 25 g protein; 130 mg cholesterol; 161 mg sodium

TURKEY MEATBALL POCKET

3 ounces ground turkey

1/2 teaspoon garlic powder

1/4 teaspoon Italian seasoning

1/8 teaspoon black pepper

1/2 whole wheat pita pocket

1/4 cup marinara sauce

1 cup mixed greens

1/2 cup thinly sliced cucumbers

11/2 teaspoons olive oil

1 teaspoon red wine vinegar

Preheat the oven to 375°F. In a small bowl, combine the turkey, garlic powder, Italian seasoning, and pepper, and mix well. Form into 1" balls; place on a baking sheet. Bake for 10 to 15 minutes, or until cooked through. Remove from the oven and place the meatballs in an open pita pocket. Place the marinara sauce in a microwaveable bowl, then microwave on high 12 to 15 seconds, or until warm. Spoon the sauce over the meatballs. Toss the mixed greens and cucumber together in a small bowl. Drizzle with olive oil and vinegar before serving.

MAKES 1 SERVING

PER SERVING: 341 calories; 17 g total fat; 3 g sat fat; 29 g carbohydrates; 5 g fiber; 21 g protein; 67 mg cholesterol; 658 mg sodium

NOTE: *This recipe is a little high in sodium (you want to aim for no more than 600 to 650 mg per meal), which you should normally avoid, but you'll be sweating a lot throughout the 2-Week Total Body Turnaround, so you can get away with it today.*

GARLIC LEMON SHRIMP

2 teaspoons olive oil

11/2 cups broccoli florets

2 cloves garlic, chopped

4 ounces peeled and deveined shrimp

1/4 cup white wine

1 teaspoon lemon juice

1/8 teaspoon black pepper

1/2 cup cooked whole grain pasta (1 ounce dry)

Heat the oil in a medium skillet on medium high; add the broccoli. Cook, stirring frequently, until tender, about 3 minutes. Turn the heat to medium, and add the garlic and shrimp. Cook for 2 minutes, tossing quickly. Stir in the wine and lemon juice, and cook an additional 1 to 2 minutes, tossing to coat. Sprinkle with pepper. Spoon the mixture over the pasta.

MAKES 1 SERVING (1¾ CUPS SHRIMP AND BROCCOLI OVER ½ CUP PASTA)

PER SERVING: 357 calories; 11 g total fat; 2 g sat fat; 32 g carbohydrates; 6 g fiber; 25 g protein; 130 mg cholesterol; 161 mg sodium

NOTE: *If your local grocery store doesn't carry peeled and deveined shrimp, ask the seafood counter to do it for you.*

DAY 2

You're a full 24 hours into the program. By now, I hope you're already starting to feel a difference in your energy and confidence. The first few steps are the hardest to take, so congratulations on getting to this point! We're going to have a lot more fun over the next couple of weeks. If you're feeling a little sore from yesterday, don't worry—that's normal, especially if you're new to exercise or haven't worked out in a while. The best thing you can do for your body is to keep moving!

CARDIO: Hills

Your cardio plan today is based on incline, or hill, training. Inclines are one of the best ways to boost your calorie burn: Walking on a 5 percent grade burns 60 percent more calories than walking on a 0 percent grade. And there's a bonus: Walking uphill also helps sculpt your legs, butt, and core, since you're using them to power you up the incline. (Any of you who live in San Francisco or another hilly locale have an advantage!)

For this workout, find a moderately steep incline that is at least ⅛ of a mile long. (If you're using a treadmill, use a grade of 5 to 7 percent.) If you can't find a hill that's long enough to take you through the longest part of the workout (2½ minutes), go as long as you can, and then continue to walk as fast as you can until you hit your target time. Turn around and walk downhill after each "walk hard" interval. Don't have access to a treadmill and live in a place that's pretty much pancake flat? Repeat yesterday's speed bursts or substitute another interval workout.

"Determination gives you the resolve to keep going in spite of the roadblocks that lie before you."
—Denis Waitley, *motivational speaker*

INTENSITY	TIME	RPE	TALK TEST
Warm up, moderate pace, flat surface (heart rate: Zone 2)	3 min.	4–5	You can speak in full sentences (slightly breathless)
Walk hard uphill (heart rate: Zone 4)	30 sec.	8–9	You can only say one or two words (very breathless)
Recover, walk downhill (heart rate: Zone 2)	30 sec.	4–5	Slightly breathless
Walk hard uphill (heart rate: Zone 4)	1 min.	8–9	You can only say one or two words (very breathless)
Recover, walk downhill (heart rate: Zone 2)	1 min.	4–5	Slightly breathless
Walk hard uphill (heart rate: Zone 4)	90 sec.	8–9	You can only say one or two words (very breathless)
Recover, walk downhill (heart rate: Zone 2)	90 sec.	4–5	Slightly breathless
Walk hard uphill (heart rate: Zone 3–4)	2 min.	7–8	You can only say short phrases or a few words (very breathless)
Recover, walk downhill (heart rate: Zone 2)	2 min.	4–5	Slightly breathless
Walk hard uphill (heart rate: Zone 3–4)	2½ min.	7–8	You can only say short phrases or a few words (very breathless)
Recover, walk downhill (heart rate: Zone 2)	2½ min.	4–5	Slightly breathless
Walk hard uphill (heart rate: Zone 3–4)	2 min.	7–8	You can only say short phrases or a few words (very breathless)
Recover, walk downhill (heart rate: Zone 2)	2 min.	4–5	Slightly breathless
Walk hard uphill (heart rate: Zone 3–4)	90 sec.	7–8	You can only say short phrases or a few words (very breathless)
Recover, walk downhill (heart rate: Zone 2)	90 sec.	4–5	Slightly breathless
Walk hard uphill (heart rate: Zone 4)	1 min.	8–9	You can only say one or two words (very breathless)
Recover, walk downhill (heart rate: Zone 2)	1 min.	4–5	Slightly breathless
Cool down, easy pace, flat surface (heart rate: Zone 1)	3 min.	2–3	Conversational pace

STRENGTH: Lower Body + Core

Today's strength plan is all about working the muscles of your lower body (hips, butt, hamstrings, quads, calves), plus your abs and lower back. If you're a little sore from yesterday's strength workout, don't worry—those muscles are getting their rest and recovery time as you focus on your lower half. Since the muscles of the lower body are generally much bigger and more powerful than those of the upper body, be sure to take your time and move through each repetition very carefully in order to maximize each exercise's effect. Do each exercise with the recommended reps in the order given, then repeat if you have time.

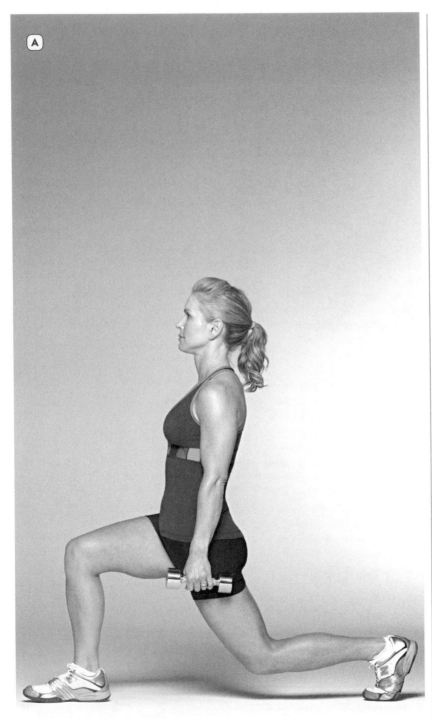

Ⓐ

FLOATING LUNGE

TARGETS: Quads, butt

A. Stand with feet together, arms at sides holding dumbbells. Step left foot behind you, lowering into a lunge for 4 counts; keep right knee over right ankle as you bend knees 90 degrees.

B. Lift left leg up and "float" it forward in 2 counts, pausing in the middle to tap foot down.

C. Lunge left foot forward in 4 counts, keeping left knee over ankle as you bend knees 90 degrees. Lift left foot and float back, lunging behind you in 2 counts. Repeat 8 times; switch legs.

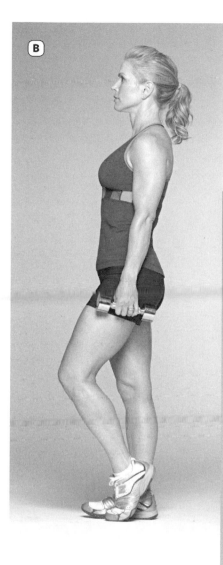

GOOD FORM TIP:
Don't push forward with your knees. Keep your front knee tracking over your shoelaces to protect your knee joint.

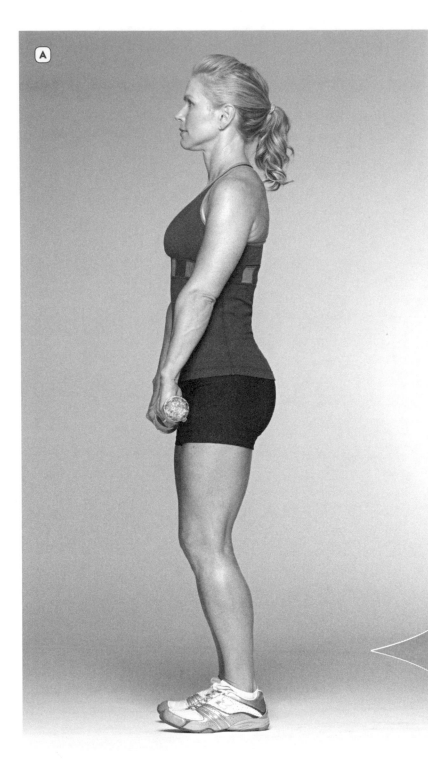

DEADLIFT

TARGETS: Hamstrings

A. Stand with feet hip-width apart, knees slightly bent, holding dumbbells with arms extended, palms facing thighs.

B. Keeping knees slightly bent, abs tight, and spine long, slowly bend forward from hips in 4 counts, lowering arms toward floor and keeping back flat as you slightly push butt behind you. Rise back to starting position in 2 counts, squeezing butt and hamstrings as you lift up. Repeat 8 to 12 times.

GOOD FORM TIP:
Keep your knees slightly soft, especially if your hamstrings are tight. Focus on pushing your butt back and using your butt and hamstrings—not your back—to stand up.

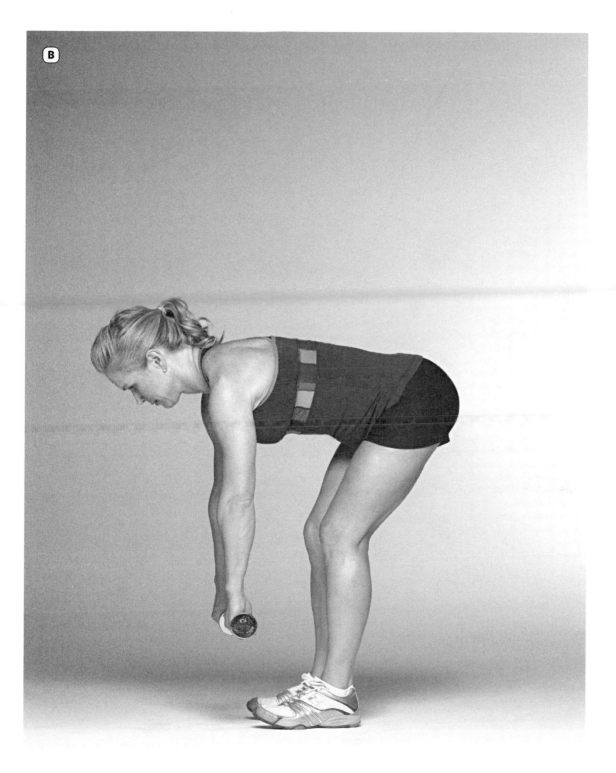

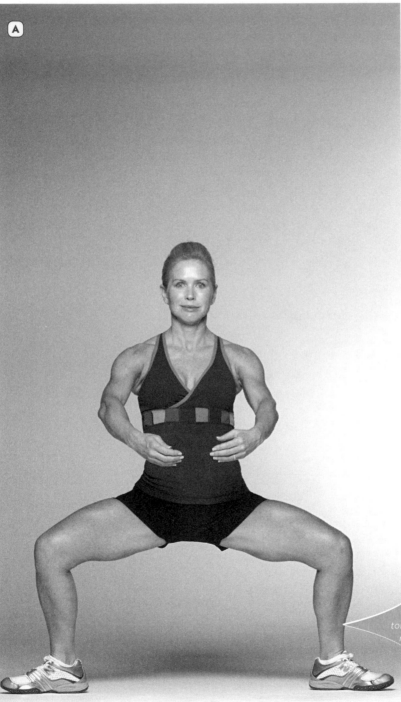

A

PLIÉ HEEL TAPS

TARGETS: Quads, butt, outer thighs, calves

A. Stand with feet shoulder-width apart, toes turned outward, and spine long. Bend knees, lowering body straight down for 4 counts.

B. Stand up in 2 counts, coming up halfway on count 1, then gently twice tapping left heel on right for 2 counts. Step back out and repeat 8 times. Switch to the other side, this time tapping right heel on left for 2 counts. Repeat 8 times.

GOOD FORM TIP: *Keep your tailbone tucked under your torso. If your hips are tight, ease into the movement—it may take some practice to move further into the plié.*

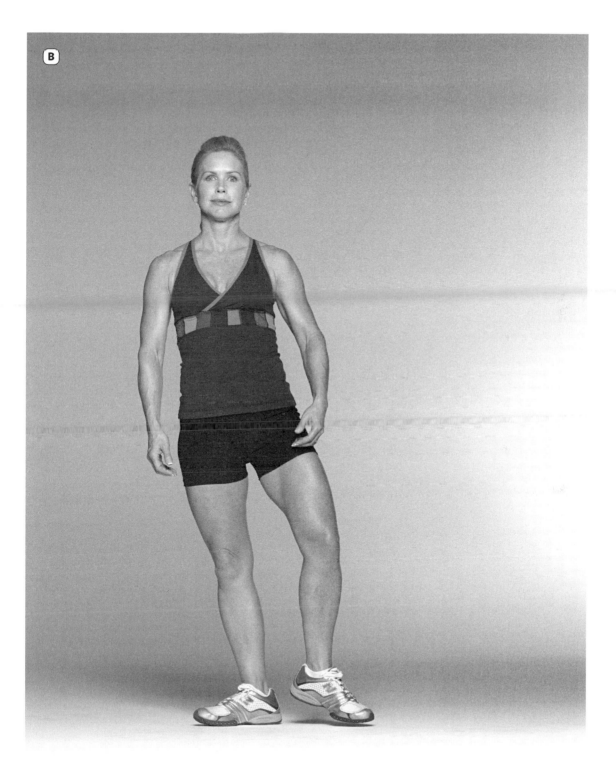

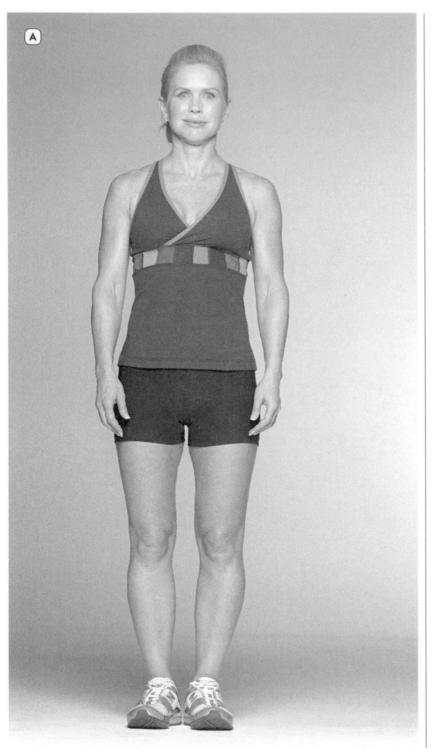

SCISSOR SQUAT

TARGETS: Quads, butt, outer and inner thighs

A. Stand with feet together, arms at sides.

B. Step left foot wide out to the left on count 1. Squat down on counts 2–4, as if sitting in a chair, keeping weight in heels.

C. (not shown) Stand up and bring feet back together, taking 2 counts.

D. (not shown) Repeat on opposite side, stepping right foot out wide to right on count 1, then squatting down on counts 2 to 4. Take 2 counts to stand up and return to start. Repeat 8 times on each side.

B

GOOD FORM TIP:
Keep your knees tracking over your shoelaces—not past your toes—when squatting to avoid putting pressure on your kneecaps. Keep your torso lifted with chin parallel to floor.

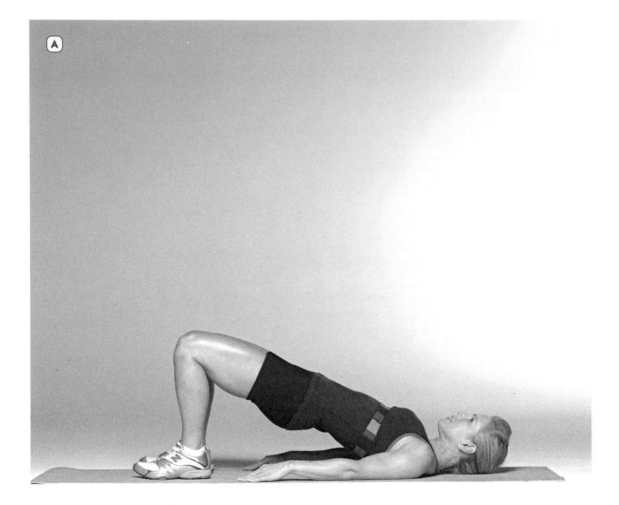

CALF ATTACK BRIDGE

TARGETS: Hamstrings, butt, calves

A. Lie face up on floor, knees bent, and feet flat on floor, about 3 to 4 inches apart. Pushing feet into floor, lift hips up for 2 counts, keeping abs tight and body in a straight line from knees to chest.

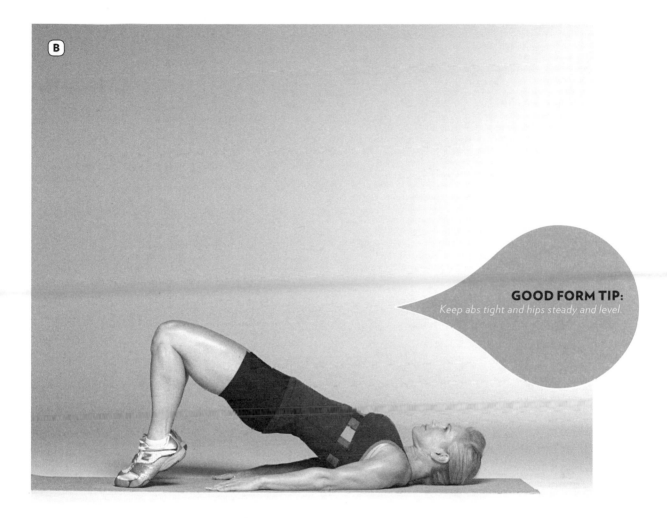

GOOD FORM TIP:
Keep abs tight and hips steady and level.

B. Holding here, lift heels, squeezing calves for 2 counts. Slowly lower heels for 4 counts. Continue to hold hips up in isometric contraction. Repeat 8 to 12 times.

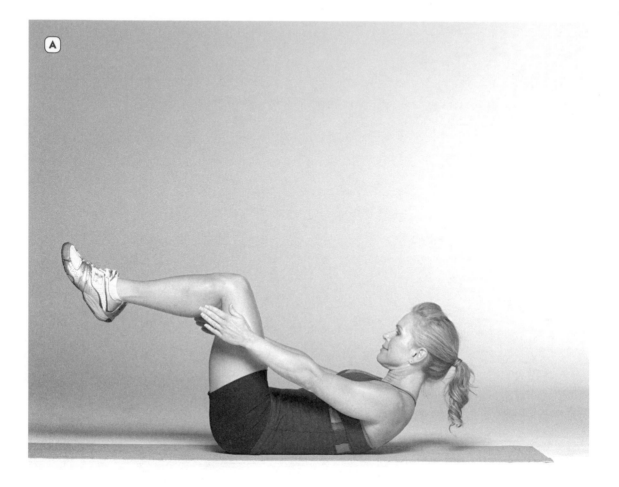

DOUBLE LEG STRETCH

TARGETS: Abs

A. Lie face up on floor, knees bent 90 degrees with knees over hips and hands reaching for shins.

B. Inhale and take 4 counts to lower arms behind head and extend legs 45 degrees to floor, forming a V-shape.

C. Exhale and pull legs back in while circling arms around the sides back to starting position in 2 counts. Repeat 8 to 10 times. Keep upper body as still as possible during the exercise.

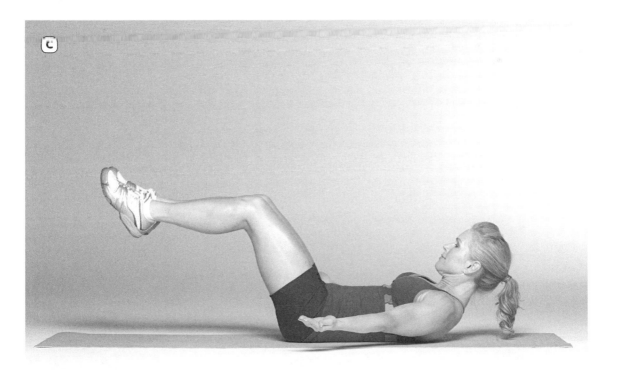

GOOD FORM TIP:
Slightly press your lower back into the floor, pulling your belly button toward your lower back.

DAY 2 TURNAROUND TIP
Remember the 2 Qs

As you progress on this journey, food is obviously an important consideration. We need food to survive on the most basic level. But we also need food to have energy for everything we do. After all, calories are really just units of energy, and what we eat absolutely affects our energy levels. I want you out there moving and going, and to do so, you need to fuel yourself for optimum energy. Today I want to talk about the 2 Qs when it comes to food: *quantity* and *quality*.

When it comes to *quantity*, my motto each and every day is *"calories in versus calories out."* On a basic level, it's all about arithmetic, since this number of calories you take in must be less than the calories you burn in order to lose weight. Bottom line, portion control is a must! Here are some eye-opening facts for you: Over the past 3 decades, fast food hamburgers have grown in size approximately 25 percent, soft drink sizes have increased more than 50 percent, and serving sizes of snacks (chips and pretzels) are up 60 percent. But the problem isn't just "super" meals. Things may be marketed as "healthy," but just because they are labeled "organic," "baked," or even "whole grain" does not mean they have no calories. Make sure you are reading the portion size on the packaging of foods you are consuming. Don't deprive, just divide!

Now let's discuss *quality*, which is just as important as quantity when it comes to energy. Food is made of lots of stuff, and the stuff in food informs our bodies how to react. Our body is a machine and it has rules. Our organs and hormones need to have certain nutrients to operate properly. Unfortunately, there's no manual that comes with our bodies. But we do know that poor-quality foods (foods with lots of additives, chemicals, preservatives, etc.) often confuse and "gum up" your genes and hormones. The result can be extra body fat and unnecessary sickness (inflammation, diabetes, etc.).

You can see how important the quality of food is when you are choosing to improve your health. You need quality foods with lots of nutrients to keep that amazing body of yours working and running at its very best! Feed good information to your body so it performs its jobs well. Give it the right tools to fulfill its duties. Quality eating is what I call clean eating—it's *intelligent* eating. It's eating from plants, animals, and trees, not from boxes and bags. It's looking for fresh food versus those steeped with preservatives. It's a nutrient-dense diet versus a nutrient-free one.

So, start looking at what you are putting into your body: This is a crucial step to turning around your health. Remember, it's *quantity* and *quality*.

I LOVE TO EAT carbs. I mean, who doesn't like to bite into a thick slice of bread or gobble up a big bowl of pasta? And guess what? Carbs are an essential part of your diet. Eaten in moderation, they will help keep you fired up all day long. To put it simply: Your brain (and the rest of your body) simply won't work without enough carbohydrates.

The controversy over carbs usually boils down to the *type* and the *amount*. Simple carbohydrates are digested very quickly, and they're found in foods like white bread, rice, pasta, cookies, sugary sodas, and many other types of processed foods. Complex carbohydrates—whole grains, fruits, vegetables, beans, and other natural food sources—take longer for the body to break down and digest.

LEARN ABOUT: CARBS

In general, the longer the carbohydrate takes to break down, the healthier it is. Nutritionists use what's called the glycemic index (GI) to decide how quickly and how high a food will boost blood sugar. The higher the number, the faster the food enters your bloodstream. Foods with a high glycemic index (candy, pasta, white bread) cause a quick spike; lower glycemic index foods (oats, whole grains) take longer. That's important as it relates to weight loss, because the body often can't break down a high-GI food fast enough, so it diverts the carbohydrates to fat stores to be broken down later and stored as fat. But with a low-GI food, your body will have enough time to break down the carbohydrates without having them stored as fat.

That said, eat too much of even the heartiest of whole grains and (in addition to getting a bellyache!) your body will store the excess amounts as fat. And not all foods with a high GI are bad for you: Watermelon, pineapple, and mango all have a moderate-to-high GI rating, but they're still filled with antioxidants, vitamins, and other healthy stuff and are a relatively low-cal way to satisfy your sweet tooth. Same thing with baked potatoes, beets, corn, and other vegetables—even though they have a high GI rating, they're still a great source of nutrients that can fill you up without a ton of calories (just watch the toppings). The Institute of Medicine recommends a daily diet with about 45 to 65 percent of its calories from carbohydrates.

My favorite carb-rich food is cereal—I eat it almost every morning! But I try to buy healthy brands that are lower in calories and sugar, and try not to eat more than the recommended serving size.

My bottom line message here: Carbs are not your enemy. They're an important source of fuel and are necessary to burn stored body fat, because your body burns fat in a carbohydrate flame—so without getting adequate carbs in your diet, you'll have a hard time burning off that body fat.

MEAL GUIDELINES:

Suggested amounts for each meal

BREAKFAST

2 grains/starchy veggies

1 dairy

1 protein

1 fruit

1 fat

A.M. SNACK

1 dairy

1 fruit

LUNCH

1 grain/starchy veggie

1 protein

2 veggies

1 fat

P.M. SNACK

1 dairy

DINNER

1 grain/starchy veggie

1 protein

2 veggies

1 fat

DAY 2 SUGGESTED MENU

BREAKFAST

1 whole-grain waffle topped with 1 cup mixed berries and 2 tablespoons chopped walnuts. Serve with 3 ounces veggie sausage and 1 cup skim milk.

PER SERVING: 480 calories; 18 g total fat; 2 g sat fat; 51 g carbohydrates; 16 g fiber; 33 g protein; 4 mg cholesterol; 830 mg sodium

NOTE: *This meal is a little high in sodium (you want to aim for no more than 600 to 650 mg per meal), which you should normally avoid, but you'll be sweating a lot throughout the 2-Week Total Body Turnaround, so you can get away with it today.*

SNACK

$^1/_2$ cup nonfat ricotta cheese topped with $^1/_4$ cup raisins and a sprinkle of cinnamon

PER SERVING: 160 calories; 0 g total fat; 0 g sat fat; 34 g carbohydrates; 1 g fiber; 6 g protein; 10 mg cholesterol; 70 mg sodium

LUNCH

Dijon Chicken and Chickpea Salad

PER SERVING: 393 calories; 14 g total fat; 2 g sat fat; 40 g carbohydrates; 10 g fiber; 30 g protein; 52 mg cholesterol; 642 mg sodium

SNACK

1 cup chocolate soymilk

PER SERVING: 90 calories; 2 g total fat; 0 g sat fat; 12 g carbohydrates; 0 g fiber; 7 g protein; 0 mg cholesterol; 180 mg sodium

DINNER

Tofu-Vegetable Marinara with Parmesan

PER SERVING: 352 calories; 16 g total fat; 2 g sat fat; 38 g carbohydrates; 8 g fiber; 18 g protein; 5 mg cholesterol; 603 mg sodium

DIJON CHICKEN AND CHICKPEA SALAD

2 teaspoons olive oil

1 teaspoon Dijon mustard

1 tablespoon cider vinegar

1 tablespoon lemon juice

$\frac{1}{8}$ teaspoon black pepper

Pinch of salt

$\frac{1}{2}$ cup no-salt-added canned chickpeas

$\frac{1}{2}$ cup chopped tomatoes

$\frac{1}{2}$ cup sliced red or yellow bell peppers

$\frac{1}{2}$ cup shredded carrots

1 cup mixed greens

3 ounces rotisserie skinless chicken breast, sliced

In a small bowl, combine the olive oil, mustard, vinegar, lemon juice, black pepper, and salt, whisking until combined. Set aside. In a medium bowl, toss together the chickpeas, tomatoes, bell peppers, carrots, and mixed greens. Drizzle with the dressing and toss until well coated. Top with the chicken breast slices.

MAKES 1 SERVING (2$\frac{3}{4}$ CUPS SALAD MIXTURE)

PER SERVING: 393 calories; 14 g total fat; 2 g sat fat; 40 g carbohydrates; 10 g fiber; 30 g protein; 52 mg cholesterol; 642 mg sodium

TOFU-VEGETABLE MARINARA WITH PARMESAN

3 ounces firm or extra-firm tofu, cubed

1$\frac{1}{2}$ teaspoons olive oil

$\frac{1}{2}$ cup sliced zucchini

1 cup sliced portobello mushrooms

$\frac{1}{2}$ cup marinara sauce

1 tablespoon chopped fresh basil

$\frac{1}{2}$ cup cooked whole grain pasta (or brown rice)

1 tablespoon grated Parmesan cheese

In a medium saucepan over medium-high heat, cook the tofu in the olive oil, stirring frequently, for about 5 minutes, or until just browned. Remove from the pan and set aside. Add the zucchini and mushrooms, and cook, stirring frequently, for about 5 minutes, or until tender. Stir in the reserved tofu and the marinara sauce and basil. Cook until warmed through. Spoon over the pasta (or rice), and sprinkle with the cheese before serving.

MAKES 1 SERVING (1$\frac{1}{4}$ CUPS MIXTURE OVER $\frac{1}{2}$ CUP COOKED PASTA)

PER SERVING: 352 calories; 16 g total fat; 2 g sat fat; 38 g carbohydrates; 8 g fiber; 18 g protein; 5 mg cholesterol; 603 mg sodium

NOTE: *This dish also works well with chicken.*

REAL 2-WEEK TURNAROUND SUCCESS STORY

Teresa
McDonald

AGE:
47

HEIGHT:
5'9"

STARTING WEIGHT:
247
pounds

AFTER 2 WEEKS:
236
pounds

RESULTS:
11 pounds,
10¾ inches
lost
(including 2 inches
off waist and
2½ inches off hips)

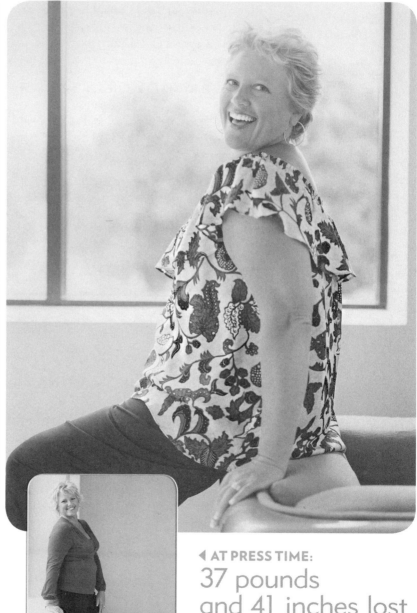

◀ **AT PRESS TIME:**
37 pounds
and 41 inches lost
in 5 months!

Like many long-time dieters, Teresa has tried pretty much every weight-loss plan that has come into vogue. "Weight Watchers, NutriSystem, the Banana Diet, the Grapefruit Diet, fasting—you name it, I've been on it," she says. A serious car accident nearly 20 years ago left her with lifelong back problems, and raising two daughters, now ages 10 and 15, gave her little time to exercise. "The weight kept coming on a little bit more every year," she notes. By the age of 47, Teresa had reached almost 250 pounds.

With a family history of weight problems—her father died of a heart attack, her mother and five siblings are all overweight—Teresa was determined to change course. "My girls are very fit and active now, but I wanted to teach them about the importance of portion control and exercise. I not only wanted to be around longer and do more with my kids, I also wanted to instill healthy habits in them."

What attracted Teresa to the 2-Week Total Body Turnaround was the structure of the plan. "Everything was laid out for me—what I could eat, what exercises I needed to do, tips on staying motivated. It was the complete package."

She got out her measuring cups and began to literally measure out each serving size. "For me, a bowl of ice cream was more like a half gallon. It was a real eye-opener to see what a portion looked like." She stocked up on fruits and vegetables, especially frozen berries, which she used to make smoothies with fat-free yogurt or sparkling soda.

"After just a couple of days, I found I wasn't even craving junk food. I fell in love with the idea of 'clean' eating." Instead, she found herself craving more fruits and vegetables and even the idea of exercise itself, doing a combination of walking outside or indoors on an elliptical machine, as well as her daily strength moves. "I'm listening to my body now and what it needs. I don't think I ever really listened before!"

When the 2 weeks were up, Teresa had lost an incredible 11 pounds and almost 11 inches. After 6 weeks of maintaining her program, she'd dropped 20 pounds and at least two dress sizes. At the 3-month mark, she was down a full 30 pounds; after a year on the program, she had lost nearly 60 pounds and 45 inches.

Equally dramatic, she reports, is the change in her energy levels. "I used to expend all of my energy taking care of everyone else, and by 6 p.m. I'd just crash on the couch and watch TV. Now I'm still going strong well into the evening hours." She's doing more with her kids—swimming, walking, hiking, and reports sleeping better, as well. Plus, her back pain and a history of severe ankle pain have greatly diminished.

"There's definitely been a shift to my entire way of thinking," she proclaims. "Even on my 'off' days, I still feel like I need to get up and move around. As this plan has progressed, it's become more about doing this for myself, as well as for my family."

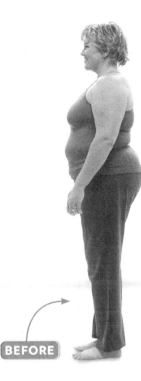

BEFORE

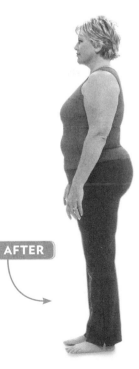

AFTER

DAY 3

■ ■ 3 ◯ ◯ ◯ ◯ ◯ ◯ ◯ ◯ ◯ ◯ ◯

Two days down, 12 to go on your journey to an amazing new life! Each day should leave you feeling stronger than before, but if you're feeling tired on occasion, that's okay too. Realize that you may be asking your body to do things it hasn't done in years, if ever. But also remember that when you're tired, sometimes the best medicine is just to get moving, even if it's only for a few minutes. This is just 2 weeks out of your life, and the workout is just 1 hour out of 24.

CARDIO: Pure Power

You've done intervals for the past 2 days, so it's time to take a bit of a break and focus on a power, or tempo, walk. Use this as an opportunity to recover and get stronger, but remember that you need to keep your mind as involved as your body. Don't just go out aimlessly for the next 30 minutes: Focus on trying to keep a pace of the highest intensity you can maintain for about 20 minutes.

INTENSITY	TIME	PACE	RPE	GOAL
Warm up (heart rate: Zone 2)	5 min.	Moderate pace	4–5	You can speak in sentences but are slightly breathless.
Power walk (heart rate: Zone 3)	20 min.	Fast pace	7	Gradually increase intensity until you are walking at the fastest pace you can sustain. You should be mostly breathless, able to speak no more than a few short phrases.
Cool down (heart rate: Zone 2)	5 min.	Moderate pace	3–4	Slow down until you are walking at a moderate pace. You should be able to speak in full sentences with some breathlessness.

STRENGTH: Total Body

I designed these total-body exercises to challenge you in new ways by engaging as many muscles as I could in one fell swoop! I love this workout because it really gets as much of your body involved as possible for 30 solid minutes. By the end, you will leave feeling totally pumped and ready to take on the world!

"The difference between the impossible and the possible lies in a person's determination."
—Tommy Lasorda, baseball legend

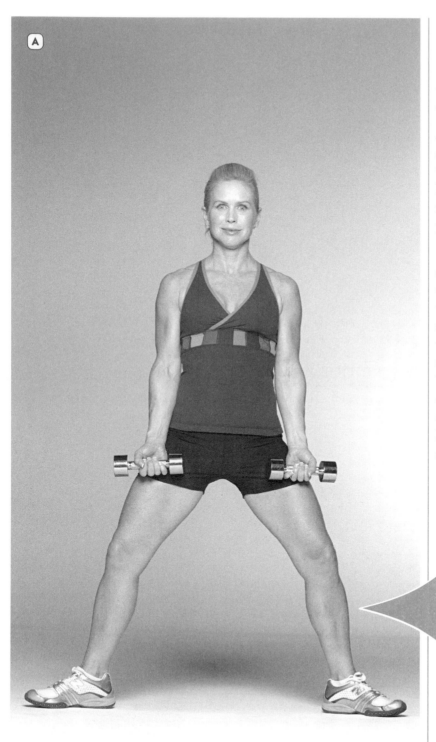

A

PLIÉ WITH BICEPS CURL

TARGETS: Biceps, butt, quads, inner thighs

A. Stand with feet shoulder-width apart, toes turned outward, holding dumbbells in front of thighs with palms facing up.

B. Slowly lower body straight down for 2 counts, bending knees 90 degrees while simultaneously curling weights toward shoulders. Slowly stand body back up for 4 counts, squeezing butt and inner thighs, as you lower arms back to starting position. Repeat 8 to 12 times.

GOOD FORM TIP:
Keep your tailbone tucked under your pelvis and your elbows close to your sides.

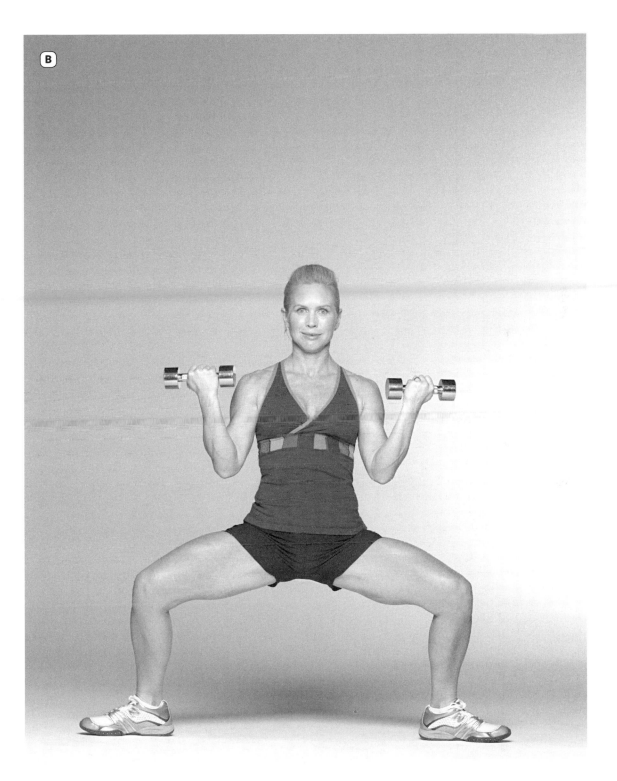

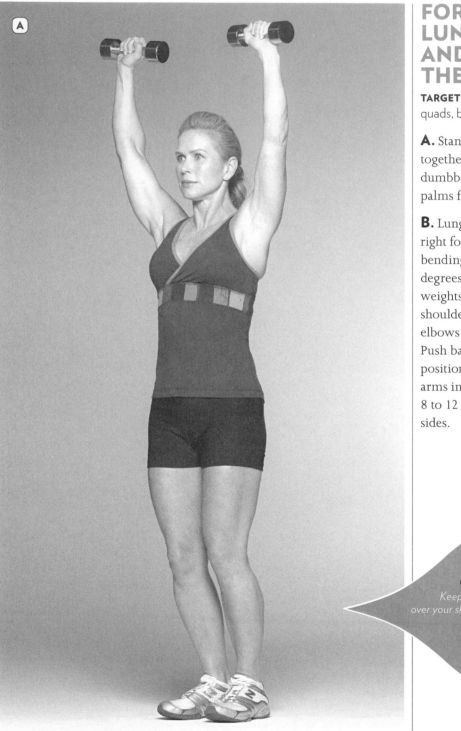

FORWARD LUNGE AND RAISE THE ROOF

TARGETS: Shoulders, quads, butt, core

A. Stand with feet together, holding dumbbells overhead, palms facing forward.

B. Lunge forward with right foot in 4 counts, bending both knees 90 degrees while lowering weights toward shoulders, bending elbows 90 degrees. Push back to starting position and straighten arms in 2 counts. Repeat 8 to 12 times; switch sides.

GOOD FORM TIP:
Keep your front knee tracking over your shoelaces to avoid putting strain on the kneecap.

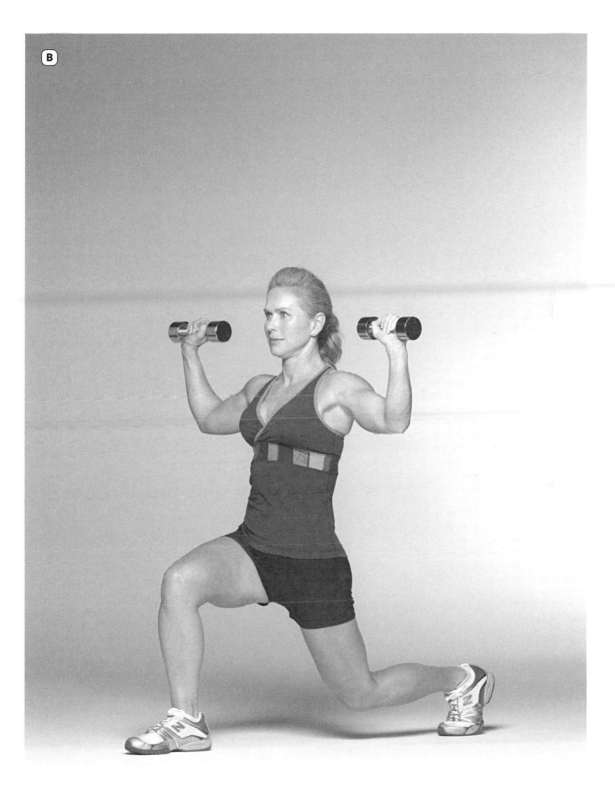

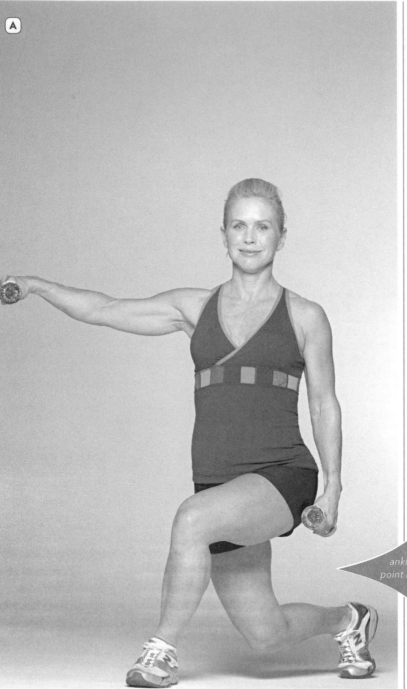

A

CURTSY LAT RAISE

TARGETS: Shoulders, butt, quads, outer thighs

A. Stand with feet shoulder-width apart, holding dumbbells at sides. Cross right leg 2 to 3 feet behind left, bending knees. At the same time, lift right arm out to side at shoulder height. Take 4 counts to perform.

B. Stand up in 2 counts, bringing right leg back to starting position as you lower arm. Repeat 8 times. Switch sides, repeat 8 times.

GOOD FORM TIP:
Keep the front knee over the ankle and facing forward (don't turn it); point back knee down. Use your shoulder to raise the arm out to the side; don't scrunch up your neck.

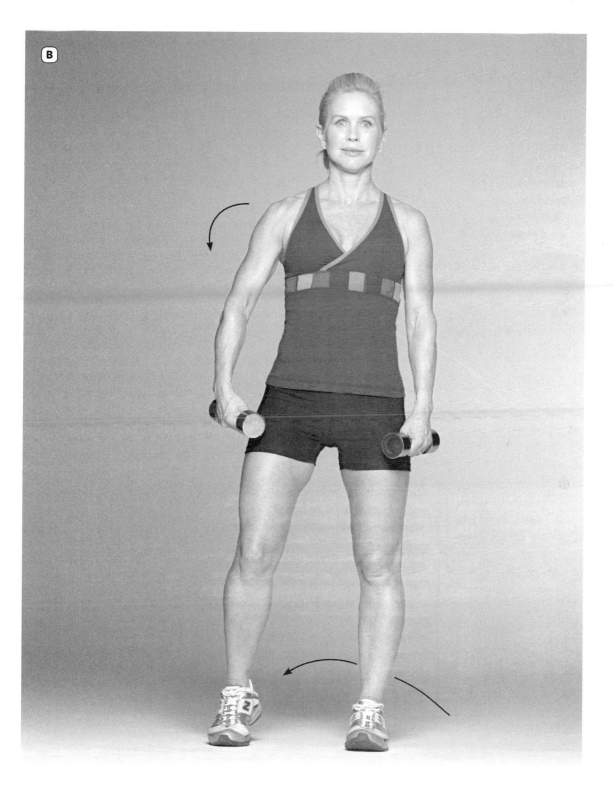

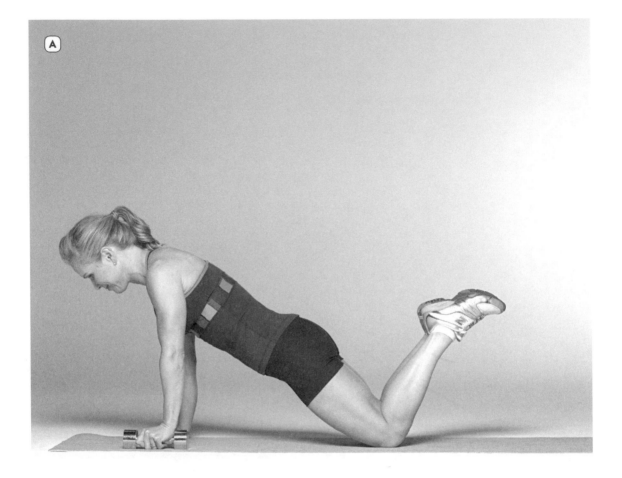

PUSHUP ROW

TARGETS: Chest, back

A. Start in modified pushup position (on knees), holding dumbbell on floor with left hand.

B. Slowly bend elbows 90 degrees as you lower chest toward floor for 4 counts, keeping abdominals tight and back straight.

C. Push back to start position for 2 counts, pulling left elbow up toward ribs. Lower weight back toward floor in 4 counts. Repeat 6 to 8 times. Switch hands and repeat the pushup 6 to 8 times, this time holding weight in right hand and lifting right elbow.

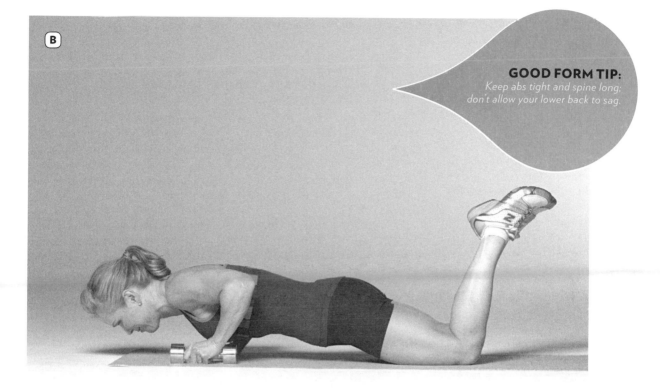

GOOD FORM TIP:
Keep abs tight and spine long; don't allow your lower back to sag.

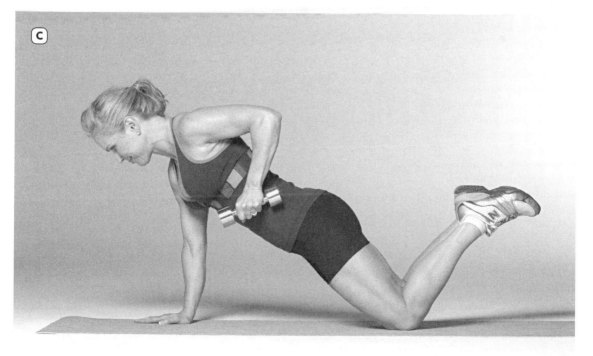

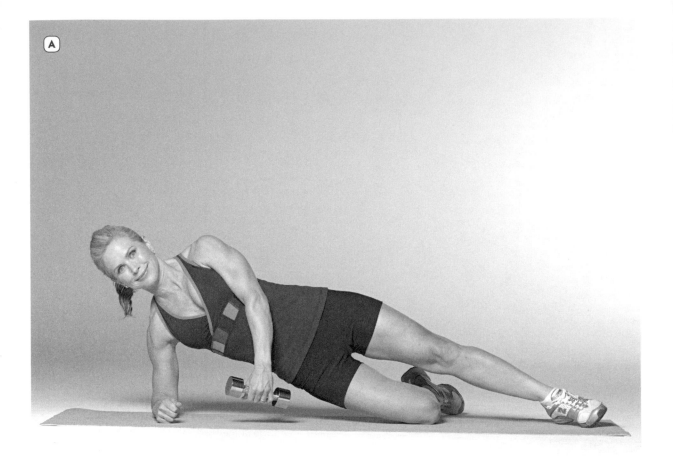

FOREARM SIDE PLANK WITH SHOULDER RAISE

TARGETS: Shoulders, obliques, abs

A. Lie on right side, hips stacked, elbow under shoulder and right forearm on floor with bottom knee on floor and top leg extended. Hold a dumbbell in left hand on floor, just in front of body. Lift hips, forming a straight line from shoulders to heels, keeping abdominals tight.

B. Lift left arm above shoulder for 2 counts and lower slowly for 4 counts, keeping hips still. Repeat 8 times. Switch sides, repeat 8 times.

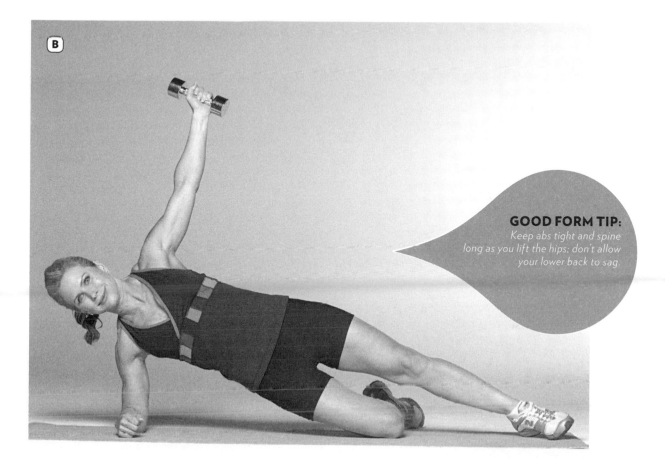

GOOD FORM TIP:
Keep abs tight and spine long as you lift the hips; don't allow your lower back to sag.

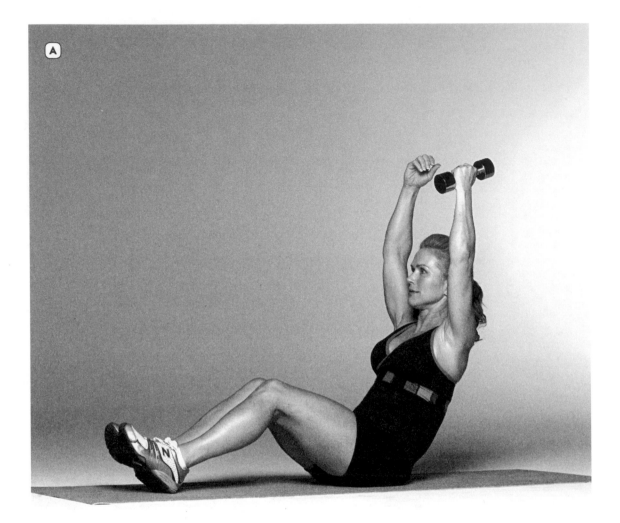

PASS THE BELL

TARGETS: Abs, shoulders

A. Sit on floor with knees bent and heels on floor in front of you. Raise both arms overhead, holding a dumbbell in left hand. Keep your back slightly rounded and abs engaged.

B. Lean back slightly and lower arms out toward shoulder height in 4 counts, keeping weight in left hand and both elbows slightly bent.

C. Lift arms back overhead in 2 counts, then switch dumbbell to right hand and repeat. Continue to "pass the bell" between hands for 8 to 10 repetitions per side.

B

GOOD FORM TIP:
*Imagine "sewing" your belly
button into your lower back to
activate your lower abs and
protect your back.*

C

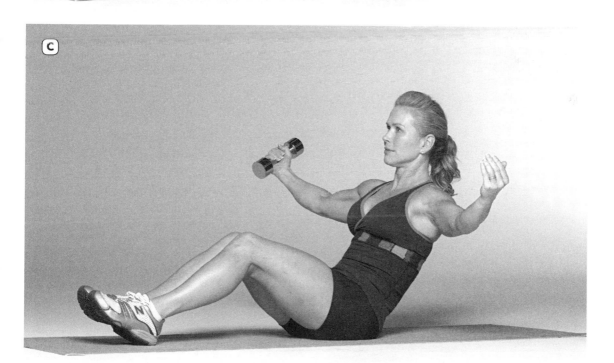

DAY 3 TURNAROUND TIP

Eat Smart When Eating Out

One of the challenges many of us face when we try to maintain a healthy lifestyle is how to eat well when eating out. On any given day, statistics say that half of all Americans will end up dining at a restaurant. But don't worry: It's safe to eat out as long as you are mentally prepared!

The secret is to realize that just because you are eating out doesn't mean you have to treat the experience like an indulgence. I understand how easy it is to slip into bad habits at restaurants. There are so many things to tempt us. The portions served are notoriously humungous, and it is easy to feel like you don't have control over the way your food is prepared. But there are a lot of tricks you can use when ordering at a restaurant that can keep your calories and fat grams down and help you stay healthy and fit. Here are a few:

- Order fish or chicken and ask for extra veggies instead of rice or potatoes. And get a side salad to start!

- Look for entrées that are baked, steamed, grilled, broiled, or poached. Avoid crusted, stuffed, and fried foods.

- If you are going to a restaurant you have never been to before, look up the menu online and preselect the healthiest choices.

- Ask for salsa as a side sauce instead of sour cream, butter, cheese, or bacon.

- Ask for a take-out container before you start eating and divide your meal in half right away. Then take half of your meal home.

- Watch your liquid calories. Avoid soft drinks, alcoholic drinks, and flavored coffees especially. If you must drink, a glass of wine is your best choice.

- Choose foods that are rich in whole grains. Ask for brown rice instead of white, whole grain bread instead of white.

- If you have a sweet tooth, split your dessert with others at the table. If no one will split with you, order lighter fare, like fresh fruit or sorbet. If you absolutely must, order the dessert but only take a couple of bites—and don't feel guilty for leaving the rest on the plate! Remember you are in control of your choices! I want you to leave that restaurant feeling as good as you did when you walked in.

IT MAY BE HARD to believe after years of being told fat is bad, but fat really can be your friend. But hold off on the double mocha chip: Like carbs, not all fat is created equal.

There are still the bad guys of the fats world, especially saturated and trans fats. Saturated fats are found in many animal sources like meat and whole-milk dairy products (cheese, milk, and yes, premium ice cream), as well as a few plant-based foods like coconut and palm oils. Saturated fats are known to boost cholesterol levels by elevating the "bad" LDL. Worse than saturated fats are trans fatty acids, a.k.a. trans fats, which are created by heating vegetable oils in the presence of hydrogen (you might know this as hydrogenation). Food manufacturers do this because it makes oils more stable and foods less likely to spoil. And that big basket of fries is usually dipped into a fryer filled with partially hydrogenated oils. There's been a big movement to ban trans fats, which is why so many companies are touting that their foods are "trans-fat-free" on their labels. But even trans-fat-free foods can have up to $1/2$ gram of the fats, which add up over time.

LEARN ABOUT: **FAT**

On to the good guys: Unsaturated fats are our heroes; they've been shown to improve cholesterol levels, reduce inflammation, lower risk of certain cancers, and even keep your brain healthy. There are two types of unsaturated fats: monounsaturated and polyunsaturated.

Monounsaturated fats (MUFAs) are common in oils like canola, olive, and peanut; nuts like pistachios, almonds, and pecans; seeds like pumpkin and sesame; and foods like avocados. (They're also found in dark chocolate—bonus! More on that on page 173.) There's been a plethora of research lately about the amazing benefits of MUFAs, everything from protecting your heart to reducing belly fat.

Polyunsaturated fats are found in foods like sunflower or corn oils, as well as walnuts and many types of fish. Omega-3 fats are a key polyunsaturated fat that has been linked with many important health benefits, from reducing arthritis to improving heart health.

In addition to the benefits above, fat helps supply the body with energy (important to help fuel your daily workouts!) and also serves as a carrier for important fat-soluble vitamins like A, D, E, and K.

Of course, like any food, fats are only going to be good for you in moderation. Because they are calorically dense (remember, 1 gram of fat has 9 calories versus just 4 calories for a gram of either carbs or protein), too much fat is going to be stored in your body as just that: adipose tissue, or fat. If you take in more calories—in any form—than you burn, you will gain weight. However, fat is a necessary nutrient on many levels. In addition to the health and nutrition benefits of MUFAs and polyunsaturated fats, having a small amount of fat in your diet (less than 25 percent) will help control your appetite and curb cravings.

MEAL GUIDELINES:
Suggested amounts for each meal

BREAKFAST
2 grains/starchy veggies

1 dairy

1 protein

1 fruit

1 fat

A.M. SNACK
1 dairy

1 fruit

LUNCH
1 grain/starchy veggie

1 protein

2 veggies

1 fat

P.M. SNACK
1 dairy

DINNER
1 grain/starchy veggie

1 protein

2 veggies

1 fat

DAY 3 SUGGESTED MENU

BREAKFAST

Apple-Pecan Oatmeal

3 vegetarian sausage links

PER SERVING: 456 calories; 12 g total fat; 1 g sat fat; 62 g carbohydrates; 10 g fiber; 26 g protein; 5 mg cholesterol; 587 mg sodium

SNACK

1/2 cup fat-free cottage cheese with 2 cups diced cantaloupe

PER SERVING: 170 calories; 1 g total fat; 0 g sat fat; 27 g carbohydrates; 3 g fiber; 15 g protein; 5 mg cholesterol; 340 mg sodium

LUNCH

Salad and sandwich combo: 3 ounces of skinless chicken breast (about 1/2 cup pulled from a rotisserie chicken) and 2 slices of tomato served on 1 slice of toasted whole-grain bread spread with 1 tablespoon lite mayonnaise. Serve with 1 cup of mixed greens and 1/4 cup each diced red bell pepper and shredded carrot, tossed with 1 tablespoon olive oil and a splash of white wine vinegar.

PER SERVING: 400 calories; 23 g total fat; 4 g sat fat; 21 g carbohydrates; 5 g fiber; 27 g protein; 63 mg cholesterol; 350 mg sodium

SNACK

Moroccan Dip with Crudités

PER 1/4-CUP SERVING: 37 calories; 1 g total fat; 0.5 g sat fat; 5 g carbohydrates; 0.5 g fiber; 3 g protein; 3 mg cholesterol; 39 mg sodium

DINNER

3 ounces grilled fish of choice served with 2 cups mixed steamed veggies, 10 olives, and 1/2 whole grain pita

PER SERVING: 310 calories; 15 g total fat; 3 g sat fat; 17 g carbohydrates; 6 g fiber; 23 g protein; 55 mg cholesterol; 620 mg sodium

APPLE-PECAN OATMEAL WITH SAUSAGE

1 cup fat-free milk, divided

$^1/_2$ teaspoon cinnamon

$^1/_4$ cup old-fashioned oats

1 small apple, peeled, cored, and chopped (about 1 cup)

2 teaspoons brown sugar

$^1/_2$ teaspoon vanilla extract

1 tablespoon chopped pecans

3 vegetarian sausage links

In a small saucepan over medium heat, heat $^1/_2$ cup milk and the cinnamon until boiling. Stir in the oats and cook for 3 to 5 minutes, or until thickened. Stir in the apple, sugar, vanilla, and pecans, and cook for 1 minute longer. Remove from heat.

In a small skillet coated with nonstick cooking spray, cook the sausage until heated through, about 5 minutes. Serve with the oatmeal and the remaining $^1/_2$ cup milk.

MAKES 1 SERVING (1 CUP)

PER SERVING: 456 calories; 12 g total fat; 1 g sat fat; 62 g carbohydrates; 10 g fiber; 26 g protein; 5 mg cholesterol; 587 mg sodium

NOTE: *Look for low-sodium vegetarian sausage.*

MOROCCAN DIP

$^3/_4$ cup plain low-fat yogurt

1 cup peeled, chopped cucumber

$^1/_4$ teaspoon hot sauce (like Tabasco)

$^1/_2$ teaspoon cumin

$^1/_2$ teaspoon garlic powder

1 tablespoon chopped fresh mint

Combine the ingredients and serve with 1 cup sliced veggies, such as carrots, red bell pepper, and cucumber.

MAKES 4 SERVINGS (1 CUP)

PER $^1/_4$-CUP SERVING: 37 calories; 1 g total fat; 0.5 g sat fat; 5 g carbohydrates; 0.5 g fiber; 3 g protein; 3 mg cholesterol; 39 mg sodium

DAY 4

▪ ▪ ▪ [4] ☐ ☐ ☐ ☐ ☐ ☐ ☐ ☐ ☐

By now you're on the path to really making some great changes in your lifestyle. Are you starting to feel the changes? "Fit Has a Feeling" was an ad campaign for Propel fitness water, and I think that sums up my feelings about exercise perfectly. When I have to wake up early, pull on my workout clothes, and head to the gym to teach my 5:30 a.m. class, I, too, will feel a little tired. But once I start to get moving, I get into a groove and feel great. I'm always playing up the physical benefits you'll get from exercise, but there are emotional ones, too.

Everybody is different, but I am a true believer in movement therapy. Any movement is good movement. Just move your body and your mood starts to change. It's like music—it creates a feeling. Maybe it's the confidence you get knowing that you are accomplishing something good for yourself. Maybe it's stress relief, being able to just be in the moment and let the outside world go. Maybe it's a stimulant, recharging your battery and giving you energy. Maybe it's beauty, because when you feel beautiful on the inside, it shows on the outside.

So go for it! Get hooked on a feeling! Often it's that feeling that brings you back for more. I may not be able to put my finger on it, but when 4:30 a.m. is my rise-and-shine time, there must be a feeling that is getting me motivated. It's deep inside, and, as tired as I may feel, I love it!

I'm not suggesting everyone needs to start getting up at 4:30 a.m. I'm just suggesting you get moving at some point in the day and pay attention to the feeling during and after your workout. I know what some of you may be thinking: "The only feeling I have when I work out is pain!" But start with baby steps and give it a few weeks. Recently I

"Clear your mind of can't."
—Samuel Johnson, British author

saw a client who had just started a regular exercise routine 6 months before. She had to really stay focused to keep it up, but when I saw her, I asked, "So, you are still working out all the time?" And she replied back, "Yeah, I am. I guess it's just a part of me now." She got hooked on a feeling, and it's not just weight loss that kept her committed—it's so much more!

CARDIO: Pyramid

Today's cardio workout is a pyramid, which features slightly longer intervals that build in intensity. It's a great way to keep you motivated and challenged throughout the full half-hour workout.

INTENSITY	TIME	RPE	TALK TEST
Warm up (heart rate: Zone 2)	3 min.	4–5	You can speak in full sentences (slightly breathless)
Increase pace (heart rate: Zone 3)	2 min.	6–7	You can speak mostly in phrases (breathless)
Slow down (heart rate: Zone 2–3)	2 min.	5–6	Somewhat breathless (brisk walk)
Speed up, pump arms (heart rate: Zone 4)	4 min.	8–9	Very breathless
Slow down (heart rate: Zone 2–3)	4 min.	5–6	Somewhat breathless (brisk walk)
Speed up, pump arms (heart rate: Zone 4)	5 min.	8–9	Very breathless
Slow down (heart rate: Zone 2–3)	2 min.	5–6	Somewhat breathless (brisk walk)
Speed up, pump arms (heart rate: Zone 4)	4 min.	8–9	Very breathless
Slow down (heart rate: Zone 2)	4 min.	5	Somewhat breathless (brisk walk, gradually moving into cooldown)

STRENGTH: Upper Body + Core

Today's workout features all-new upper-body moves to work your back, shoulders, arms, and chest. You'll also tone your abs with exercises that target these muscles both directly and indirectly. Remember to really take your time with each repetition: Slowing down the exercise is what is going to help you get the results you want.

Ⓐ

FLY AWAY (WIDE AND HIGH)

TARGETS: Back, shoulders

A. Stand with right foot in front of left, leaning forward slightly but keeping spine long and abs tight. Hold dumbbells near to right leg, elbows slightly bent and palms facing each other.

B. Lift arms up and back, keeping elbows bent and squeezing shoulder blades together for 2 counts. Lower back to start position for 4 counts. Repeat 6 times and switch legs, left foot forward, repeating 6 more times.

GOOD FORM TIP: *Pull the weights back and squeeze your shoulder blades together; focus on using your back, not your neck. Press your shoulders away from your ears.*

Ⓐ

SUSPENDED BICEPS CURL

TARGETS: Biceps

A. Stand with arms extended out to sides at shoulder height, holding dumbbells with palms facing up, elbows slightly bent. Curl weights toward shoulders in 2 counts.

B. Reverse the move in 4 counts, lowering arms back to sides. Repeat 8 to 12 times.

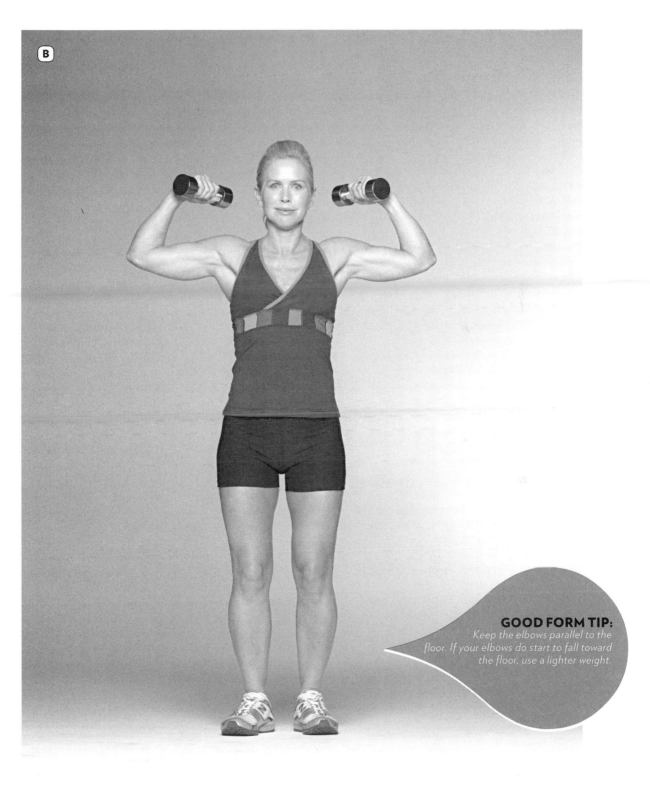

B

GOOD FORM TIP:
Keep the elbows parallel to the floor. If your elbows do start to fall toward the floor, use a lighter weight.

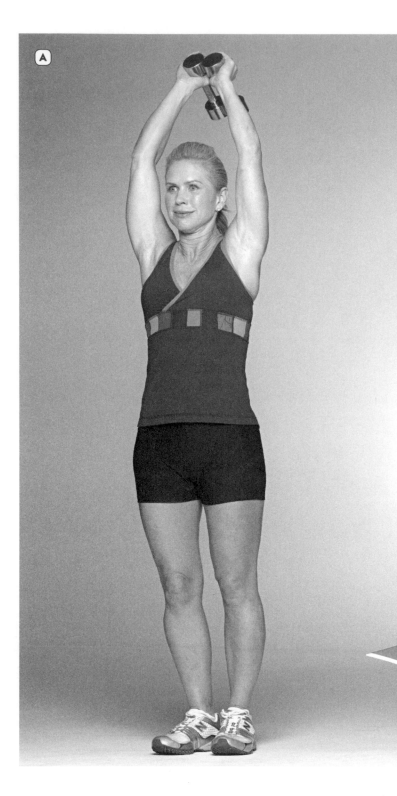

STANDING TRICEPS TONER

TARGETS: Triceps

A. Stand with feet hip-distance apart, arms extended over head, holding one or two dumbbells with both hands.

B. Slowly bend elbows and lower weight behind head for 4 counts. Lift weight back above head for 2 counts, squeezing triceps and keeping arms next to your ears. Repeat 8 to 12 times.

GOOD FORM TIP: *Keep your elbows close to your ears; focus on using the back of your arms.*

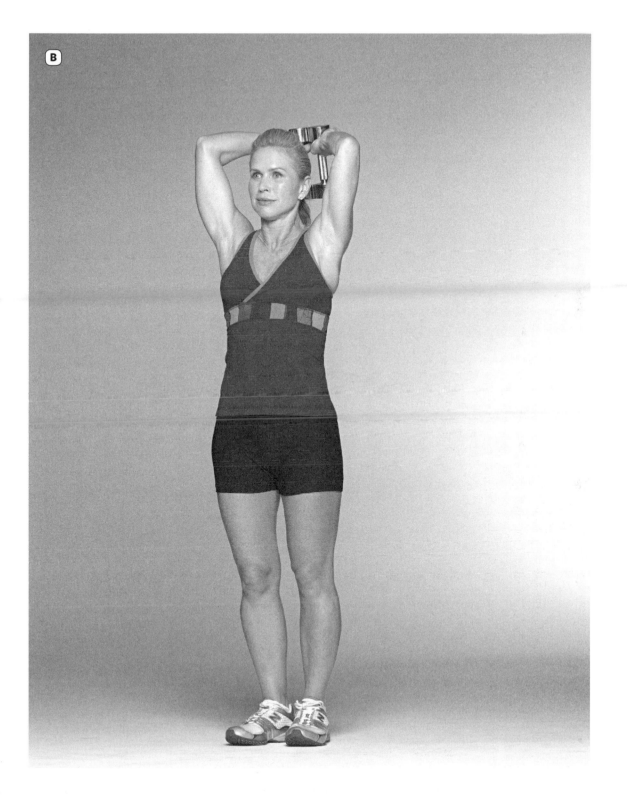

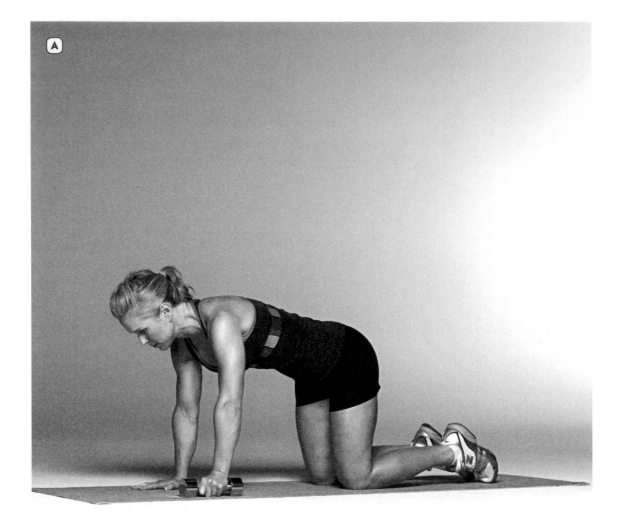

KNEELING SHOULDER SHAPER

TARGETS: Shoulders

A. Starting on all fours in kneeling position, hold dumbbell in left hand.

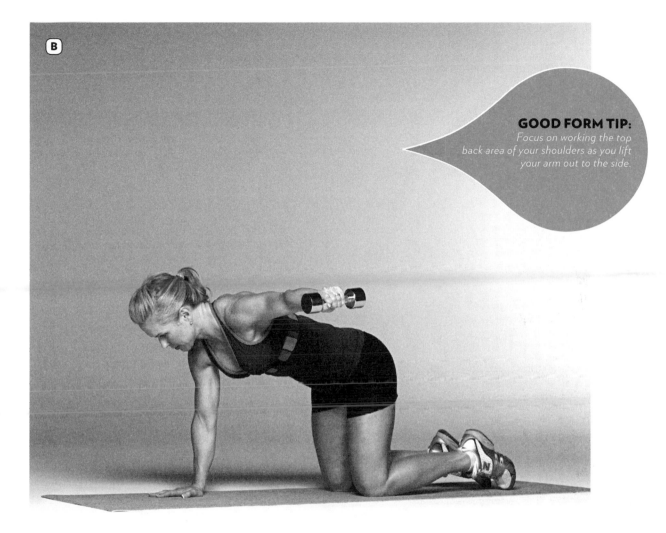

GOOD FORM TIP:
Focus on working the top back area of your shoulders as you lift your arm out to the side.

B. Keeping abdominals tight and a slight bend in the left elbow, reach dumbbell out to side slowly for 2 counts. Lower back to start position for 4 counts. Repeat 8 to 12 times; then switch sides and repeat.

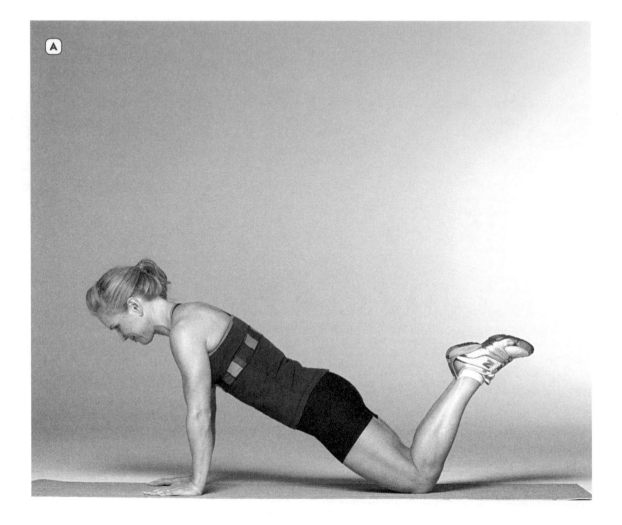

AIRPLANE PUSHUP

TARGETS: Chest, triceps, shoulders, back, abs

A. Start in modified pushup position, on knees with hands on floor shoulder-distance apart.

B. Bend elbows 90 degrees, lowering chest toward floor in 4 counts; keep abs tight and body in a straight line.

C. Push back up to start position in 2 counts, reaching left arm forward and right leg back. Balance here for a moment, then repeat, lifting right arm and left leg. Do 6 to 8 repetitions on each side.

B

GOOD FORM TIP:
Keep your abs tight and your spine long to prevent your lower back from sagging.

C

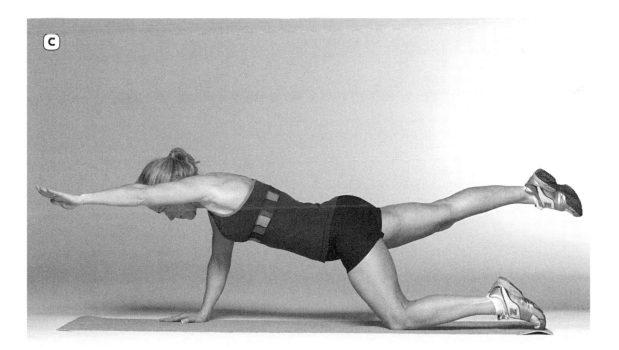

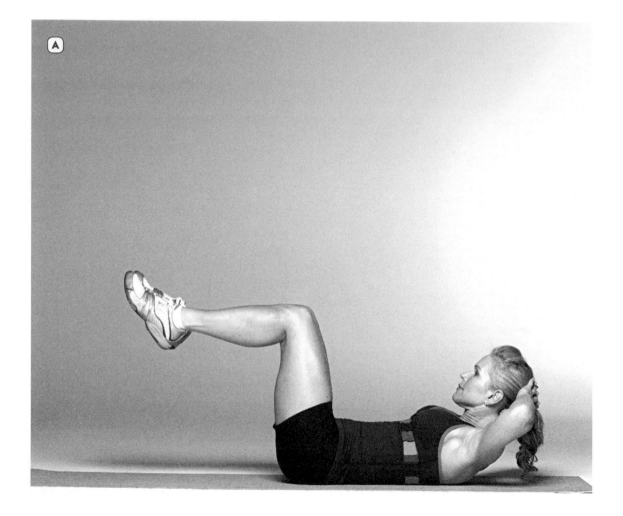

TABLE-TOP CRUNCH WITH REACH

TARGETS: Abs

A. Lie face up on floor with knees bent 90 degrees, feet lifted with shins parallel to floor, and fingers behind head. Curl your upper body up off the floor in 2 counts, using abdominal muscles.

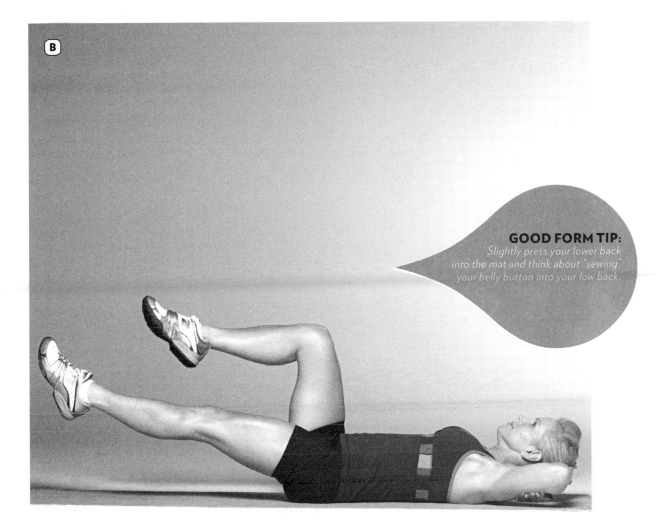

GOOD FORM TIP:
Slightly press your lower back into the mat and think about "sewing" your belly button into your low back.

B. Slowly lower upper body back toward floor in 4 counts, straightening left leg toward floor on the 4th count. Bend knee back to start and repeat, this time lowering right leg. Repeat 8 to 10 times per side.

DAY 4 TURNAROUND TIP
Adding Muscle to Your Routine

I stressed the importance of strength training earlier, and how it helps you increase your muscle mass so your body works more efficiently. In addition to boosting your metabolism and giving you more energy, strength training helps everyday activities feel easier. When you become stronger, you usually become more active in your daily life. The mental benefits are there, too. Studies have shown that lifting weights also aids in improving your self-esteem and body image. The better you feel, the more you'll want to keep moving and make healthier lifestyle choices—and that is exactly what we want to keep doing!

Lifting weights at the gym or using dumbbells at home are great ways to build strength, but they aren't the only way to build muscles. In fact, you don't need any equipment at all to reap strength benefits. Some of my favorite exercises, like pushups, squats, and lunges, use your own body weight to provide the resistance you need to strengthen your muscles. Just remember that to build muscle and jumpstart your metabolism, you should do several strength-training sessions each week. You can either do a total body workout or one that works different parts of the body (for example, your upper body or your lower body). Just remember that you do want to try to give those muscles a chance to rest and rebuild in between workouts.

As you begin adding strength training to your workout routine, keep these points in mind:

- Do the exercises slowly. Make your muscles do the work, not momentum, and be sure to use your full range of motion from the start to the finish. Don't jerk the muscles or go halfway.

- Breathe. It's important to breathe fully when you lift weights, because your body needs a good deal of oxygen to help your muscles and brain do their jobs. Remember to breathe out during the most strenuous part of the movement. Whatever you do, do not hold your breath! Not only can you get lightheaded, you may also put too much pressure on your back, chest, and abdomen.

- Keep your lower abdominal muscles tight. Think about pulling in your navel—like you were about to squeeze into a pair of tight jeans. Engaging your deep abdominals means every part of the exercise will feel easier, plus you'll help protect your lower back. By standing tall and keeping everything tight, you'll get a better workout and prevent injury.

ONCE UPON A TIME, white bread ruled the sandwich world and whole-wheat pasta was unheard of. Things sure have changed: Nowadays whole-grain breads far outnumber the plain white offerings in the supermarket, and there's a plethora of other types of whole-grain offerings up and down the aisles.

Why the fuss about whole grains? Of course, there's the fiber benefit: Whole grains are high in fiber, and fiber is like a big broom for the body's digestive system.

There are two types of fibers: soluble and insoluble. Soluble fibers bind to fatty substances and carry them out as waste, which helps lower LDL ("bad") cholesterol. They also help regulate blood sugars so you stay fuller, longer. Insoluble fibers help push food through the intestinal tract, so you stay, well, regular.

LEARN ABOUT: GRAINS

In addition, whole grains contain protective antioxidants in amounts that are close to if not higher than those found in fruits and vegetables, as well as some other unique antioxidants. Recent studies have found a diet rich in whole grains may help reduce heart disease, cancer, and diabetes.

Quick lesson about the anatomy of a whole grain: All grains start out whole before they head for the mill. If they keep all three parts (endosperm, bran, and germ), they're still whole. White flour is basically whole-wheat flour with the nutritious part taken out; white rice is basically brown rice with the nutritious part taken out.

I also encourage you to think outside the Wheaties box. Many types of grains are whole grains, including barley, corn on the cob, and oats. Experiment with "exotic" whole grains, like amaranth, quinoa, and wheatberries. You'll be surprised at how much your local grocery store carries already.

Also, be aware that multigrain foods aren't always whole grains. Multigrain only means different types of grains were used; they can still be either refined or whole. Look on the label: One of the first few ingredients should have the word "whole" in front of the grain. (Oats get a pass, because they are always whole grain.)

On the 2-Week Total Body Turnaround, you'll have 4 servings of grains a day. Make them whole grains for maximum benefits.

MEAL GUIDELINES:

Suggested amounts for each meal

BREAKFAST

2 grains/starchy veggies

1 dairy

1 protein

1 fruit

1 fat

A.M. SNACK

1 dairy

1 fruit

LUNCH

1 grain/starchy veggie

1 protein

2 veggies

1 fat

P.M. SNACK

1 dairy

DINNER

1 grain/starchy veggie

1 protein

2 veggies

1 fat

DAY 4 SUGGESTED MENU

BREAKFAST

Breakfast sandwich: Toast 2 slices of multigrain bread and fill with 3 ounces Canadian bacon and $\frac{1}{5}$ of a medium avocado. Serve with 1 cup of nonfat or low-fat yogurt mixed with 1 cup of sliced strawberries.

PER SERVING: 490 calories; 11 g total fat; 3 g sat fat; 81 g carbohydrates; 7 g fiber; 22 g protein; 24 mg cholesterol; 760 mg sodium

NOTE: *This meal is a little high in sodium (you want to aim for no more than 600 to 650 mg per meal), which you should normally avoid, but you'll be sweating a lot throughout the 2-Week Total Body Turnaround, so you can get away with it today.*

SNACK

1 part-skim string cheese with 1 cup grapes

PER SERVING: 200 calories; 6 g total fat; 4 g sat fat; 30 g carbohydrates; 1 g fiber; 8 g protein; 15 mg cholesterol; 150 mg sodium

LUNCH

Simple Salad "Niçoise"

PER SERVING: 349 calories; 11 g total fat; 1 g sat fat; 32 g carbohydrates; 6 g fiber; 28 g protein; 53 mg cholesterol; 565 mg sodium

SNACK

1 cup skim milk

PER SERVING: 80 calories; 0 g total fat; 0 g sat fat; 12 g carbohydrates; 0 g fiber; 8 g protein; 0 mg cholesterol; 100 mg sodium

DINNER

Tomato Chicken Thighs with Zucchini and Lentils

PER SERVING: 360 calories; 17 g total fat; 3 g sat fat; 29 g carbohydrates; 11 g fiber; 24 g protein; 55 mg cholesterol; 375 mg sodium

SIMPLE SALAD "NIÇOISE"

¹/₂ cup cooked whole grain pasta

3 ounces chunk light tuna, packed in water, drained

¹/₂ cup chopped tomatoes

¹/₂ cup green beans, steamed and cut into 1" lengths

1 tablespoon chopped Kalamata or niçoise olives

1 clove garlic, chopped

1 tablespoon balsamic vinegar

2 teaspoons olive oil

Pinch of salt and pepper

In a small bowl, combine the pasta with the tuna, tomatoes, green beans, olives, and garlic. Toss with balsamic vinegar, olive oil, and salt and pepper.

MAKES 1 SERVING (2 CUPS)

PER SERVING: 349 calories; 11 g total fat; 1 g sat fat; 32 g carbohydrates; 6 g fiber; 28 g protein; 53 mg cholesterol; 565 mg sodium

NOTE: *If you're a vegetarian, don't worry! Simply substitute ³/₄ cup chickpeas or other white beans for the tuna.*

TOMATO CHICKEN THIGHS WITH ZUCCHINI AND LENTILS

¹/₈ cup dry green or brown lentils

1 bay leaf

1 tablespoon chopped garlic, divided

¹/₈ teaspoon salt

¹/₈ teaspoon black pepper

1 tablespoon olive oil

1 cup chopped tomatoes

1 cup sliced zucchini

1 skinless, boneless chicken thigh (3–3.5 ounces), sliced

1 tablespoon chopped fresh basil

In a medium saucepan, combine the lentils, bay leaf, and 1 teaspoon of the garlic. Cover the lentils with 1 to 2 inches of water, and bring to a boil. Reduce the heat, cover, and simmer for 25 minutes, or until the lentils are tender, draining any liquid if necessary. Discard the bay leaf; stir in the salt and pepper. Meanwhile, heat the oil in a medium skillet over medium-high heat. Add the remaining garlic and cook, stirring frequently, for 30 seconds. Add the tomatoes and zucchini, and cook for about 2 to 3 minutes, or until barely tender. Add the chicken slices and continue cooking with the vegetables for another 5 minutes. Cover, and reduce heat to a simmer for 5 to 10 minutes more, or until the chicken is cooked through. Spoon the chicken and vegetables over the lentils to serve. Sprinkle with the basil.

MAKES 1 SERVING (1¹/₄ CUPS)

PER SERVING: 360 calories; 17 g total fat; 3 g sat fat; 29 g carbohydrates; 11 g fiber; 24 g protein; 55 mg cholesterol; 375 mg sodium

REAL 2-WEEK TURNAROUND SUCCESS STORY

Laurie Champ

AGE:
46

HEIGHT:
5'6"

START WEIGHT:
184 pounds

AFTER 2 WEEKS:
175 pounds

RESULTS:
9 pounds, 11 inches lost
(including 3¾ inches from waist and 2 inches from hips)

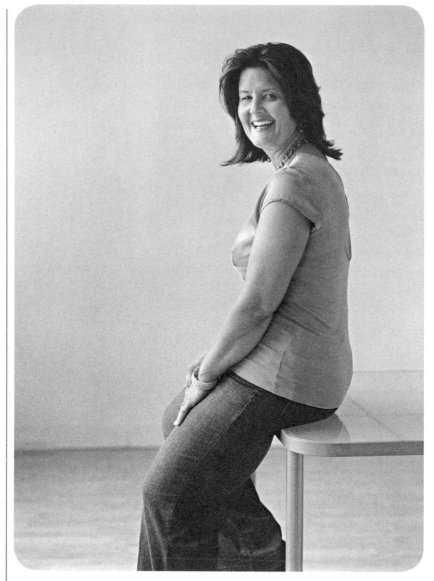

After 27 years of marriage and raising three children (ranging in age from 14 to 23), Laurie and her husband, Tim, are partners in every sense of the word. That holds true when it comes to weight loss as well. "We've been on a lot of diets together, where we've taken off the weight but put it back on," says Laurie. "Neither of us are super overweight, but we want to be around for when our grandkids and great grandkids come into this world."

Before the duo started their 2-Week Total Body Turnaround, they sat down and picked out which types of foods they wanted to eat, then hit the grocery store to stock up on necessities. Every day, Tim cooked the family meals and the pair walked together and did their strength workouts.

By the end of the 2 weeks, Laurie had dropped 9 pounds and 11 inches— almost 4 of them from her waistline alone! "The first thing I noticed shrinking was my stomach," she says. "You get that belly bloat with menopause. I noticed it getting smaller in just a few days." (Tim weighed in 12 pounds less after his 2 weeks were up.)

Although a back injury temporarily halted her progress, she's still down about 13 pounds and well on her way to her goal weight of being 40 pounds lighter. (She also credits the core-strengthening moves with helping her recover from her injury more quickly.) "This program has really been an amazing jumpstart for me. Seeing those results in such a short amount of time really motivates you to keep moving forward." She's dropped from a size 12 to a 10, and plans to get into a size 8 soon.

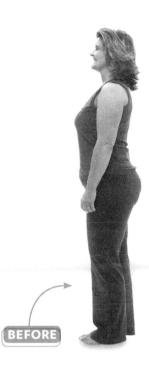

BEFORE

In addition to losing pounds and inches, Laurie says she's also noticed significant gains in her energy levels and is sleeping better at night "I always thought I was a fairly energetic person, but after losing even just a few pounds, I realized that what I thought was an '8' on a scale of 1 to 10 was more like a '5.' But now I have more energy all day long." She had the same experience with her strength gains: "I thought I was strong, but when I started lifting weights, I realized I was using muscles that hadn't been worked in a long time!"

She also found that she wasn't constantly thinking about food or feeling hungry. "In the past, by 10 a.m., I couldn't wait for lunch. Now I feel more satisfied all day long." Favorite new foods include a tablespoon of peanut butter on a whole-wheat English muffin and grilled salmon. And her new rule of thumb emphasizes moderation: "My birthday was right at the end of my second week, and I had a sliver of pie that my co-workers bought me at work. I made it up by going for an extra-long walk that night!" Keeping the idea of "Motivation Monday" is also key: "If you have a bad weekend, eating-wise, you can always start anew. The important thing is not to give up."

Most of all, says Laurie, she realizes that the ultimate responsibility for her actions lies with her. "One of Chris's tips that stuck with me is that your body and talents are God's gifts to you. But what you do with that gift is up to you. When I think about that, I realize this isn't a temporary solution but a way of life."

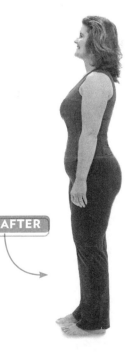

AFTER

DAY 5

■ ■ ■ ■ 5 ○ ○ ○ ○ ○ ○ ○ ○ ○

As you progress through the 2-Week Total Body Turnaround, remember that your genes don't always signal your destiny. I've had so many clients tell me that because their parents were overweight, they were doomed to be that way as well. I say: No way! Genetics loads your gun, but environment pulls your trigger. It's what you do, what you eat, what you think that shapes your life. You might have to fight a slower metabolism or naturally large bone structure, but you determine your ultimate shape and appearance.

CARDIO: Speed Ladder

This is one of my favorite workouts, because it allows you to challenge yourself with intervals that get harder but shorter. It can take you to a level that you never thought possible—but don't worry! It will be over before you know it.

INTENSITY	TIME	RPE	TALK TEST
Warm up (heart rate: Zone 2)	4 min.	4–5	You can speak in full sentences (slightly breathless)
Speed up (heart rate: Zone 2)	5 min.	5	Slightly breathless (brisk walk)
Speed up (heart rate: Zone 3)	4 min.	6	Somewhat more breathless (pace is slightly faster than before)
Slow down (heart rate: Zone 2)	2 min.	5	Slightly breathless (brisk walk)
Speed up (heart rate: Zone 3)	3 min.	7	Breathless (pace is slightly faster than last speed burst)
Slow down (heart rate: Zone 2)	2 min.	5	Slightly breathless (brisk walk)
Speed up (heart rate: Zone 4)	2 min.	8	Very breathless (pace is slightly faster than last speed burst; you can take this into a slow jog)
Slow down (heart rate: Zone 2)	2 min.	5	Slightly breathless (brisk walk)
Speed up (heart rate: Zone 4)	1 min.	9	Very breathless (Take this into a jog if you can, or walk as fast as possible)
Cool down (heart rate: Zone 2)	5 min.	4–5	Slightly breathless

STRENGTH: Lower Body + Core

An all-new set of burn-and-firm moves for your abs, legs, and butt! We're working multiple muscles at once here, so you get a bigger bang for your buck. Remember, take it slow for best results!

POWER LUNGE

TARGETS: Quads, butt

A. Stand with feet together, arms at sides holding dumbbells. Step left leg back and lower into lunge position for 4 counts, keeping right knee over ankle as you bend knees 90 degrees.

B. Lift left leg and bring left knee in front of body to hip height in 2 counts. Repeat 8 times. Switch legs and repeat.

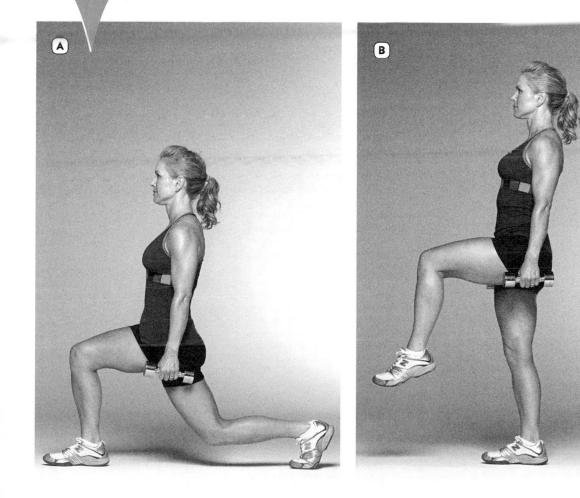

Ⓐ

STILETTO SQUATS

TARGETS: Quads, butt, calves

A. Stand with feet shoulder-width apart, arms in front at chest height. Squat down, as if sitting in a chair behind you, for 4 counts, keeping weight in heels.

B. Lift heels, keeping arms in front of you for balance.

C. Rise back up to standing for 2 counts, keeping heels lifted. Lower arms and lower heels to floor. Repeat 8 to 12 times.

GOOD FORM TIP:
When squatting back, keep your knees tracking over your shoelaces (not past your toes) to avoid putting pressure onto kneecaps. Keep torso lifted, chin parallel to the floor.

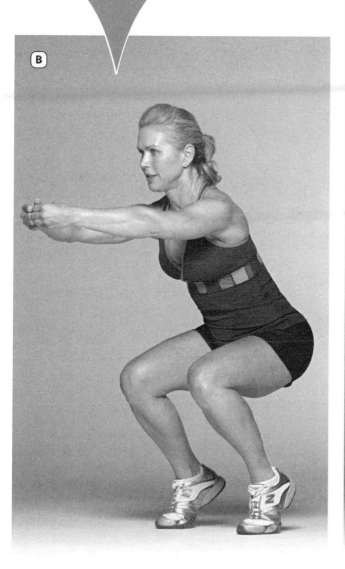

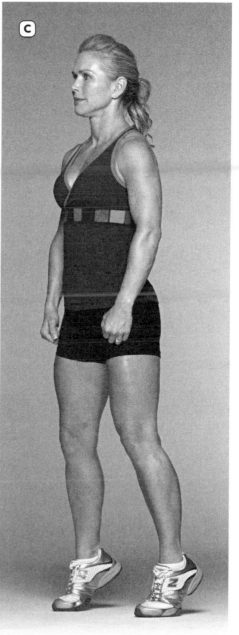

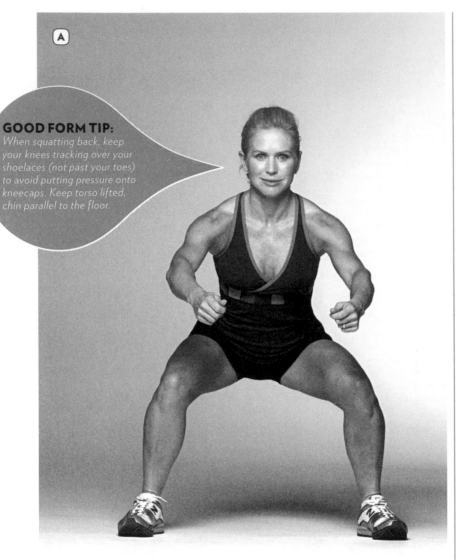

GOOD FORM TIP:
When squatting back, keep your knees tracking over your shoelaces (not past your toes) to avoid putting pressure onto kneecaps. Keep torso lifted, chin parallel to the floor.

CLOCK SQUATS

TARGETS: Quads, butt

A. Stand with feet wider than shoulder-width apart. Imagine yourself standing on a big clock, with your right foot on the center and your left foot on the "9." Lower into a squat for 4 counts, keeping weight in heels.

B. Rise up for 2 counts, lifting left foot up as you pivot right foot 90 degrees, so left foot is on "12" on the final count.

C. Repeat squat, bringing left foot to "3" on the 2nd count as you stand up.

D. Repeat squat, bringing left foot to "6" position on the 2nd count as you stand up.

E. Repeat squat, this time pivoting back to start position (left foot on "9") on the 2nd count as you stand up. Repeat the entire series, this time turning counterclockwise as you lift right foot. Then repeat the entire series 2 more times in each direction.

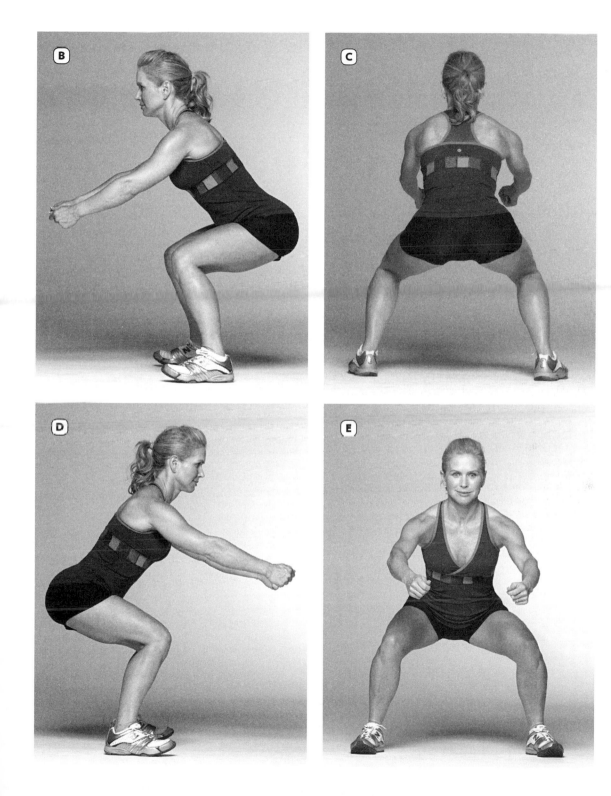

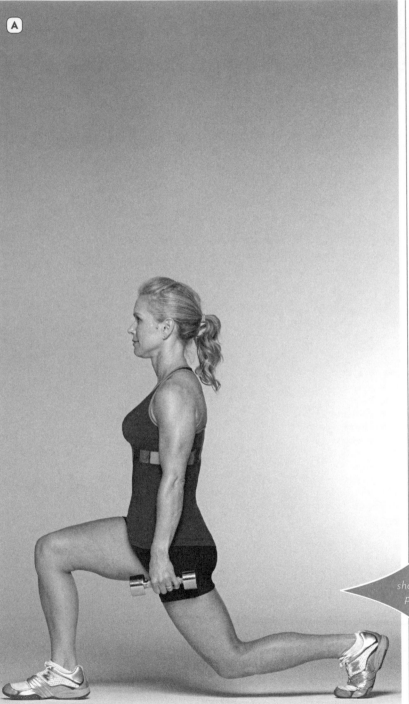

A

SPLIT-STANCE LUNGE

TARGETS: Quads, butt

A. Stand tall with legs about 3 feet apart, right foot in front of left, holding dumbbells with arms at sides. Lift left heel as you lower left knee down into a lunge for 4 counts.

B. Push up through the front foot as you stand in 2 counts, keeping back heel raised. Repeat 8 to 12 times and switch feet.

GOOD FORM TIP:
Keep front knee tracking over your shoelaces (not past your toes) to avoid putting pressure onto kneecap. Also, keep torso straight so as not to bend forward.

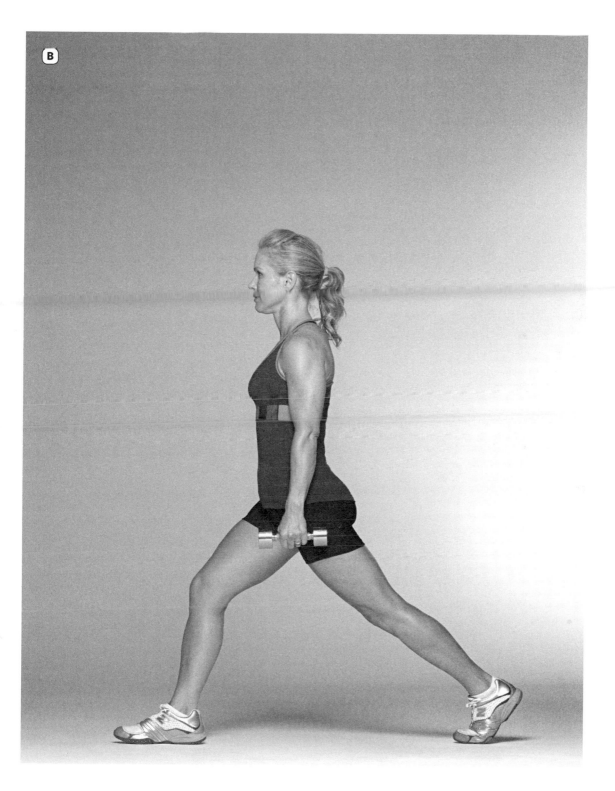

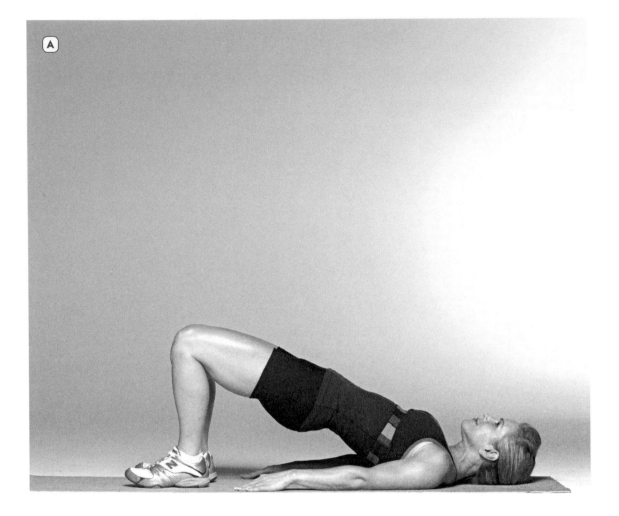

BRIDGE

TARGETS: Hamstrings, butt

A. Lie face up on floor, knees bent, feet flat on floor. Pushing feet into floor, lift hips up for 2 counts, keeping abs tight and body in a straight line from knees to chest.

B. Slowly lower body back to floor for 4 counts. Repeat 8 to 12 times.

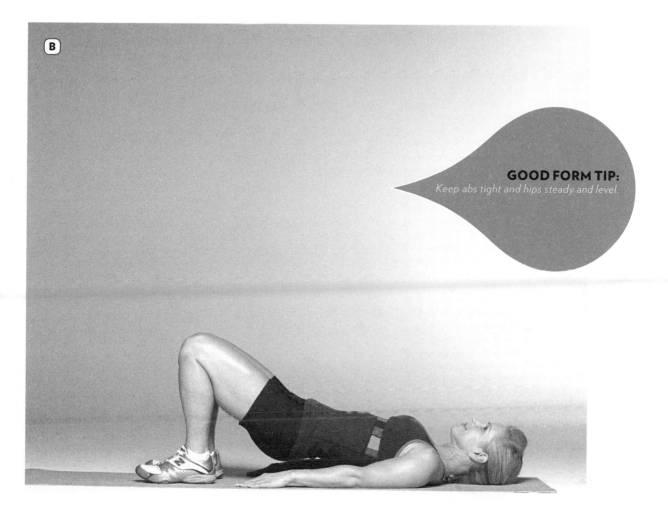

B

GOOD FORM TIP:
Keep abs tight and hips steady and level.

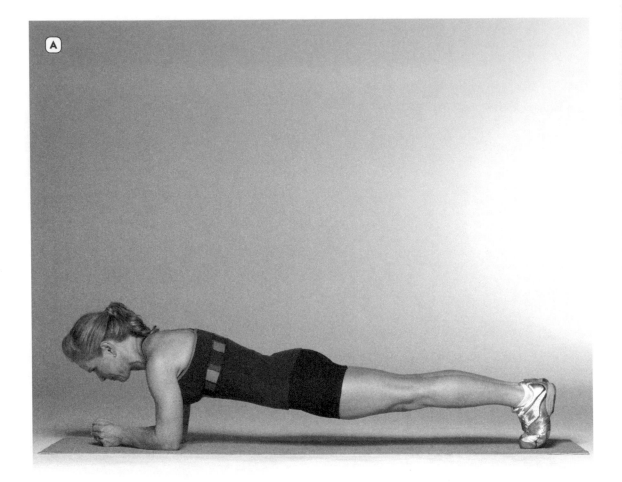

HIP DROP

TARGETS: Abs, obliques

A. Lie face down on floor, legs extended, with elbows and forearms on floor. Lift hips, keeping abs tight while forming a straight line from head to heels.

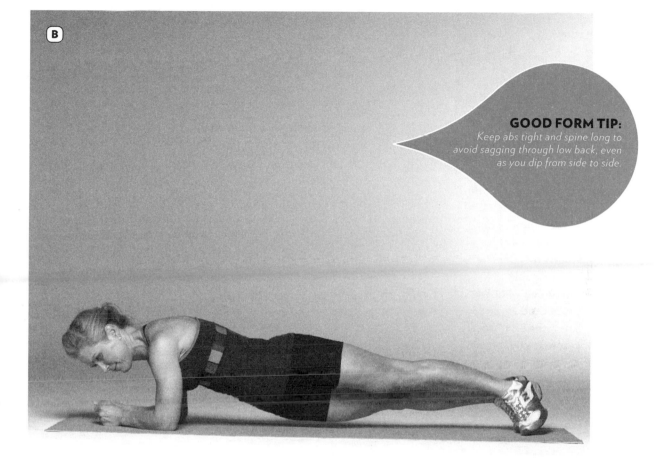

GOOD FORM TIP:
Keep abs tight and spine long to avoid sagging through low back, even as you dip from side to side.

B. Tip slightly to the right, keeping back straight, as you lower right hip to floor in 4 counts. Return to start position in 2 counts. Tip toward left side for 4 counts. Come back to start in 2 counts. Continue for 8 to 10 repetitions on each side.

DAY 5 TURNAROUND TIP
Feel Proud

I recently had the opportunity to meet Ali Vincent, the first female winner of the hit show *The Biggest Loser*. Ali lost more than 112 pounds on her journey in front of a national audience, but her experience was not entirely dissimilar to yours. From the minute the show began, it was all about working hard to meet her goals.

Ali told me she'd been a "professional dieter" in the past: Every time she would fall off a diet with a point system or specific meal plan, she'd think, "Forget it!" Her weight gain happened in her adult life—it slowly started creeping up after college in increments of 5 pounds at a time, until one day she realized she'd gained more than 100 pounds. She kept thinking she could lose it, but didn't do anything about it, until one day she couldn't take it any more.

While you probably don't have to resort to extreme measures like *The Biggest Loser* to get results, we are doing some of the same things here: watching portion sizes, picking from certain food groups. You are making the choice and learning how to shape your own meals. The workout plan I've given you is hard. It's demanding. And you have to make it all happen while dealing with everything and everyone around you.

The bottom line for Ali is that she will never go back to her old self. Since the show ended, she's adapted the fundamentals of eating right and exercising to her new lifestyle. I play the song "Proud" by Heather Small almost weekly in my spin class. It's *The Biggest Loser* theme song, and I find the lyrics so inspirational. I'm endlessly passionate about helping people lose weight and create a healthy lifestyle. I know you are going to have that "a-ha!" moment on this program, when you realize that this was the jumpstart you needed to take control of your health. So I ask you: "What will you do today to make you feel proud?"

> "What have you done today to make you feel proud? It's never too late to try."
> —Heather Small, *singer*

IN SMALL DOSES, SODIUM is one of the most important minerals for your body: It plays a key role in maintaining fluid balance throughout the body. Along with chloride and bicarbonate, it helps maintain the acid-base balance in the body. It's essential for the passage of metabolic materials through cell walls. And (along with potassium) it aids in nerve stimulation and muscle contraction.

But the key phrase is "small doses." The USDA Dietary Guidelines recommend a maximum of 2,300 milligrams of sodium per day—that's about 1 teaspoon of salt! Currently, the average sodium intake is about 4,000 milligrams a day, nearly twice the recommended level. Although some foods do naturally contain sodium, most of what we get in our diets comes from processed foods, which often contain salt and sodium to enhance flavor and prevent spoilage. Pickles, canned soups, hot dogs, frozen dinners—you name it, they're high in salt.

LEARN ABOUT: **SODIUM**

So what's the problem with too much salt? A large study called DASH (Dietary Approaches to Stop Hypertension) from the National Heart, Lung, and Blood Institute found that when people cut their sodium levels, they also reduced high blood pressure. The biggest changes came when people consumed just 1,500 milligrams of sodium a day. Following a low-sodium diet (along with eating plenty of fruits, vegetables, and whole grains) was estimated to reduce heart disease by 15 percent and stroke by 27 percent.[3]

It's not hard to cut the amount of salt in your diet. For one, skip the processed foods as much as possible, or choose those that are low sodium or sodium free. Use herbs and spices while cooking, and eat fresh and frozen veggies rather than canned ones. And beware of hidden sources of salt: Bouillon cubes, marinades, soy sauce, and steak sauce can all be high in sodium.

You'll see in our suggested menus, by the way, that we recommend no more than 600 to 650 milligrams of sodium in each meal (and no more than 150 to 200 milligrams of sodium in each snack) to stay under the 2,300-milligram-a-day level. However, you'll also see that there are a few meals that go beyond that range. As usual, you can always make exceptions to any nutrition rule as long as you keep things balanced overall. In addition, because you'll be sweating a lot during this 2-week program, a little extra sodium during this time period isn't likely to be a problem!

MEAL GUIDELINES:
Suggested amounts for each meal

BREAKFAST

2 grains/starchy veggies

1 dairy

1 protein

1 fruit

1 fat

A.M. SNACK

1 dairy

1 fruit

LUNCH

1 grain/starchy veggie

1 protein

2 veggies

1 fat

P.M. SNACK

1 dairy

DINNER

1 grain/starchy veggie

1 protein

2 veggies

1 fat

DAY 5 SUGGESTED MENU

BREAKFAST

1 whole-wheat English muffin spread with 1 tablespoon peanut butter. Serve with 3 ounces Canadian bacon, 1 apple, and 1 cup skim milk.

PER SERVING: 430 calories; 12 g total fat; 3 g sat fat; 61 g carbohydrates; 9 g fiber; 23 g protein; 19 mg cholesterol; 690 mg sodium

NOTE: *This meal is a little high in sodium (you want to aim for no more than 600 to 650 mg per meal), which you should normally avoid, but you'll be sweating a lot throughout the 2-Week Total Body Turnaround, so you can get away with it today.*

SNACK

1 cup vanilla soymilk with 1 peach

PER SERVING: 140 calories; 3 g total fat; 1 g sat fat; 20 g carbohydrates; 1 g fiber; 7 g protein; 0 mg cholesterol; 170 mg sodium

LUNCH

Open-Faced Mushroom-Onion Veggie Burger

PER SERVING: 310 calories; 16 g total fat; 2 g sat fat; 28 g carbohydrates; 8 g fiber; 17 g protein; 3 mg cholesterol; 567 mg sodium

SNACK

1/2 cup nonfat cottage cheese

PER SERVING: 60 calories; 0 g total fat; 0 g sat fat; 1 g carbohydrates; 0 g fiber; 12 g protein; 5 mg cholesterol; 290 mg sodium

DINNER

Seared Chicken Fajita Salad

PER SERVING: 360 calories; 14 g total fat; 2 g sat fat; 30 g carbohydrates; 12 g fiber; 30 g protein; 49 mg cholesterol; 464 mg sodium

OPEN-FACED MUSHROOM-ONION VEGGIE BURGER

1 teaspoon olive oil

¼ cup sliced sweet onion

¼ cup sliced red bell pepper

¼ cup sliced baby portobellos

1 tablespoon balsamic vinegar

1 veggie burger patty (I used Boca Original to analyze)

½ crusty whole-wheat roll or whole-wheat English muffin, toasted

1½ teaspoons mayonnaise

½ teaspoon spicy mustard

¼ cup mixed greens

Heat 1 teaspoon of the olive oil in a medium skillet over medium heat. Add the onion, pepper, and mushrooms and cook, stirring frequently, for about 5 to 7 minutes, or until tender. Remove from the pan, drizzle with the balsamic vinegar, and set aside. Add the veggie burger to the same pan and cook, turning once, for about 8 to 10 minutes, or until heated through. Spread the roll or muffin with the mayonnaise and mustard. Top with the veggie burger, mixed greens, and vegetable mixture.

MAKES 1 SERVING

PER SERVING: 310 calories; 16 g total fat; 2 g sat fat; 28 g carbohydrates, 8 g fiber; 17 g protein; 3 mg cholesterol; 567 mg sodium

SEARED CHICKEN FAJITA SALAD

1 skinless, boneless chicken breast (3 ounces)

½ cup canned no-salt-added black beans, rinsed and drained

¼ cup diced avocado

2 tablespoons minced red onion

1 teaspoon chopped fresh cilantro

2 cups mixed greens

1 tablespoon lime juice

1 clove garlic, chopped

¼ teaspoon cumin

1½ tablespoons red wine vinaigrette dressing

Heat a skillet coated with nonstick cooking spray over medium-high heat. Add the chicken breast and cook, turning once, for about 3 to 5 minutes per side, or until cooked through. Remove from the pan and set on a cutting board. Meanwhile, in a medium bowl, combine the beans, avocado, onion, cilantro, and mixed greens; toss to combine. In a small bowl, whisk the lime juice, garlic, cumin, and vinaigrette dressing. Slice the chicken into thin slices. Toss the salad with the dressing and top with the chicken.

MAKES 1 SERVING

PER SERVING: 360 calories; 14 g total fat; 2 g sat fat; 30 g carbohydrates; 12 g fiber; 30 g protein; 49 mg cholesterol; 464 mg sodium

DAY 6

We wouldn't be women if we didn't find flaws in our bodies. I have yet to meet a woman who feels she is perfect. In fact, most of the time it's quite the contrary. Get her going and she will nitpick herself body part by body part. But hopefully as we age we can all find good in what our bodies have done for us and continue to do.

I was watching *Today* and saw Emme, the plus-size model, discussing body image and food addiction. Her book, *What Are You Hungry For?*, is about helping young kids and parents become aware of some underlying emotional and physical needs that may be lacking, therefore forcing food to fill the void. Often overeating is a result of unmet needs and not true hunger.

Although my kids are older now, I still think about body image. My daughter is a dancer, and body size and weight is a very real and visual part of her world. Thank goodness she shows no signs of food problems, but I see it all around her. I am really passionate about helping young women understand that they are beautiful not because they are tall, thin, or have great hair—rather, it's about their minds, their emotions, and their hearts.

I preach exercise—that's what I do. But many young girls don't exercise due to poor body image. It's the chicken-before-the-egg syndrome: Do we get them to love themselves, therefore giving them the confidence to exercise, or do we get them to exercise, therefore teaching them to have confidence in their abilities? I don't think there is a right answer, but I do know it's important to teach girls about positive body image. I started by motivating my kids to move, because they start to see that their bodies are more than a visual display. Their bodies are what help them perform the dance, or swim the lap, or run the mile. Their bodies are what give them freedom to feel good. I know my

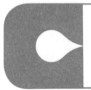

"It's not who you are that holds you back, it's who you think you're not." —Unknown

daughter is happiest when she is dancing, which she's been doing since she was 2 years old.

When I was a teen, I put a lot of pressure on myself to be perfect. I wanted to be the smartest, the most popular, the skinniest. Wisdom has taught me that perfection isn't happiness. I have come to accept my body and be proud of what I can do. I've had three kids, sun damage, and yes, I have some cellulite. At age 43, I can't complain. I can still kickbox, jump, run, bike, dance, lift weights, and do crazy drills in my classes.

My goal with my kids has been to encourage accomplishment but accept imperfection! As you begin Day 6, remember that everything you do during these 2 weeks and beyond is about trying your best and being proud of what you can achieve.

CARDIO: Mini-Bursts

Everyone's heard the term "power walk," but this workout gives it new meaning. It combines moving at a pace that's fast enough to challenge you, but not so fast that you can't keep it up for a good 20 minutes. Add on a few mini speed bursts to boost the challenge: They only last 30 seconds, so go ahead and try jogging! You'll never know if you can do it until you try.

INTENSITY	TIME	PACE	RPE	GOAL
Warm up (heart rate: Zone 1–2)	5 min.	Moderate pace	2–4	You can have a conversation but are starting to get breathless.
Power walk (heart rate: Zone 3) with mini-bursts (heart rate: Zone 4)	20 min.	Fast pace	7 (8–9 for mini bursts)	Gradually increase intensity until you are walking at the fastest pace you can sustain. Every few minutes, try jogging or walking as fast as you can for 30 seconds, then return to fast walking pace. Try to do at least 5–7 of these mini speed bursts.
Cool down (heart rate: Zone 1–2)	5 min.	Moderate pace	3–4	Slow down until you are walking at a moderate pace. You should be able to speak in full sentences with some breathlessness.

STRENGTH: Total Body

Your final strength workout for the week! I can't stress enough the importance of resistance training to help you get results. These total-body moves will help strengthen and tone all of your trouble zones, and because you're working several muscle groups at once, they'll keep your mind engaged along with your body.

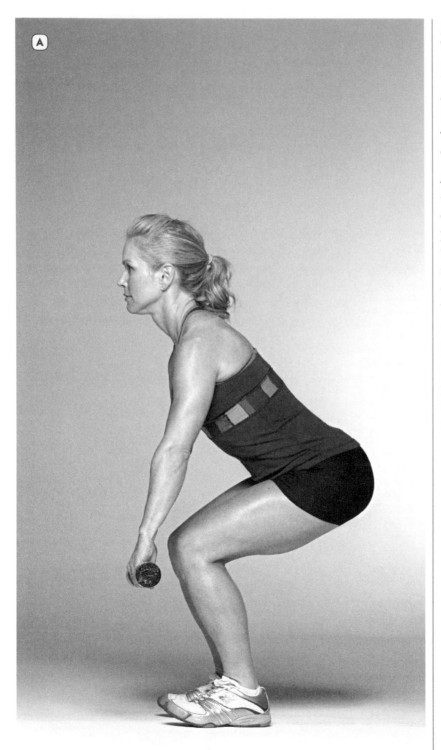

SQUAT WITH STRAIGHT ARM PRESSBACK

TARGETS: Shoulders, arms, quads, butt

A. Stand with feet about 4 inches apart, holding dumbbells at sides with palms facing behind you. Slowly lower into squat position for 4 counts, keeping body weight over heels as arms move forward.

B. Stand back up in 2 counts while pressing palms behind you. Repeat 8 to 12 times.

B

GOOD FORM TIP:
Keep abs tight and spine long.
Use backs of shoulders to press, keeping
arms straight.

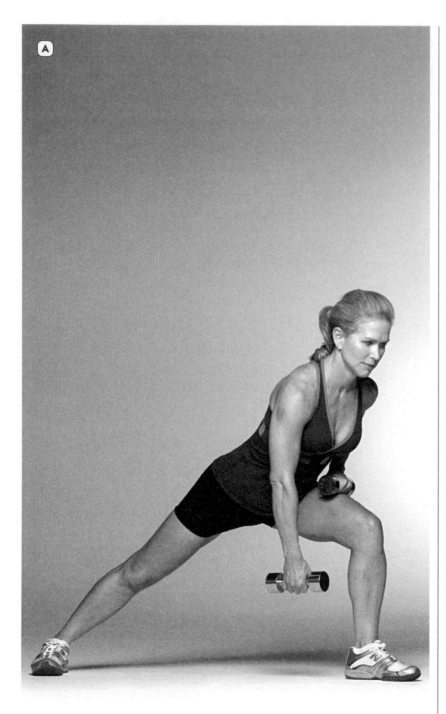

DIAGONAL LUNGE WITH ROW

TARGETS: Quads, butt, back

A. Stand with feet wider than shoulder-width apart, left foot turned out 45 degrees, holding dumbbells with arms extended at sides. Slowly bend left knee, sitting back into left butt in 4 counts while straightening right leg, reaching right dumbbell toward left ankle. (Keep knee in line with shoelaces.)

B. Push back up to start position in 2 counts, keeping left knee slightly bent, and squeezing through left butt while pulling right elbow across body and behind you in a row; keep elbow close to sides (you'll feel this in the middle of your back). Repeat 8 times. Switch to the other side and repeat 8 times.

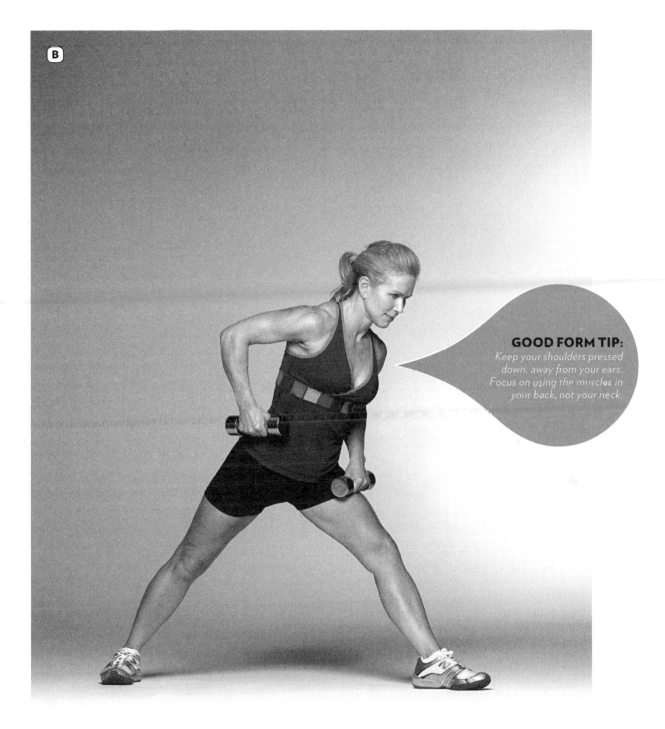

GOOD FORM TIP:
Keep your shoulders pressed down, away from your ears. Focus on using the muscles in your back, not your neck.

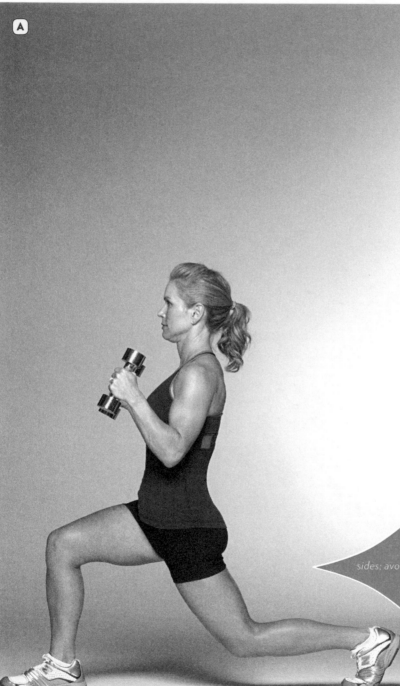

A

HAMMER TIME

TARGETS: Arms, quads, butt

A. Stand with feet 2 to 3 inches apart, holding dumbbells at sides. Lunge back with left foot in 2 counts, bending both knees 90 degrees (keep right knee over right ankle) while curling weights toward shoulders with thumbs facing up.

B. Slowly rise back up in 4 counts and return to starting position while lowering arms. Repeat 8 times. Switch sides and repeat 8 times.

GOOD FORM TIP:
Keep your elbows close to your sides; avoid swinging from your shoulders as you lunge back.

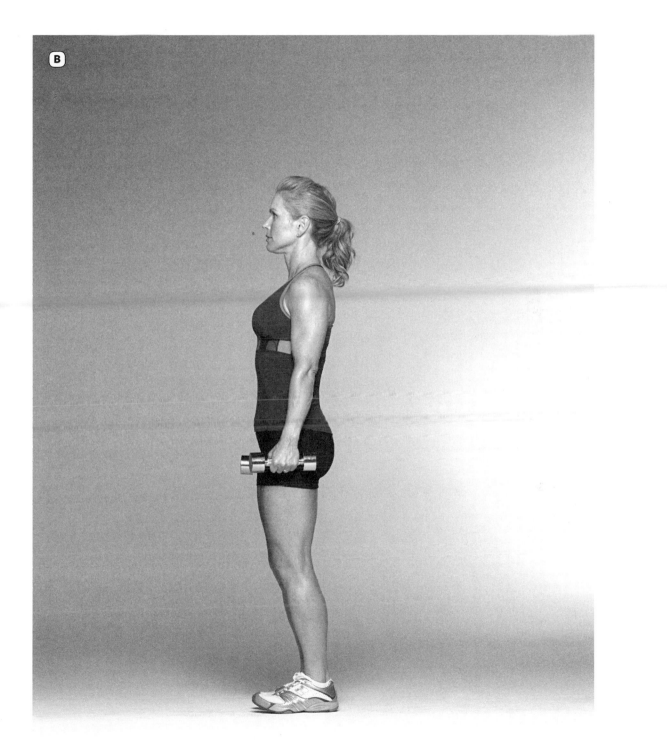

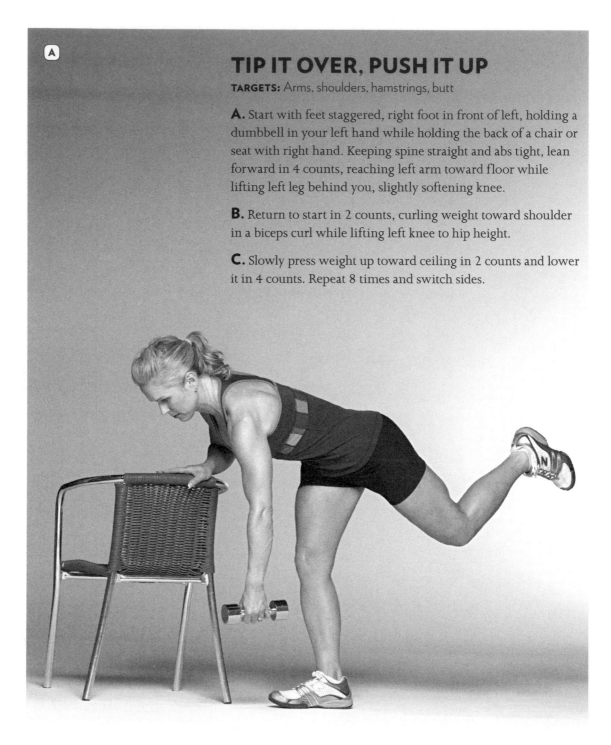

TIP IT OVER, PUSH IT UP

TARGETS: Arms, shoulders, hamstrings, butt

A. Start with feet staggered, right foot in front of left, holding a dumbbell in your left hand while holding the back of a chair or seat with right hand. Keeping spine straight and abs tight, lean forward in 4 counts, reaching left arm toward floor while lifting left leg behind you, slightly softening knee.

B. Return to start in 2 counts, curling weight toward shoulder in a biceps curl while lifting left knee to hip height.

C. Slowly press weight up toward ceiling in 2 counts and lower it in 4 counts. Repeat 8 times and switch sides.

GOOD FORM TIP:
Keep your abs tight and your spine long so your lower back doesn't sag. Stand by pulling up through your hamstrings and butt, not your lower back.

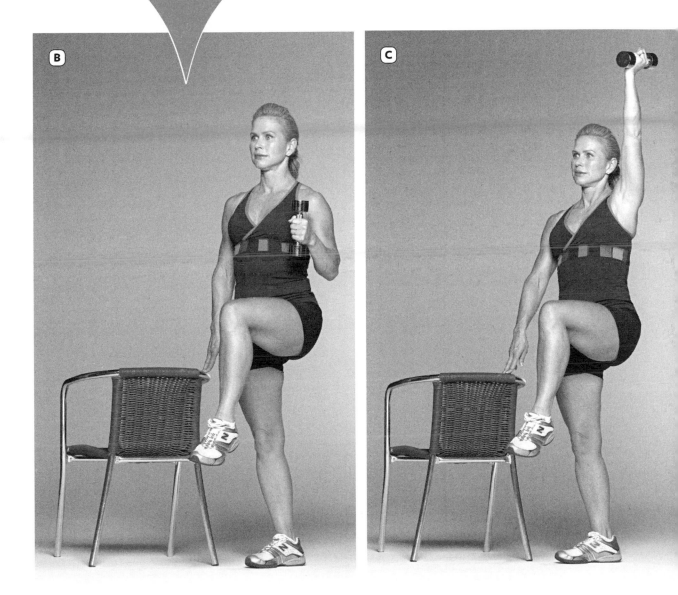

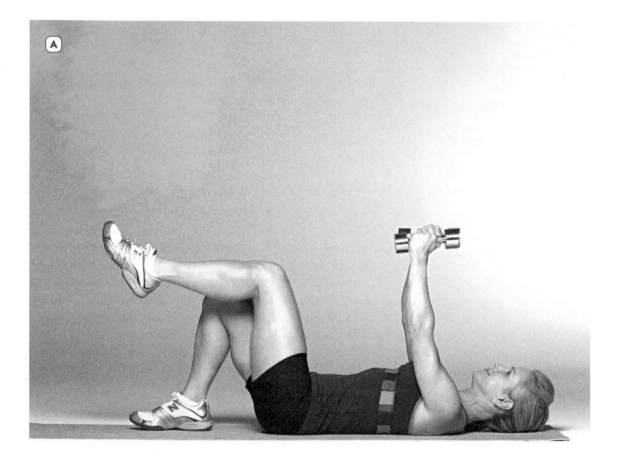

BEACH BALL HUG

TARGETS: Chest, abs, hips

A. Lie face up on floor, knees bent and feet flat on floor, holding dumbbells above chest with arms extended, elbows slightly bent, palms facing each other. Lift left leg, keeping knee bent 90 degrees, shin parallel to floor.

B. Slowly lower arms out to sides in 4 counts, keeping elbows slightly bent while simultaneously "reaching" left foot out to straighten leg. Pull knee back to start in 2 counts while lifting arms back above chest, squeezing your chest muscles as if you're hugging a beach ball. Repeat 6 times with left leg, then do the exercise 6 times with right leg.

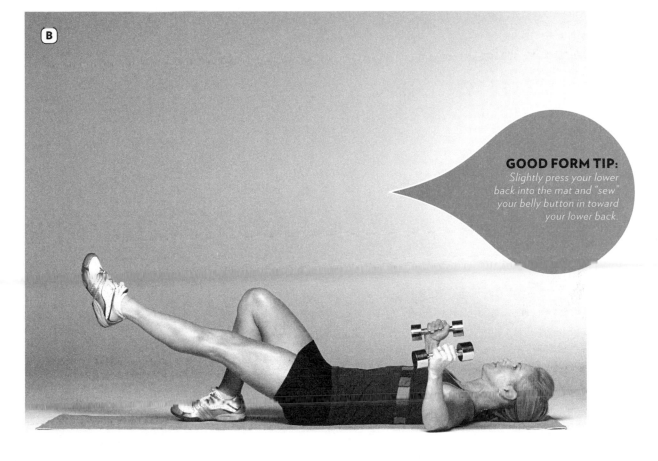

GOOD FORM TIP:
Slightly press your lower back into the mat and "sew" your belly button in toward your lower back.

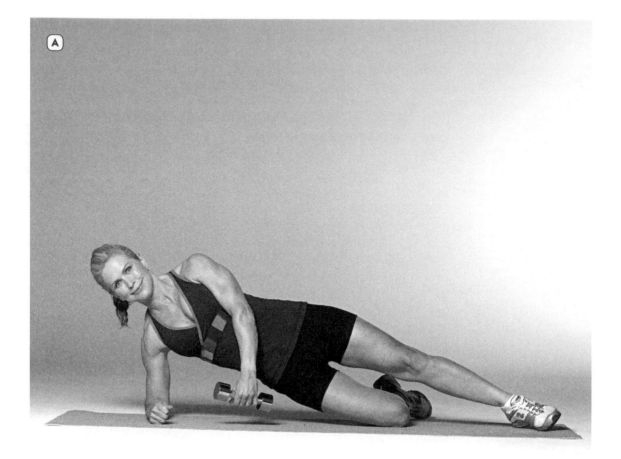

FOREARM SIDE PLANK WITH SHOULDER RAISE

Note that you already know how to do this move from Day 3.

TARGETS: Shoulders, abs, obliques

A. Lie on right side, hips stacked, elbow under shoulder and right forearm on floor with bottom knee on floor and top leg extended. Hold a dumbbell in left hand on floor, just in front of body. Lift hips, forming a straight line from shoulders to heels, keeping abdominals tight.

B. Lift left arm above shoulder for 2 counts and lower slowly for 4 counts, keeping hips still. Repeat 8 times. Switch sides; repeat another 8 times.

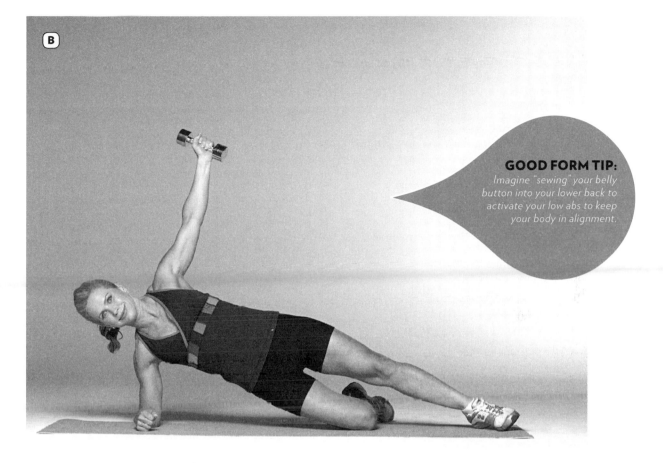

B

GOOD FORM TIP:
Imagine "sewing" your belly button into your lower back to activate your low abs to keep your body in alignment.

DAY 6 TURNAROUND TIP

Be Thankful

I love Thanksgiving time—the turkey, seeing friends and family, even the pumpkin pie (in moderation, of course!). Celebrating our thankfulness once a year as a nation is teriffic, but being thankful is a habit we should all incorporate into our lives every day.

We all have many things to be thankful for, whether we choose to acknowledge them or not. Our society often focuses on the things that are wrong with our appearance. But what about what is right with our bodies, how they work and the amazing things they can accomplish? If you can train your mind to focus on all the many positive things about your body, your whole attitude will be transformed.

Here's a little exercise I share with clients to help adjust their attitudes when they are in the habit of constantly cutting themselves down. Take 5 minutes and write down at least 15 things you are thankful for when it comes to your body. Don't say you can't think of anything: It can be as simple as "I can see clearly" or as specific as "I can run a mile." No matter what shape your body is in or what fitness level you are currently at, you can find things you are thankful for. It might take some practice for you to start focusing on them, but when you do start looking at yourself in a positive light, you will feel motivated to improve your health and to take care of yourself.

I'm grateful to my body because

_____

_____

_____

_____

_____

Now that you have your list (and hopefully you wrote down even more than 15 things!), tape it to your mirror. For the rest of the 2-Week Total Body Turnaround, review this list every time you are looking in the mirror to remind yourself about just how incredible your body is—and start believing it!

WHEN YOU THINK ABOUT calcium, you probably think about your bones and teeth. But this important mineral is also responsible for many other functions in the body, including blood clotting, transmitting nerve impulses, and regulating your heart rhythm.

Almost all (99 percent) of the calcium in your body is stored in your bones and teeth, with the remainder in blood and other tissues. Your body needs calcium to survive, and it either gets it from calcium-rich foods (more on that in a minute), or in an emergency, by pulling it from the bones.

The calcium/healthy-bone link has been well established. Bones are constantly being built up and broken down. Before the age of 30, if you get enough calcium and are active, your bone production will exceed bone destruction; after that, the breakdown usually wins out. That's why so many women are at risk for osteoporosis. We all lose bone as we age, and postmenopausal women are especially at risk, because estrogen levels, which are important in maintaining bone health, start to decline at menopause. An estimated 8 million women and 2 million men have osteoporosis, with an additional 34 million more at risk.[4]

It's clear that getting enough calcium in your diet is crucial to helping prevent osteoporosis. Dairy products are among the best sources of calcium, but remember to choose low-fat or fat-free options to keep your calories in check. On the 2-Week Total Body Turnaround, you'll consume 3 servings a day of foods like yogurt, cottage cheese, and fat free milk.

But if dairy upsets your stomach, no worries: There are also plenty of nondairy foods that provide plenty of calcium, including dark green vegetables like broccoli, spinach, and kale. Just remember that plant-based foods generally have less bioavailability, which means it's a little harder for your body to absorb the calcium. In addition, lots of foods are fortified with calcium, from orange juice to tofu to cereals.

Unfortunately, most of us don't come anywhere close to the Recommended Daily Allowance (RDA) of about 1,000 milligrams a day. That's why many nutritionists recommend that, in addition to trying to get calcium through your diet, you take a calcium supplement (500 to 600 mg twice a day for a total of 1,000 to 1,200 mg). Split the dose, because the body can only absorb about 600 mg at a time.

There's another important reason to love calcium: Studies have shown it may play an important role in weight loss. One study found subjects who followed a diet that included 800 mg of calcium supplements lost significantly more weight than those who had only about half the calcium in their diet; those who had gotten their calcium through dairy products (3 servings a day, or about 1,200 to 1,300 mg of calcium) lost even more.[5]

LEARN ABOUT: **CALCIUM**

MEAL GUIDELINES:
Suggested amounts for each meal

BREAKFAST
2 grains/starchy veggies

1 dairy

1 protein

1 fruit

1 fat

A.M. SNACK
1 dairy

1 fruit

LUNCH
1 grain/starchy veggie

1 protein

2 veggies

1 fat

P.M. SNACK
1 dairy

DINNER
1 grain/starchy veggie

1 protein

2 veggies

1 fat

DAY 6 SUGGESTED MENU

BREAKFAST

1 whole-grain pita filled with 5 scrambled egg whites and $1/4$ cup shredded colby. Serve with 1 banana and 1 cup nonfat or low-fat yogurt.

PER SERVING: 510 calories; 3 g total fat; 2 g sat fat; 75 g carbohydrates; 7 g fiber; 46 g protein; 10 mg cholesterol; 650 mg sodium

SNACK

1 apple with 1 slice reduced-fat Cheddar

PER SERVING: 160 calories; 6 g total fat; 4 g sat fat; 20 g carbohydrates; 3 g fiber; 6 g protein; 20 mg cholesterol; 240 mg sodium

LUNCH

Beef Tostadas

PER SERVING: 325 calories; 18 g total fat; 4 g sat fat; 20 g carbohydrates; 4 g fiber; 22 g protein; 53 mg cholesterol; 645 mg sodium

SNACK

1 cup skim milk

PER SERVING: 80 calories; 0 g total fat; 0 g sat fat; 12 g carbohydrates; 0 g fiber; 8 g protein; 0 mg cholesterol; 100 mg sodium

DINNER

Tofu Stir-Fry with Peanut Sauce

PER SERVING: 387 calories; 13 g total fat; 2 g sat fat; 50 g carbohydrates; 12 g fiber; 23 g protein; 0 mg cholesterol; 689 mg sodium

BEEF TOSTADAS

3 ounces 95% lean
ground beef

2 teaspoons taco
seasoning

1 tablespoon olive oil

$^1/_2$ cup chopped onion

$^1/_2$ cup chopped green or
red bell pepper

$^1/_2$ cup sliced mushrooms

$^1/_2$ cup broccoli florets

2 small (4") corn tortillas,
warmed

$^1/_4$ cup fat-free sour
cream (optional)

In a nonstick skillet, combine the beef and taco seasoning and cook, stirring frequently, until crumbled and cooked through. Drain any fat; remove from the skillet and set aside.

Heat the olive oil over medium-high heat in the same skillet. Add the onion and pepper, and cook 2 minutes. Stir in the mushrooms and broccoli and sauté about 5 minutes, or until tender. Return the beef to the pan; cook until heated through, stirring occasionally. Top the warmed tortillas with the beef-veggie mixture and top with sour cream, if desired.

MAKES 1 SERVING

PER SERVING: 325 calories; 18 g total fat; 4 g sat fat; 20 g carbohydrates, 4 g fiber; 22 g protein; 53 mg cholesterol; 645 mg sodium

TOFU STIR-FRY WITH PEANUT SAUCE

3 ounces firm tofu, cubed

$^3/_4$ cup sugar snap peas

$^1/_2$ cup asparagus, sliced
on the diagonal

$^1/_4$ cup sliced mushrooms

1 tablespoon creamy
peanut butter

2 tablespoons vegetable
broth

$^1/_2$ teaspoon brown sugar

1 teaspoon white wine
vinegar

2 teaspoons lite soy sauce

Pinch of red-pepper
flakes

$^1/_2$ cup julienned
(matchsticks) carrots

$^1/_2$ cup cooked whole-
grain spaghetti

In a medium nonstick skillet coated with cooking spray, cook the tofu over medium heat, stirring frequently, for about 5 minutes, or until browned. Remove from the pan and set aside. Add the peas, asparagus, and mushrooms, and cook, stirring frequently, for about 3 to 5 minutes, or until crisp-tender. In a small bowl, combine the peanut butter, broth, sugar, vinegar, soy sauce, and pepper flakes, stirring to combine. Pour the sauce over the vegetables and simmer for 1 minute. Add the tofu, carrots, and pasta, stirring to coat, and cook until heated through.

MAKES 1 SERVING (1$^3/_4$ CUPS VEGETABLES AND $^1/_2$ CUP PASTA)

PER SERVING: 387 calories; 13 g total fat; 2 g sat fat; 50 g carbohydrates; 12 g fiber; 23 g protein; 0 mg cholesterol; 689 mg sodium

NOTE: *This recipe is a little high in sodium (you want to aim for no more than 600 to 650 mg per meal), which you should normally avoid, but you'll be sweating a lot throughout the 2-Week Total Body Turnaround, so you can get away with it today.*

DAY 7

■ ■ ■ ■ ■ ■ 7 ☐ ☐ ☐ ☐ ☐ ☐ ☐

Hooray! You've made it to the end of your first week. Congratulations! You're halfway toward your 2-Week Total Body Turnaround. And you are doing an amazing job. This is not an easy program, I know! But with great efforts come great rewards. Think about how far you have come in just 7 days. Then think about how much stronger and more powerful you're still going to become. Your possibilities are endless. After all, this is your jump-start—a kick in the butt, a spark in your engine. It's all about shaking things up to make your mind realize that you are capable of more than you give yourself credit for.

More good news: Today is considered a "rest" day in your plan. Now before you burst into applause and make a beeline for the sofa, keep in mind that this is no ordinary day of rest. We're going to focus on something called active recovery.

You've worked really hard over the last 6 days and deserve a break. Even more importantly, your body *needs* a break in order to continue to burn calories and get fit. The exercises we've been doing on the 2-Week Total Body Turnaround actually cause microscopic tears in the muscle fibers. It's the rebuilding process of these fibers at the cellular level that actually makes you stronger, but your body needs some downtime to do that. Still, you don't want to put the brakes on all of the forward momentum you've built up these past few days. Enter the idea of active rest.

The concept behind active rest is pretty much as simple as it sounds: The idea is to work hard enough to remove some of the waste products (like lactic acid and other molecular by-products of exercise) from your muscles and speed the rebuilding process, but not so hard that you end up producing more waste products. In other words, you want to have some level of

"Little by little, one walks far."
—Peruvian proverb

light activity, but not so much that you're stressing those muscles again. That can mean going for a brisk walk, doing some light stretches, even playing with your kids. You just want to keep your body moving at a point below an aerobic level. Scientists say lactic acid production begins at about 65 percent of your maximum heart rate, or an RPE of about 4 or 5 (you can still chat with a friend but might be slightly breathless). In addition to helping speed the rebuilding process, this light cardio will also help keep your heart healthy.

Think NEAT

The time that you spend exercising isn't the only way that you get fit. Think of it like this: Your body doesn't have an on-off switch. Everything you do throughout the day contributes to your fitness level. Researchers recently validated this idea with a unique study that found the more you move, the more calories you burn—even if the movement is as little as tapping your feet, standing up as you talk on the phone, or pacing around the room. In fact, the researchers found that people who are the most active, regardless of doing a formal "workout," burned 350 more calories a day than those who sit still. Multiply that over a year and that equals almost 37 pounds!

It comes down to something called nonexercise activity thermogenesis, or NEAT. Scientists at the Mayo Clinic found that obese people sit, on average, 150 more minutes a day than people who are naturally lean. The study was one of the largest of its kind, and it's pretty fascinating. They asked 20 people—10 lean and 10 obese—to wear specially designed undergarments (engineered with the same motion-sensing technology as a jet fighter) 24 hours a day for 10 days, and go about their normal routines. (For the curious: They got fresh undergarments every morning.) The only exceptions: No swimming and no eating any food not prepared by the research group. The garments were designed to keep track of every movement, even a toe tap, and log that data every half second. They then overfed the lean people by 1,000 calories a day to make them gain weight and underfed the obese people by 1,000 calories to make them lose weight, then monitored them for another 10 days to compare results. Here's what they found: Even after the lean people gained weight, they still stood, walked, and even fidgeted more than the overweight group. The conclusion: Obese people may be "NEAT-deficient," meaning they just may not have the same drive to move about.[6]

That may be all well and good in a scientific study, but what's that

GOOD TO KNOW

mean in the real world? I was curious to find out, so as part of an article for *Prevention* magazine I did a test with a group of women to see whether you really could burn more calories without actually "exercising." I asked five women to wear a device called the Body Bug, which measures the amount of calories you burn throughout the day. Here's what I found: By being really conscious about every movement they made, they burned as many as 500 extra calories a day, without ever breaking a sweat! Here's a look at some things they did to increase the number of calories burned:

- Do crunches in bed: One tester found she burned 20 calories in less than 5 minutes (not to mention strengthened her abs and revved her energy levels) just by drawing her knees into her chest 25 to 50 times.

- Dance around while getting dressed: One of the women put on the radio and shimmied her way through the morning household tasks (getting dressed, packing lunch for her family). Net burn: 55 calories an hour!

- Walk, climb, move! By doing little bits of activity—climbing the stairs at work to use the restroom on another floor; taking a 5-minute walk before work and then a 15-minute walk at lunch; doing an extra lap around the grocery store—you can burn up to 375 calories by the end of the day.

- Stand up: Don't sit when you can be on your feet. You'll burn about 40 percent more calories. So, for those of you who might remember the R.E.M. song, just "Stand." On the phone. At your desk. During your child's dance class or soccer match or at the playground.

- Laugh. Okay, this one sounds a little silly, but research has shown that laughing for 10 to 15 minutes (like when you're watching *The Office*) burns about 40 calories. Not impressive by itself, but over a year that adds up to 4 pounds. And that's nothing to laugh at![8]

TIP: If you missed a workout day earlier this week, guess what—that was your rest day! So substitute whatever exercises you were scheduled to do for today. It's important to stay on track to meet your goals!

DAY 7 TURNAROUND TIP
The Halfway Point

Congratulations! You have completed half of the 2-Week Total Body Turn-around.

Here's what Sue P., from our test panel, reported at the halfway point:

"So many times I've started a diet only to quit by dinnertime. Exercise programs are the same—it's so easy to come home from work and feel tired, which means just flipping on the TV. How am I doing? GREAT!!! Here's a list of my accomplishments:

"I've done all of the exercises so far.

"I went to a wine class and only smelled the wine (I became the designated driver!).

"I went to an open house and drank water. I had a salad right before I went, so I wasn't hungry. I had just as much fun, and no one felt I was antisocial by not eating!

"I learned how to get the incline up and do the intervals on a treadmill!

"I looked in the mirror while weight training to check my form.

"I'm not eating from the office candy dish.

"I'm logging my foods in at prevention.com. I started to take multivitamins because I found I'm a little low in some vitamins even though I'm eating well.

"I just keep thinking about my goal. I will probably never love exercising, but I feel like I have more energy, so I'll keep doing it. I love eating, but I'm finding it's easy to eat healthy and I'm not depriving myself by missing wine and cake. I'm looking forward to seeing all of my results!"

I hope all of you feel as proud of what you have achieved as Sue P. did.

YOU'VE WORKED HARD FOR the past week and you deserve a reward! And believe me, nothing says "good job" like a piece of chocolate. We're practically hard-wired to crave the stuff. And best of all, it's actually *good* for you! Studies have shown that phytochemicals called flavonoids, found in the cacao bean, may help improve heart health, lower blood pressure, reduce inflammation, increase HDL, and reduce LDL.

For the most health benefits, look for dark chocolate with at least 70 percent cocoa (most milk chocolates have only about 50 percent cocoa). Plus, the dairy added to milk chocolate may make it harder to absorb—so ounce-for-ounce, dark is a better choice. The higher the cocoa content, the more antioxidants, but darker is also a little less sweet.

LEARN ABOUT: **CHOCOLATE**

Sadly, there is too much of a good thing, which means you can't go too crazy with the chocolate. Along with those healthy flavonoids come plenty of fat, sugar, and calories. One ounce is a good snack-size to aim for. It'll cost you about 150 calories . . . but it's worth every bite.

MEAL GUIDELINES:

Suggested amounts for each meal

BREAKFAST

2 grains/starchy veggies

1 dairy

1 protein

1 fruit

1 fat

A.M. SNACK

1 dairy

1 fruit

LUNCH

1 grain/starchy veggie

1 protein

2 veggies

1 fat

P.M. SNACK

1 dairy

DINNER

1 grain/starchy veggie

1 protein

2 veggies

1 fat

DAY 7 SUGGESTED MENU

BREAKFAST

Broccoli-Cheddar Scramble

PER SERVING: 430 calories; 10 g total fat; 5 g sat fat; 54 g carbohydrates; 10 g fiber; 37 g protein; 28 mg cholesterol; 784 mg sodium

SNACK

Slices from 1 orange dipped in 1 cup nonfat or low-fat yogurt

PER SERVING: 200 calories; 1 g total fat; 0 g sat fat; 34 g carbohydrates; 3 g fiber; 15 g protein; 5 mg cholesterol; 190 mg sodium

LUNCH

Chicken salad: Combine 1 cup mixed greens, 3 ounces diced grilled chicken breast, 1/2 cup halved grape tomatoes, 1/2 cup sliced cucumber, 1 tablespoon pine nuts, 1 tablespoon olive oil, and a splash of balsamic vinegar.

PER SERVING: 350 calories; 23 g total fat; 3 g sat fat; 9 g carbohydrates; 3 g fiber; 29 g protein; 75 mg cholesterol; 90 mg sodium

SNACK

1 part-skim string cheese

PER SERVING: 80 calories; 6 g total fat; 4 g sat fat; 1 g carbohydrates; 0 g fiber; 7 g protein; 15 mg cholesterol; 150 mg sodium

DINNER

Spiced Salmon with Spinach-Feta Couscous

PER SERVING: 366 calories; 17 g total fat; 3 g sat fat; 32 g carbohydrates; 7 g fiber; 24 g protein; 52 mg cholesterol; 498 mg sodium

BROCCOLI-CHEDDAR SCRAMBLE

1/2 cup chopped broccoli (fresh or frozen)

1/2 cup chopped mushrooms

1/3 cup chopped red or green bell peppers

3/4 cup egg whites

1/4 cup shredded reduced-fat Cheddar cheese

1/2 whole-wheat English muffin, toasted

1 tablespoon low-fat cream cheese

1 1/4 cups strawberries

1/2 cup freshly squeezed orange juice

In a nonstick skillet coated with cooking spray, cook the broccoli, mushrooms, and peppers, stirring frequently, for about 5 minutes, or until tender. Add the egg whites and cook for 2 to 3 minutes, or until set. Sprinkle the cheese on top of the eggs to melt. Cover for a few seconds. Spread the English muffin with the cream cheese. Serve with strawberries and orange juice.

MAKES 1 SERVING

PER SERVING: 430 calories; 10 g total fat; 5 g sat fat; 54 g carbohydrates; 10 g fiber; 37 g protein; 28 mg cholesterol; 784 mg sodium

NOTE: *This recipe is a little high in sodium (you want to aim for no more than 600 to 650 mg per meal), which you should normally avoid, but you'll be sweating a lot throughout the 2-Week Total Body Turnaround, so you can get away with it today.*

SPICED SALMON WITH SPINACH-FETA COUSCOUS

1/2 teaspoon brown sugar

1/4 teaspoon cumin

1/4 teaspoon coriander

1/4 teaspoon garlic powder

1/8 teaspoon cinnamon

1/8 teaspoon salt

1 salmon fillet (3 ounces), skinned

1 teaspoon olive oil

2 cups fresh baby spinach

1 teaspoon pine nuts, chopped

2 teaspoons crumbled reduced-fat feta cheese

1/2 cup cooked whole-wheat couscous

Preheat the oven to 375°F. Combine the first 6 ingredients in a small bowl. Rub over both sides of the salmon. Place the salmon on a baking sheet coated with cooking spray and bake for 15 minutes, or until cooked through and fish flakes easily when tested with a fork. Meanwhile, heat the olive oil in a nonstick skillet over medium heat. Add the spinach and cook for about 2 to 3 minutes, or until wilted. Toss the spinach, pine nuts, and feta cheese with the couscous until combined. Serve the salmon with the couscous.

MAKES 1 SERVING

PER SERVING: 366 calories; 17 g total fat; 3 g sat fat; 32 g carbohydrates; 7 g fiber; 24 g protein; 52 mg cholesterol; 498 mg sodium

REAL 2-WEEK TURNAROUND SUCCESS STORY

Linda
Agnes

AGE:
40

HEIGHT:
5'6"

START WEIGHT:
179.2
pounds

AFTER 2 WEEKS:
167.2
pounds

RESULTS:
12 pounds,
16 inches
(including 4½ inches
from waist and
2½ inches from hips)

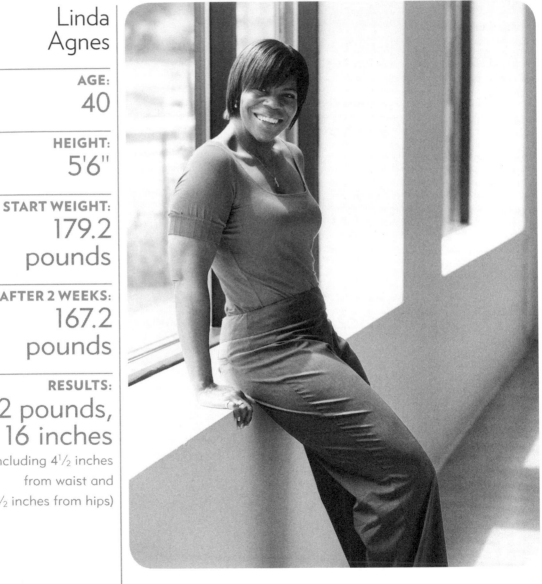

Linda had always considered herself to be an active person, working out up to 6 days a week, running or lifting weights for at least an hour at a time. But after undergoing a hysterectomy 3 years ago, followed by surgery on her hip 1 year later, her activity level plummeted. Within 2 years, she'd gained more than 40 pounds, fueled by a combination of chips, candy, fries, microwaveable dinners, and nightly takeout. Her energy levels took a nose-dive as well, and between her job as an administrative manager and raising two teenagers, she found herself simply exhausted by the early evening hours. "I'd sack out on the couch and couldn't move," she recalls.

Desperate for a change, she signed up to take the 2-week challenge. The first 2 days, she says, were the hardest. "I just started to cry when I realized how emotionally dependent I had become on food and how stressed out I really was." But, she reports, something happened on Day 3: "My brain suddenly cleared. After 3 days of working out and eating clean, it felt like I woke up from some kind of coma and was starting anew. It felt like I was finally moving on a solid foundation."

Her energy levels took a noticeable reversal. "Whereas I would typically shut down by 9 o'clock, I found myself having energy to spare after 10." Her diet took a turn for the better, as well. "I went from eating garbage every day to eating totally clean—lean proteins like fish, chicken, turkey, or tuna, fresh veggies, fruits, and whole grains, all in significantly reduced portions."

The results of her efforts were dramatic: By the end of the first week, Linda had lost more than 8 pounds; after 2 weeks, she was down 12 (her husband, who followed the plan with her, shed 20). And her belly went from bloated to almost completely flat. Co-workers commented on her healthy glow and rapidly changing physique.

Moreover, the pain and pressure she'd been feeling in her hip dramatically diminished. "My joints used to hurt all the time, and my surgeon told me I'd have to have a second surgery on my right hip—but since I started the program I've strengthened that area and it hasn't given out on me once. It's just felt really good to move—and I don't think I will have to have another operation!"

Today she's down 5 more pounds and is well on her way to her goal weight of 140 pounds by the end of the year. Although a busy schedule has meant she's had to cut down her workout time to about 30 minutes a day, she continues to make healthy choices for her meals, substituting the occasional low-cal frozen treat for a big bowl of ice cream or a small piece of steak instead of the whole porterhouse.

"I intend to follow this program for the rest of my life. This has ignited a positive change in my life, both physically and mentally. I know exactly what I need to do now to get results, and I know I will get there."

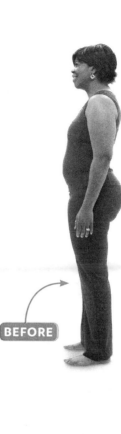

BEFORE

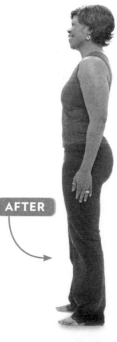

AFTER

WEEK 2

Think about how far you've come in just 7 days! Be proud of all that you have accomplished, the strength you've started to build, the challenges you have held for yourself, the way you've eaten "clean" and healthy. Now think about what it is you want to achieve in the next week. Use this halfway point to give yourself a big pat on the back, and then get fired up for all that you can do for yourself—your mind, your body, your life   in the next 7 days.

In Week 2, you'll see that your cardio exercises will get a little more intense and your strength-training exercises a little more challenging. We've either added weight or a balancing component to most of the strength moves; you'll see these changes highlighted in bold text in the exercise descriptions. We've also added a new Core Challenge exercise to each day's routine.

To simplify your busy days, your meal plan will be a repeat of Week 1. Now let's get ready for Week 2!

DAY 8

■ ■ ■ ■ ■ ■ ■ 8 ☐ ☐ ☐ ☐ ☐ ☐

Now that you're in the rhythm of the 2-Week Total Body Turnaround and have been doing the strength and cardio for a full week, it's time to kick things up a notch. Don't panic! I know this plan has been plenty challenging so far. But in order to keep your muscles from plateauing and to keep your aerobic fitness going strong, we need to increase the intensity a bit. You can do it! Of course, you need to work within your own fitness level, but know that improvement can happen at any level, whether you're a beginner or advanced. It's all relative to your own body. Own your fitness: If the exercises in Week 1 were extremely challenging, then work on repeating them. But if you're up to trying one of the balance moves, go for it. There are no hard-and-fast rules here—you are ultimately responsible for your results, so if you don't feel up to all of the advanced moves, try picking just a few to try. The bottom line is just like I tell my kids: "You only grow and learn when you face a challenge."

CARDIO: Speed Bursts

Today's cardio workout is similar to Day 1, only this time you have a bit less time to recover. One important way to improve cardiovascular fitness is by shortening recovery time, so you can get right back into that challenge phase. You'll also do a few more intervals to really fire up your fat-blasting machine! You may find you need to take your walk into a jog in order to hit the high end of the intensity. Remember to always use both your rate of perceived exertion (RPE) and the talk test to adjust the intensity level to your own needs.

"Success is the sum of small efforts, repeated day in and day out."

—Robert J. Collier, writer/author

INTENSITY	TIME	RPE	GOAL
Warm up (heart rate: Zone 2)	5 min.	4–5	You can speak in full sentences (slightly breathless)
Speed burst (heart rate: Zone 4)	1 min.	8–9	You can only say short words (very breathless)
Recover (heart rate: Zone 2)	1 min.	4–5	You can speak in full sentences (slightly breathless)
Repeat speed burst/recovery combo 10 more times for a total of 11 intervals (heart rate: Zone 4/2), going directly from final recovery into cooldown			
Cool down (heart rate: Zone 1)	3 min.	3	You can speak easily

STRENGTH: Upper Body + Core

As I mentioned a little earlier, your strength moves will also become a little more challenging this week. I'd like to see you work on improving your balance as you build strength. Balance is so important, and it's an area we rarely focus on— who has time when you're already busy working on so many other things? But it's easy to incorporate balance drills such as standing on one leg while you do an upper body exercise like a biceps curl. And good balance is important in so many things, from being able to slip on your shoes while you're standing up to catching yourself if you trip. As a bonus, many balance moves also work your core muscles, because you have to really engage your abs to keep yourself steady—so you're really getting a core workout the entire time. Plus, you're also working your butt—single-leg moves work your butt twice as hard because all of your body weight is on one side!

I also want you to really focus on working your abdominals. Everyone wants flat abs, of course, but a strong core (your abdominals and lower back muscles) is also important for keeping you strong all over, because virtually every exercise you do engages your core muscles at one point or another. So we're adding on one more core-focused move for each of the remaining days of the plan.

Most of these exercise are a variation on what you did last week, so don't worry: I'm not asking you to learn too many new moves. (The changes to your Week 1 exercises are highlighted in bold type.) Try to do these more challenging versions, but if you really can't complete the exercise without proper form, do the moves you did last week. Today's exercises are similar to Day 1, plus that extra all-new move for your abs.

BALANCING TANK TOP TONER

TARGETS: Arms, back, shoulders

A. Stand holding dumbbells in front of thighs, palms facing legs. **Lift right foot, balancing on left leg.**

B. Bending elbows, lift weights to chin on count 1 in a reverse curl (palms will now face forward).

C. (not shown) Straighten arms forward on count 2, reaching up and out. Slowly lower straight arms back to start position, taking 4 counts. Do 6 reps, then switch feet, **balancing on right leg.**

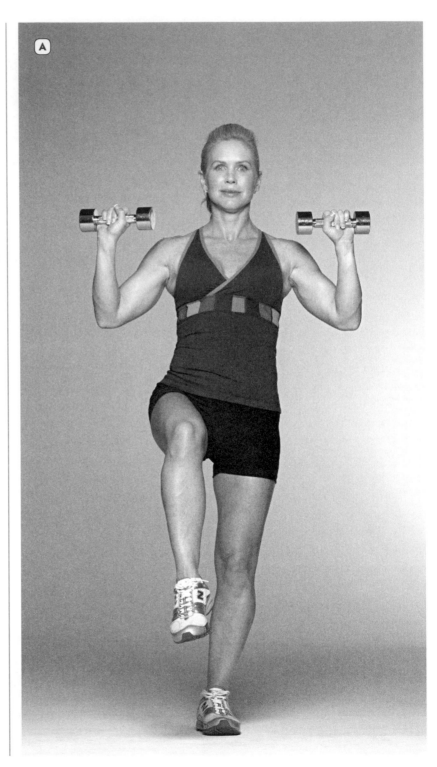

A

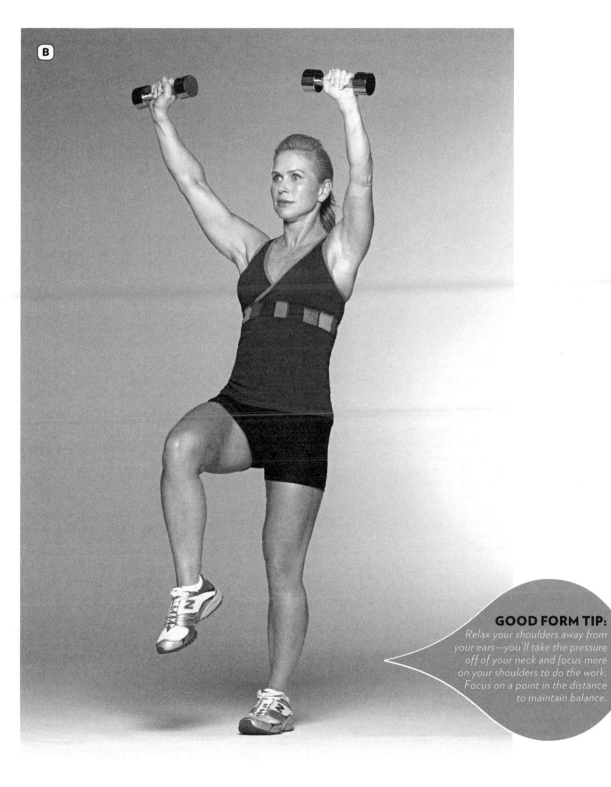

B

GOOD FORM TIP:
Relax your shoulders away from your ears—you'll take the pressure off of your neck and focus more on your shoulders to do the work. Focus on a point in the distance to maintain balance.

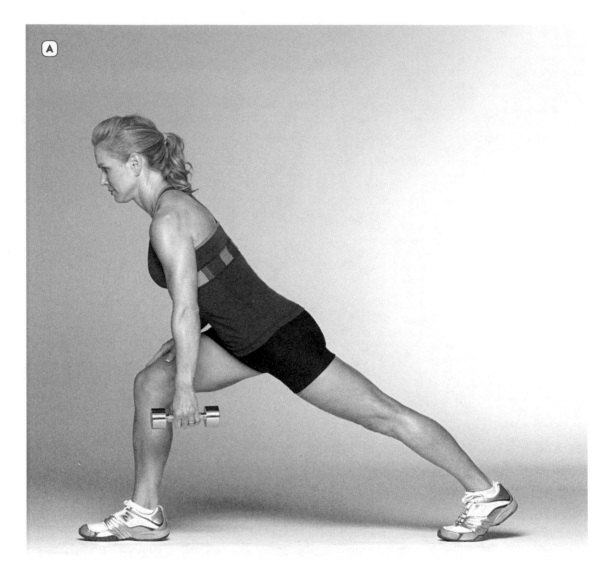

SINGLE-ARM ROW

TARGETS: Back

A. Stand with feet staggered, right foot in front of left, leaning forward slightly with long spine, abs tight. **Hold a slightly heavier dumbbell than used in Day 1 workout** in left hand next to inside of right thigh, right hand resting on top of right thigh. Keep your back straight and abs tight, and think about maintaining a long spine.

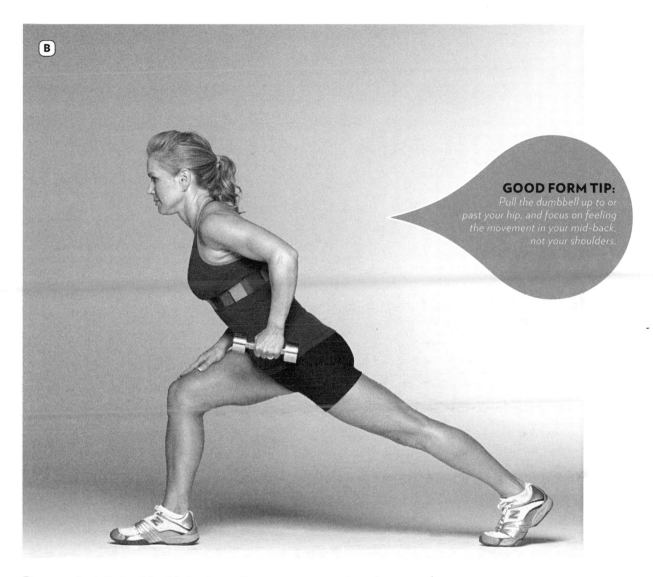

GOOD FORM TIP:
Pull the dumbbell up to or past your hip, and focus on feeling the movement in your mid-back, not your shoulders.

B. Using the left shoulder blade, draw elbow up toward ceiling for 2 counts (your hand should end up near hip bone; do not shrug your shoulder). Take 4 counts to lower to start position. Repeat 8 to 12 times and switch positions, with left leg in front and weight in right hand.

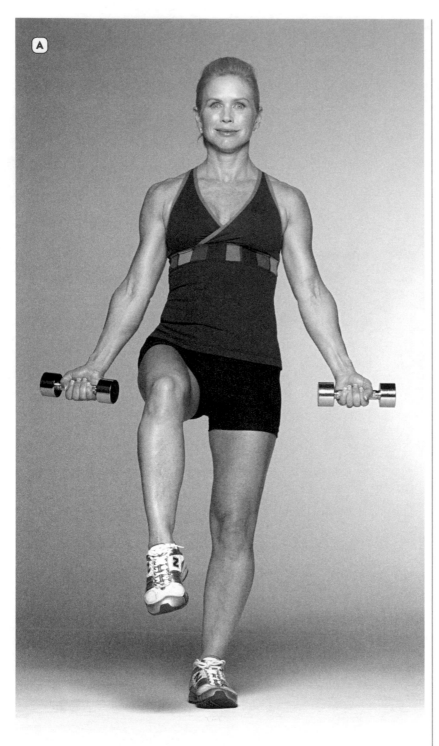

BALANCING BICEPS CURL

TARGETS: Biceps

A. Stand holding dumbbells at sides, palms facing up and arms straight. **Lift right foot off floor, balancing on left leg.**

B. Curl weights up toward shoulder by bending elbows and contracting biceps for 2 counts. Lower slowly back to start position in 4 counts. Do 6 reps. Switch feet, **balancing on right leg,** and do 6 reps.

GOOD FORM TIP:
Keep your elbows close to your sides and your torso upright and still. You'll work more of your biceps and less of your shoulders. Focus on a point in the distance to maintain balance.

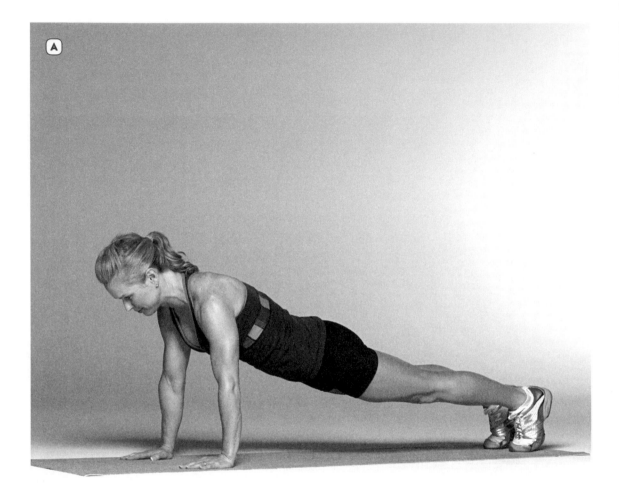

FULL PUSHUP SHOULDER TAP

TARGETS: Chest, triceps, shoulders

A. Start in full pushup position, hands shoulder-width apart on floor and legs extended, balancing on toes and forming a straight line from head to heels.

B. Lower chest slowly to floor for 4 counts, keeping abs tight and body in a straight line.

C. Push back up to start position for 2 counts, tapping left hand to right shoulder on 2nd count. Repeat, this time tapping right hand to left shoulder on 2nd count. Do a total of 6 to 8 on each side.

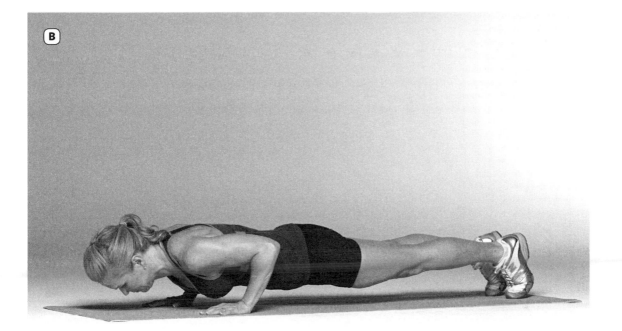

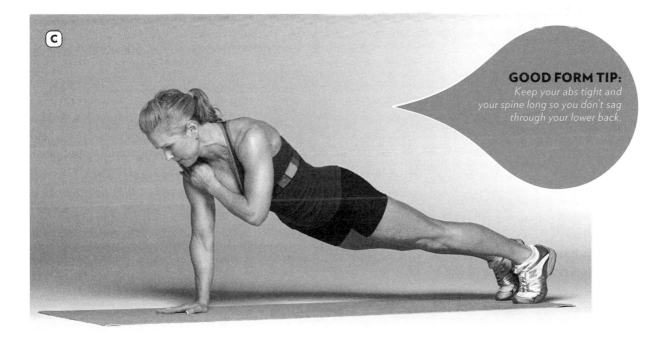

GOOD FORM TIP:
Keep your abs tight and your spine long so you don't sag through your lower back.

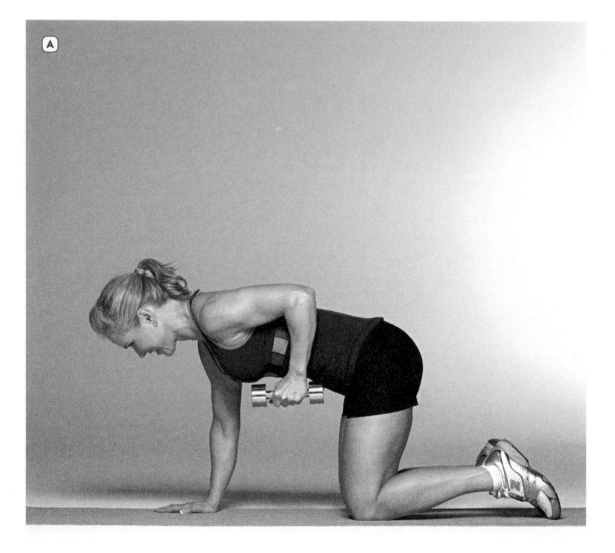

BALANCING TRICEPS KICKBACK

TARGETS: Triceps, core

A. Start on all fours, holding dumbbell in left hand and abdominals tight, keeping back flat. Lift elbow next to ribs to begin.

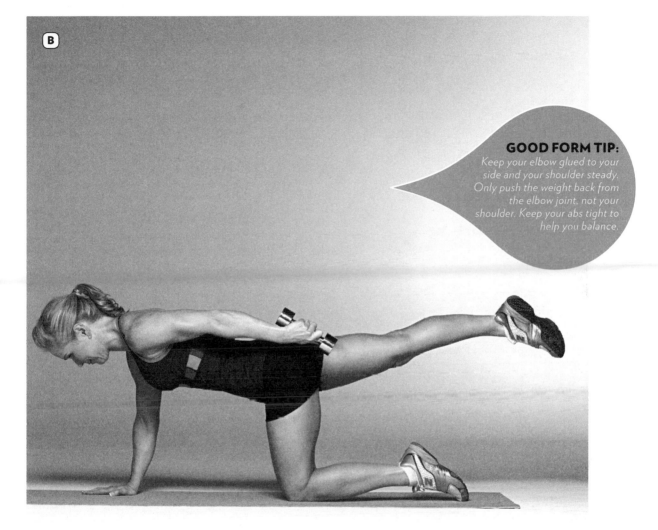

GOOD FORM TIP:
Keep your elbow glued to your side and your shoulder steady. Only push the weight back from the elbow joint, not your shoulder. Keep your abs tight to help you balance.

B. Extend arm, pressing dumbbell back for 2 counts until arm is straight. **At the same time, extend right leg straight behind you.** Slowly bend arm to bring weight back toward body in 4 counts while bending knee and lowering leg. Repeat. Do not let shoulder move during the exercise; focus on straightening and bending just the elbow joint. Repeat 8 to 12 times. Switch sides, and repeat another 8 to 12 times, **extending left leg back while straightening right arm.**

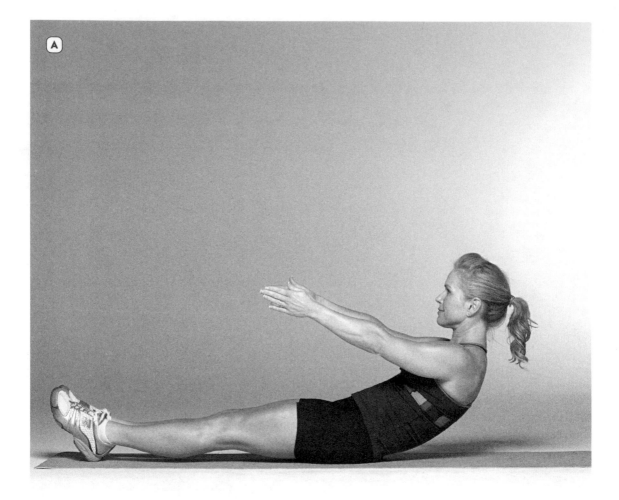

FULL BODY ROLLUP

TARGETS: Abs

A. Lie face up on the floor, legs slightly bent and arms extended next to head, shoulders relaxed, palms facing each other. Pressing your shoulders down, slowly roll up off the floor in 4 counts, keeping abs pulled in and arms extended.

B. Finish by reaching forward toward your toes. Slowly roll back down to floor to starting position, taking about 6 to 8 counts to lower. Repeat 6 to 8 times.

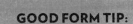

B

GOOD FORM TIP:
Keep your heels on the mat as you roll up; use just your abs to move you up, not your hip flexors.

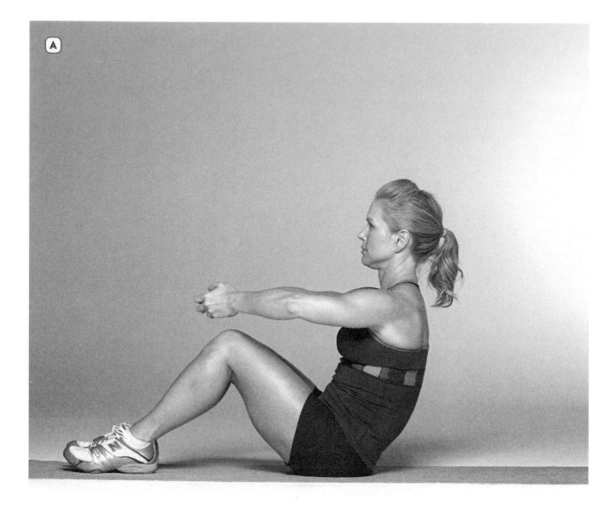

NEW EXERCISE! **CORE CHALLENGE**

DUMBBELL OBLIQUE TWIST

TARGETS: Obliques

A. Sit on floor with knees bent and feet flat on floor. Hold one dumbbell in both hands with arms extended in front of body. Lean back slightly, rounding back and engaging abs.

B. Twist to left in 4 counts, reaching dumbbell to left side. Take 2 counts to bring dumbbell back to center of chest. Repeat, twisting to right in 4 counts. Repeat 10 to 12 times total.

GOOD FORM TIP:
*Round your back into a C-curve
and keep your lower abs engaged to
protect your lower back. Twist from your
obliques, not just your shoulders.*

DAY 8 TURNAROUND TIP
Beware Food Rationalizations

How many times do you eat something when you don't really even want it? Maybe you eat it because it's free, or because you feel obligated, or it's just right in front of you. The list goes on and on. Rationalizing food choices in your mind can leave you with a lot more calories in your daily diet, and all of those extra bites can make or break your weight-loss program. Attitude and awareness are key. Let's explore a few of these food rationalizations that can lead to diet disaster.

THE LOGIC: It's free, therefore I should eat it.

THE SOLUTION: Whether it's free samples at the grocery store or your office or the old "buy one, get one free" at the market, guess what? Free calories count! Watch out—you can end up eating about 500 calories just while grocery shopping. Ask yourself: Would I eat this if I had to pay for it?

THE LOGIC: I don't want to be rude.

THE SOLUTION: If you're at a dinner party or a friend's house for coffee, you feel obligated to eat what is served. But the reality is, you don't have to. It's all in how you say "no." Be polite and pass on the things that you know won't help you lose weight. If you simply can't pass, take a very small portion and just eat a bite. That way your tastes are satisfied and your host won't feel slighted.

THE LOGIC: I need to clean my plate—there are starving kids in Africa.

THE SOLUTION: This was something ingrained in my head when I was a kid. But cleaning your plate is not going to help solve world hunger—it's only going to add inches to your hips. Whether your extras go into the garbage or into your stomach doesn't change the starvation problem in other countries. If you want to help with world hunger, get involved with organizations that help with that cause.

Portion control is more successful when done before eating. If you think, "Oh, I'll just eat half," you'll usually end up polishing it off because you can't resist and then beat yourself up for your lack of control. Remove the temptation from the get-go—after all, even Adam and Eve gave into temptation. It's human nature.

And don't be afraid to take your food home or have leftovers. I was a waitress in high school and college, and we would put away many side dishes, leftover desserts, soups, etc., to reuse the next day—always safe but definitely saved!

THE LOGIC: It's a special occasion.

THE SOLUTION: Even if it's your birthday or anniversary, going face down in a big piece of chocolate cake will set you back. Don't deprive yourself entirely: Have a small portion, but be reasonable. You'll get through the day without feeling guilty.

THE LOGIC: I deserve it!

THE SOLUTION: If you've had a particularly bad day, don't let food be your compensation. Instead, treat yourself with a bubble bath, a massage, a good book, or, best of all, a walk, alone or with a friend!

THE LOGIC: Food makes it fun.

THE SOLUTION: We tend to associate good times with food—family picnics, a day at the beach, holiday gatherings. But you can have fun with activities, too: In my family, we have a pool tournament at Christmas and water races on the Fourth of July. Plan family activities that take the focus off what you eat, whether it's playing games, looking at old photos, or making a movie. Enjoy the gathering, and of course offer up some healthy food choices, but don't make food the focus.

WHAT OUR TEST PANELISTS TOLD US

"I am still 100 percent invested in the program. It's not always easy, but I am doing it. I think the weekend was the hardest with my husband home, but he did his chores and I did my exercises, then we went golfing and fishing. He is eating healthier with me. And I'm not as sore this week!"
—**Roxanne S., 50**

ALL FOODS, IN THEIR most fundamental state, are used for energy. After all, whatever you eat is digested by your body into the simplest form in order to pass into the bloodstream, where it can be absorbed: Carbs are broken down into simple sugars and converted into glucose, fats into fatty acids, and protein into amino acids.

Glucose is your body's first choice for fuel: Any excess glucose not immediately required is stored as glycogen in the liver and muscles. Fatty acids are your main alternative energy sources—particularly in lower-intensity exercise like walking—but it takes longer for your body to convert them into energy. Fatty acids are stored as, yes, fat, whether it's around the major abdominal organs (that visceral fat we talked about

LEARN ABOUT: **ENERGIZING FOODS**

in Part I) or under the skin, and for women especially (no shock here) in the hips, butt, and thighs. Unlike glycogen, which can only be stored in relatively small amounts, your body has an unlimited capacity to store fat. Good for times of famine, bad for those of us dealing with modern-day obesity issues. Finally, amino acids from protein are used primarily for tissue growth and repair, and are not usually used as a major source of fuel. That said, your body is able to break down muscle tissue to provide energy in an emergency. But since you want to preserve as much of your calorie-burning lean muscle mass as possible, this is definitely not a strategy that you want to pursue. Remember that excess amounts of both glucose and amino acids can also be converted to fat, which means eat too much of anything—bagels, steak, even low-fat yogurt—and it will eventually show up on your thighs.

When it's time to create energy, your body converts glucose, fatty acids, and sometimes amino acids to a molecule called adenosine triphosphate, or ATP. ATP is then used by the body through a metabolic process for all of its energy needs. And that doesn't necessarily mean going out and walking a mile. Even at rest, the body uses a lot of energy simply to maintain its normal state: About 60 to 70 percent of our total energy expenditure is to maintain basic functions like breathing, blinking, circulation, body temperature, and digestion. The rest is on movement, whether it's playing with your kids, doing the dishes, or lifting weights. How much energy you need depends on how vigorous the activity is and how long you do it.

The bottom line to all this biology is that at the most basic level, foods that supply plenty of energy are going to have lots of carbs (the easiest fuel for the body to use) and, depending on when you're eating it, a little protein. A light, mostly carb snack (a handful of pretzels, a banana) is great in the hour or two before a workout, since it can be broken down quickly. Avoid sugary snacks and sodas, which (in addition to being high in calories) are broken down so quickly that they'll spike your blood sugar levels but then leave you crashing. Remember, even though a banana is high on the glycemic index, it has only about 100 calories and a satisfying amount of fiber and is far more nutritious than candy or soda. In fact, bananas are rich in vitamin B_6, which helps regulate glucose levels, and are a good source of potassium, which prevents muscle fatigue and helps control high blood pressure. They're also very portable (they come in their own convenient packaging!), inexpensive, and available year-round.

For longer-lasting energy, add a bit more protein to the mix, which will slow down the rate of absorption and give you more fuel for the long run. Try low-fat cheese and some whole-grain crackers, or an apple and a handful of nuts.

Certain vitamins, minerals, and other nutrients play a role in converting food to energy and in keeping the body in working order. One recent study found women with adequate levels of vitamin C in their bodies burned 40 percent more fat during exercise and exercised about 15 percent more efficiently than those with low levels of the vitamin.[9] Aim for about 200 milligrams a day through fruits like kiwifruit, oranges, grapefruits, strawberries, and cantaloupe, or vegetables like red or green bell peppers, broccoli, and Brussels sprouts.

Another key energy source is iron, which is used by red blood cells to transport oxygen throughout the body. Premenopausal women need 18 milligrams a day, and are often deficient (since women with heavy periods can lose significant amounts of iron). A lack of iron can leave you feeling lethargic and easily fatigued. Lean beef is, of course, always a good source of iron, but so are clams, oysters, turkey, lamb, chicken, pork, and shrimp. I don't eat beef, so instead I have tons of fish, chicken, and turkey. On the vegetarian side, look for soybeans or tofu, fortified whole-grain cereals, lentils, spinach, kale, and beans (kidney, chickpeas, lima, navy, and black). Eat an iron-rich food with an orange and you'll get both the C and the iron, plus vitamin C aids in iron absorption.

A quick note on energy drinks, bars, and snacks: Most of us really don't need them. Energy bars can easily pack on 200 calories or more, and those highly caffeinated energy drinks give you only a short-lived burst (not to mention an upset stomach), plus all of that caffeine is a diuretic. Good old-fashioned water will give you all the hydration you need, unless you're going to be exercising for more than an hour or in particularly hot conditions. In that case, a sports drink like Gatorade can provide carbs for fuel, plus fluid for hydration and electrolytes to replace minerals lost through sweat. Just remember that even 8 ounces of Gatorade has 50 calories.

MEAL GUIDELINES:
Suggested amounts for each meal

BREAKFAST
2 grains/starchy veggies

1 dairy

1 protein

1 fruit

1 fat

A.M. SNACK
1 dairy

1 fruit

LUNCH
1 grain/starchy veggie

1 protein

2 veggies

1 fat

P.M. SNACK
1 dairy

DINNER
1 grain/starchy veggie

1 protein

2 veggies

1 fat

DAY 8 SUGGESTED MENU

BREAKFAST

1 cup whole-grain cereal topped with 1 cup skim milk and 2 tablespoons sliced almonds. Serve with 3 ounces Canadian bacon and $1/2$ grapefruit.

PER SERVING: 450 calories; 13 g total fat; 2 g sat fat; 67 g carbohydrates; 9 g fiber; 24 g protein; 19 mg cholesterol; 620 mg sodium

SNACK

1 sliced pear with $1/4$ cup crumbled blue cheese

PER SERVING: 220 calories; 10 g total fat; 6 g sat fat; 28 g carbohydrates; 6 g fiber; 8 g protein; 25 mg cholesterol; 470 mg sodium

LUNCH

Turkey Meatball Pocket

PER SERVING: 341 calories; 17 g total fat; 3 g sat fat; 29 g carbohydrates; 5 g fiber; 21 g protein; 67 mg cholesterol; 658 mg sodium

SNACK

1 cup nonfat or low-fat yogurt

PER SERVING: 140 calories; 0 g total fat; 0 g sat fat; 19 g carbohydrates; 0 g fiber; 14 g protein; 4 mg cholesterol; 190 mg sodium

DINNER

Garlic Lemon Shrimp

PER SERVING: 357 calories; 11 g total fat; 2 g sat fat; 32 g carbohydrates; 6 g fiber; 25 g protein; 130 mg cholesterol; 161 mg sodium

TURKEY MEATBALL POCKET

3 ounces ground turkey

$1/2$ teaspoon garlic powder

$1/4$ teaspoon Italian seasoning

$1/8$ teaspoon black pepper

$1/2$ whole wheat pita pocket

$1/4$ cup marinara sauce

1 cup mixed greens

$1/2$ cup thinly sliced cucumbers

$1 1/2$ teaspoons olive oil

1 teaspoon red wine vinegar

Preheat the oven to 375°F. In a small bowl, combine the turkey, garlic powder, Italian seasoning, and pepper, and mix well. Form into 1" balls; place on a baking sheet. Bake for 10 to 15 minutes, or until cooked through. Remove from the oven and place the meatballs in an open pita pocket. Place the marinara sauce in a microwaveable bowl, then microwave on high 12 to 15 seconds, or until warm. Spoon the sauce over the meatballs. Toss the mixed greens and cucumber together in a small bowl. Drizzle with olive oil and vinegar before serving.

MAKES 1 SERVING

PER SERVING: 341 calories; 17 g total fat; 3 g sat fat; 29 g carbohydrates; 5 g fiber; 21 g protein; 67 mg cholesterol; 658 mg sodium

NOTE: *This recipe is a little high in sodium (you want to aim for no more than 600 mg per meal), which you should normally avoid, but you'll be sweating a lot throughout the 2-Week Total Body Turnaround, so you can get away with it today.*

GARLIC LEMON SHRIMP

2 teaspoons olive oil

$1 1/2$ cups broccoli florets

2 cloves garlic, chopped

4 ounces peeled and deveined shrimp

$1/4$ cup white wine

1 teaspoon lemon juice

$1/8$ teaspoon black pepper

$1/2$ cup cooked whole-grain pasta (1 ounce dry)

Heat the oil in a medium skillet on medium high; add the broccoli. Cook, stirring frequently, until tender, about 3 minutes. Turn the heat to medium, and add the garlic and shrimp. Cook for 2 minutes, tossing quickly. Stir in the wine and lemon juice, and cook an additional 1 to 2 minutes, tossing to coat. Sprinkle with pepper. Spoon the mixture over the pasta.

MAKES 1 SERVING ($1 3/4$ CUPS SHRIMP AND BROCCOLI OVER $1/2$ CUP PASTA)

PER SERVING: 357 calories; 11 g total fat; 2 g sat fat; 32 g carbohydrates; 6 g fiber; 25 g protein; 130 mg cholesterol; 161 mg sodium

NOTE: *If your local grocery store doesn't carry peeled and deveined shrimp, ask the seafood counter to do it for you.*

SUCCESS STORY

Michelle Knapek

AGE:
46

HEIGHT:
5'1½"

START WEIGHT:
133 pounds

AFTER 2 WEEKS:
127 pounds

RESULTS:
6 pounds, 11¾ inches lost

(including 3 inches
from waist and
1 inch from hips)

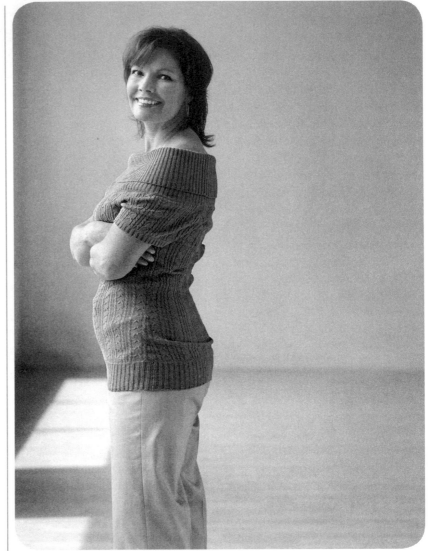

With her daughter's wedding rapidly approaching and a scale that remained stuck despite a few attempts at weight loss, Michelle knew she had to change something. "I'm pretty active—I bike and walk a lot—but it seemed like nothing was working for me," she says. Her menopausal symptoms (sleepless nights, constant headaches, bloating), which had been plaguing her for months, didn't make things easier. "My girlfriends from high school and I were all noticing that it's just not as easy to lose weight like it was in the past. It felt like the fat was just sticking around."

A few days into her 2-Week Total Body Turnaround, however, she began to see a difference. "The first thing I noticed was that the puffiness in my face and body went down. Then I found I was sleeping better. And the greatest change was that it nearly completely alleviated all of those miserable menopausal symptoms!"

The workout paid off in other ways, as well. She noticed more muscle definition in her arms, and her belly looked flatter. By the end of 2 weeks, she'd lost 6 pounds and nearly 12 inches off her body, including a remarkable 3 inches off her waist.

Michelle credits the combo of strength and cardio for her changes. "I always moved around a lot, but I didn't really lift weights. I was shocked at how much difference I saw in muscle tone in such a short time."

And even with a work schedule as a career counselor that she classified as "the busiest in 9 years," she says fitting in the time to exercise was surprisingly easy. "I thought it was going to be incredibly time-consuming, but the time went by so quickly," she notes. Michelle's strategy was to do her strength in the morning and cardio in the evening. "Sometimes it would be after 8:00 at night, but it was still manageable."

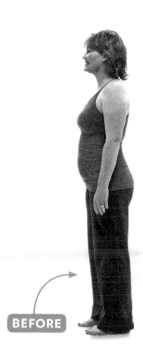

BEFORE

Being on the plan compelled her to squeeze in her cardio, even if the weather didn't look like it was going to cooperate. "Whereas in the past I would pass on a walk because it looked like it might rain, now I went out no matter what—and more often than not, the skies held out or maybe it just drizzled lightly. Since it was only for a half hour, it was totally doable." She also found that despite being active in the past, she hadn't really pushed herself to her limits. "I thought it would be really difficult, but it wasn't hard to get my intensity up and then recover, and I think that really helped me save time versus going to the gym for 90 minutes."

Adding more vegetables to her diet and making healthier meal choices also contributed to her success. She found a new, satisfying midday snack: lima beans with a drop of butter and a little salt, which she heated up at work. Other favorite foods include natural applesauce mixed with ground-up flaxseed as a sweet treat, plus chicken breast or salmon on salad, and lots of fruit or vegetables at every meal.

After the 2 weeks were up, she added on even more activities— swimming in the lake near her house, going for bike rides, even running up a flight of stairs for interval training—and kept up her healthy food choices.

As for her daughter's wedding, not only did she have more energy to manage the pre-wedding craziness of houseguests and entertaining, but she felt stronger and more confident than ever in her fitted gown. "I was so comfortable with my appearance—I didn't have to worry about how I looked. I really reshaped my body. And I didn't even have to put on Spanx!"

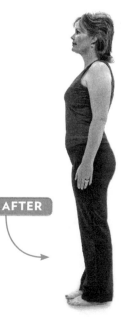

AFTER

DAY 9

■ ■ ■ ■ ■ ■ ■ ■ **9** ☐ ☐ ☐ ☐ ☐

Now that you're well into the 2-Week Total Body Turnaround, you might be thinking about what will happen when the 14 days are over. Will you return to whatever state you were in before you picked up this book? What if you stumble, veer off course, have a really bad day, and dive headfirst into a bag of chips? Take heart: Even the best athlete occasionally stumbles, and all of us have come up against challenges that can make us question whether or not we can go on. The key is to always keep your goals in mind, and remember why you are choosing to embark on a path to a healthier lifestyle. Even one absolutely awful day of eating won't make you split your pants: Remember there are 3,500 calories in a pound, so you'd have to consume 17,500 calories in a day to gain 5. Don't let a single bad day make you give up on your hopes and dreams. I tell my kids: There is no such thing as a mistake, only a learning experience. I ask you every time you "flub up" to forgive yourself and then think about what triggers the behavior. I've learned over the years where my weakness comes into play. For example, often after a long couple of days on the road, I come home and find comfort in my own kitchen. I am now aware of it, so I actually now think of the one thing I'd like to eat when I get home that is not restaurant food, and I give myself one snack, instead of being a vacuum through the pantry. So remember, you can do this. Forgive yourself and move on.

CARDIO: Hills

As on Day 2, your cardio is all about hills. Remember that you'll need to find a moderately steep incline that is at least ⅛ of a mile long. (If you're using a treadmill, use a grade of 5 to 7 percent.) If you can't find a hill that's long enough to take you through the longest part of the workout (2½ minutes), go as long as you can, and then continue to walk as fast as you can until you hit your target time. Turn around and walk downhill after each "walk hard" interval. And if you can't find a hill or don't have a treadmill, do speed bursts or another interval routine.

INTENSITY	TIME	RPE	TALK TEST
Warm up, moderate pace, flat surface (heart rate: Zone 2)	3 min.	4–5	You can speak in full sentences (slightly breathless)
Walk hard uphill (heart rate: Zone 4)	30 sec.	8–9	You can only say one or two words (very breathless)
Recover, walk downhill (heart rate: Zone 2)	30 sec.	4–5	Slightly breathless
Walk hard uphill (heart rate: Zone 4)	1 min.	8–9	You can only say one or two words (very breathless)
Recover, walk downhill (heart rate: Zone 2)	1 min.	4–5	Slightly breathless
Walk hard uphill (heart rate: Zone 4)	90 sec.	8–9	You can only say one or two words (very breathless)
Recover, walk downhill (heart rate: Zone 2)	90 sec.	4–5	Slightly breathless
Walk hard uphill (heart rate: Zone 3–4)	2 min.	7–8	You can only say short phrases or a few words (very breathless)
Recover, walk downhill (heart rate: Zone 2)	2 min.	4–5	Slightly breathless
Walk hard uphill (heart rate: Zone 3–4)	2½ min.	7–8	You can only say short phrases or a few words (very breathless)
Recover, walk downhill (heart rate: Zone 2)	2½ min.	4–5	Slightly breathless
Walk hard uphill (heart rate: Zone 3–4)	2 min.	7–8	You can only say short phrases or a few words (very breathless)
Recover, walk downhill (heart rate: Zone 2)	2 min.	4–5	Slightly breathless
Walk hard uphill (heart rate: Zone 3–4)	90 sec.	7–8	You can only say short phrases or a few words (very breathless)
Recover, walk downhill (heart rate: Zone 2)	90 sec.	4–5	Slightly breathless
Walk hard uphill (heart rate: Zone 4)	1 min.	8–9	You can only say one or two words (very breathless)
Recover, walk downhill (heart rate: Zone 2)	1 min.	4–5	Slightly breathless
Cool down, easy pace, flat surface (heart rate: Zone 1)	3 min.	2–3	Conversational pace

STRENGTH: Lower Body + Core

More balance challenges here to work your lower body and abs! Try to do at least a few reps of this harder variation. You'll never know if you don't try! This is your opportunity to push yourself. If you finish an exercise and are still comfortable, you need to increase the amount of weight you are lifting. Going too light is one of the biggest reasons many women don't see results from strength training. You've got to reach muscle fatigue and tear up muscle fibers in order to build new muscle. If the weight feels too easy, or you're just not focusing, you're wasting your time. Connect your mind to the workout and focus, especially on the moves with a balance challenge. You'll establish a core connection that helps you stay centered and improves your results.

Ⓐ

KNEE LIFT FLOATING LUNGE

TARGETS: Quads, butt

A. Stand with feet together, arms at sides holding dumbbells. Step left foot behind you, lowering into a lunge for 4 counts; keep right knee over right ankle as you bend knees 90 degrees.

B. Lift left leg up to hip height as you "float" it forward in 2 counts.

C. Lunge left leg directly in front of you in 4 counts; keep left knee over ankle as you bend knees 90 degrees. **Then lift left knee to hip height and float back,** lunging behind you in 2 counts. Repeat 8 times; switch legs.

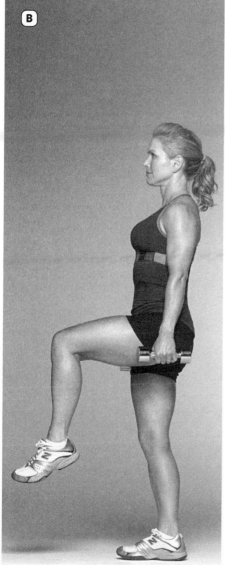

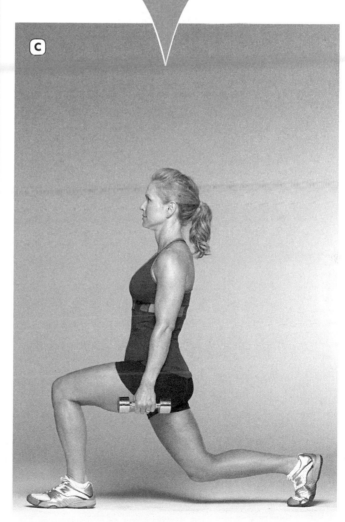

GOOD FORM TIP:
Don't push forward with your knees. Keep your front knee tracking over your shoelaces to protect your knee joint.

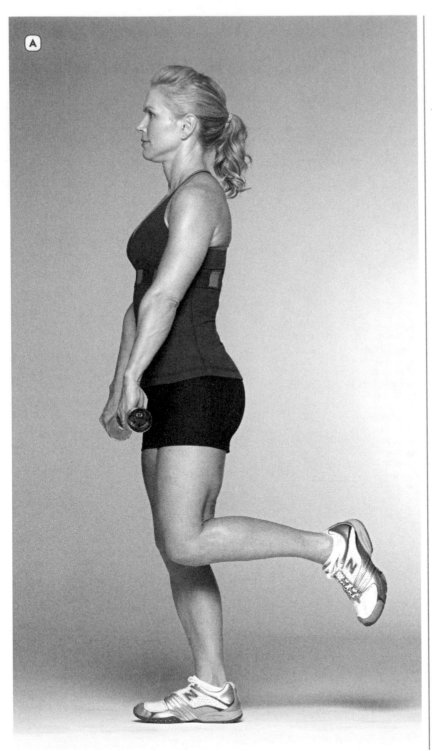

SINGLE-LEG DEADLIFT

TARGETS: Hamstrings

A. Stand with feet hip-width apart, knees slightly bent, holding dumbbells with arms extended, palms facing thighs. **Lift left leg behind you, balancing on right leg.**

B. Keeping right knee slightly bent, abs tight, and spine long, slowly bend forward from hips in 4 counts, lowering weights toward floor as left leg extends behind you. Rise back to starting position in 2 counts, pulling through right leg and butt as you lift up. Do 8 reps; switch legs and repeat.

B

GOOD FORM TIP:
Keep your knees slightly soft,
especially if your hamstrings are
tight. Push your butt back and
use your butt and hamstrings—
not your back—to stand up.
Gaze at a single spot on the
floor to help you balance.

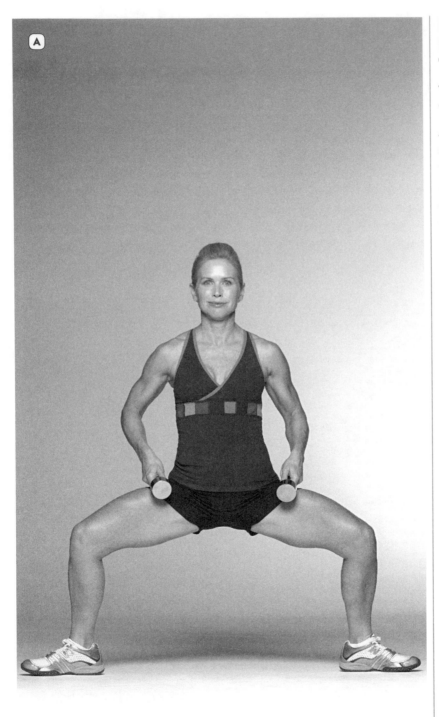

DUMBBELL PLIÉ HEEL TAPS

TARGETS: Quads, butt, outer thighs, calves

A. Stand with feet shoulder-width apart, toes turned outward and spine long, **holding dumbbells on top of thighs.** Bend knees, lowering body straight down for 4 counts.

B. Stand up in 2 counts, coming up halfway on count 1, then gently tapping left heel twice on right for count 2. Step back out and repeat 8 times. Switch sides and repeat, this time tapping with right heel on left for final 8 reps.

GOOD FORM TIP:
Keep your tailbone tucked under your torso. If your hips are tight, ease into the movement— it may take some practice to move further into the plié.

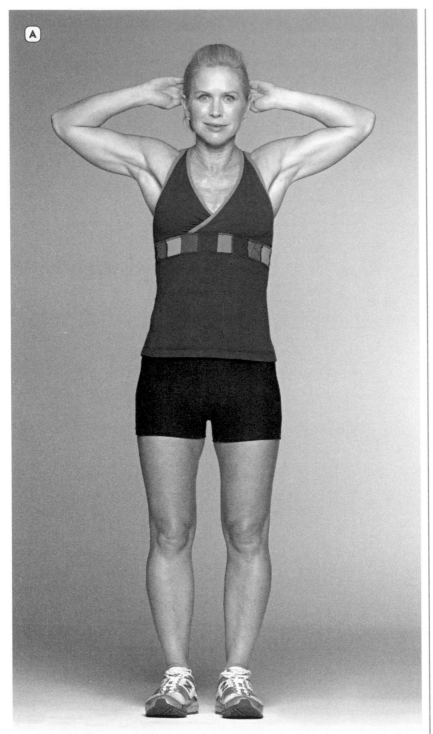

HANDS-UP SCISSOR SQUAT

TARGETS: Quads, butt, outer and inner thighs

A. Stand with feet together, **hands behind head with elbows out to sides.**

B. Step left foot wide out to the left on count 1. Squat down on counts 2–4, as if sitting in a chair, keeping weight over heels and **hands behind head (engage abs to help with balance).**

C. (not shown) Stand up slowly and bring feet back together, taking 2 counts.

D. (not shown) Repeat on opposite side, stepping right foot out wide to right on count 1, then squatting down on counts 2–4. Take 2 counts to stand up and return to start. Repeat 8 times each side.

B

GOOD FORM TIP:
*Keep your knees tracking over
your shoelaces—not past your
toes—when squatting to avoid
putting pressure on your kneecaps.
Keep your torso lifted with chin
parallel to floor.*

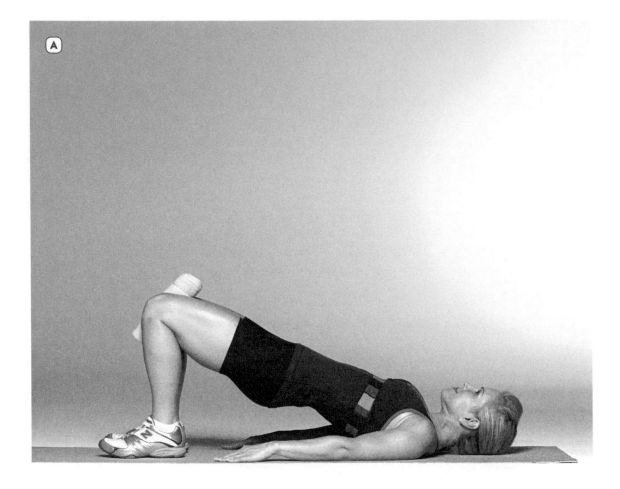

CALF AND INNER THIGH ATTACK BRIDGE

TARGETS: Hamstrings, butt, calves

A. Lie face up on floor, knees bent and feet flat on floor, about 3 to 4 inches apart. **Place a rolled-up towel or a pillow between your knees.**

B. Pushing feet into floor, lift hips up for 2 counts, **squeezing towel or pillow**; keep abs tight and body in a straight line from knees to chest. Holding here, lift heels, squeezing calves and thighs for 2 counts. Slowly lower heels for 4 counts. Continue to hold hips up in isometric contraction. Repeat 8 to 12 times.

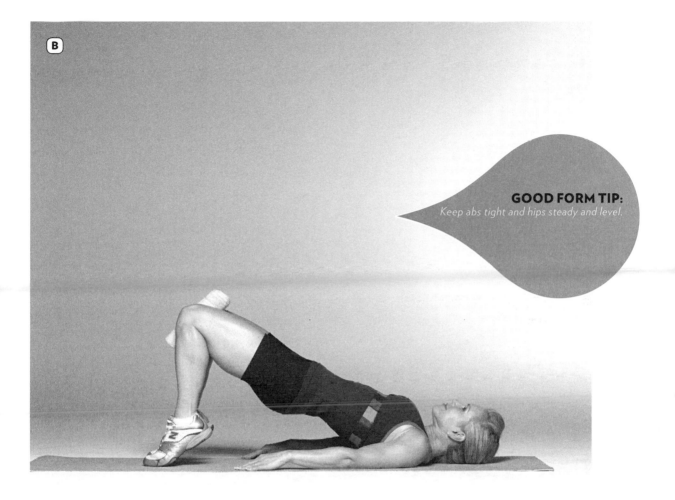

GOOD FORM TIP:
Keep abs tight and hips steady and level.

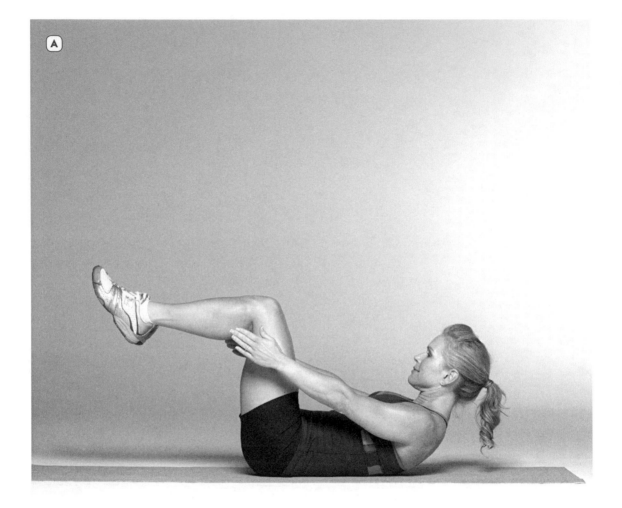

DOUBLE LEG STRETCH

TARGETS: Abs

A. Lie face up on floor, knees bent 90 degrees with knees over hips and hands reaching for shins.

B. Inhale and take 4 counts to bring arms behind head and extend legs 45 degrees to floor, forming a V-shape.

C. Exhale and pull legs back in while circling arms around the sides back to starting position in 2 counts. Repeat 8 to 10 times. Keep upper body as still as possible during the exercise.

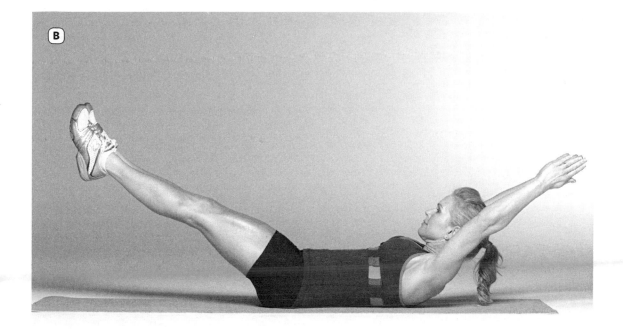

B

C

GOOD FORM TIP:
Slightly press your lower back into the floor, pulling your belly button toward your lower back.

NEW EXERCISE!
CORE CHALLENGE

READ THE PAPER

TARGETS: Abs, obliques

A. Sit on floor with knees bent and heels on floor. Hold arms in front of body, as if holding a closed newspaper.

B. Slowly lower upper body toward floor, rounding your back, stopping about halfway down, and twist to left, as if opening the paper on your left side, in 4 counts. With a big exhale, take 2 counts and pull yourself back to start position, using your obliques (the muscles in the sides of your torso). Repeat on right side. Do 8 to 12 times total.

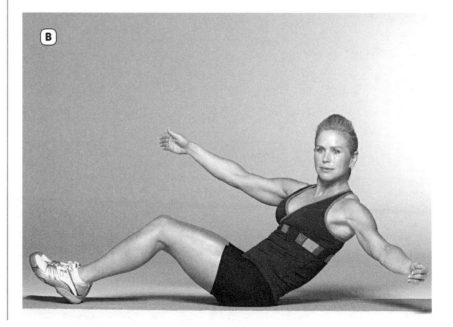

GOOD FORM TIP:
Round your back into a C-curve and keep your abs engaged to protect your lower back. Twist from your obliques, not just your shoulders.

DAY 9 TURNAROUND TIP
Remind Yourself!

When I work with new clients, I ask them to put sticky notes around the house to remind them what they want to accomplish that day. I have them write down reminders like:

"Think before you open" (on the pantry)

"Do 10 pushups before bed" (on the bathroom mirror)

"Stand tall: Keep your shoulders back and down"

"Pull in your abs"

It may sound a bit silly, but writing something down and placing it so that you stare right at it really can make a difference. I remember reading an article about a year ago about a mall in England that actually posted colorful signs by the escalator and stairs designed to encourage and inspire shoppers to walk up the stairs rather than ride the escalator. They found that the number of people who took the stairs rather than the escalator rose from 4 to 10 percent after the signs were added. In addition, the article noted that the Centers for Disease Control and Prevention (CDC) undertook an effort to beautify their indoor stairwells with music and art in order to make them more attractive to their own workers. They reported an increase in the stair use in their own building by 20 percent! These amazing statistics show that little changes in our minds and environment can make big differences. Sometimes it is as easy as reminding ourselves of what is healthy for our bodies!

While climbing one flight of stairs isn't going to substitute for consistent daily exercise, taking the stairs when you can does add into your physical activity levels. And if you make a habit of always taking the stairs, you are cumulatively adding more activity to your days. The better you start to feel physically, the more you'll be motivated to keep moving. And here's a bonus the next time you hit the mall and walk with those shopping bags: Climbing stairs while carrying 25 pounds burns almost 9 calories a minute!

SOMETIMES IT MAY FEEL like your appetite is a roller coaster, hitting hunger highs one moment, and dips the next. Things would be a lot easier if your appetite were nice and smooth, like a ride in a stretch limo. Luckily, what and when you eat can have a big impact on your hunger levels to even out some of those peaks and valleys.

Our bodies usually let us know when we're hungry. Your tummy rumbles, or you may get hunger pangs, which are just signs of your empty stomach contracting. But a more important indication of hunger is your glucose levels. When your blood sugar levels dip, the liver sends a signal to the brain, which lets your body know it's time to eat. Ignore these signals for too long and your self-control becomes a lot harder. When you've eaten enough,

LEARN ABOUT: **STABILIZING FOODS**

your body releases hormones that tell your brain it's time to stop. Hopefully, you listen.

To keep your appetite in check, don't skip meals and include at least three meals and two healthy snacks each day. Try to eat about every 3 to 4 hours, which will prevent your blood sugar levels from dipping too low and sending you on the hunt for something to eat, pronto. Start with a good breakfast. Research shows that old adage about it being the most important meal of the day is true. At the National Weight Control Registry (a listing of dieters who have successfully lost at least 30 pounds and kept the weight off for at least a year), nearly 80 percent say they eat breakfast every day.[10] Put off eating too long and you'll completely lose control of your hunger by the time lunchtime rolls around.

Foods that take longer to digest can also help stabilize sugar levels and keep you feeling fuller, longer. I call these my stabilizing stars. On my list:

- **Eggs:** A breakfast favorite for good reason, eggs are a great way to start off your day. They're a good source of protein (1 large egg has about 6 grams), which takes the body time to break down and digest. One recent study found that women following a low-fat diet who ate two eggs for breakfast at least 5 days a week for 8 weeks lost 65 percent more weight and averaged an 83 percent greater reduction in waist circumference than those who had a bagel breakfast with the same amount of calories.[11] Another study found women who ate an egg-based breakfast ate an average of 420 calories less over 36 hours than those who ate a bagel breakfast with the same number of calories.[12] Not a fan of eggs? Have some low-fat or fat-free milk or yogurt, which also contain protein.

- **Almonds:** Noshing on a small amount of these nuts, which are a good source of monounsaturated fats, can keep you satisfied for hours. One study found that among men and women who were on a low-fat diet, those who ate a few ounces of the nuts reduced their waistlines about $6^{1}/_{2}$ inches in 24 weeks, nearly 50 percent more than those who didn't eat the nuts, although they all consumed the same amount of total calories.[13] Another study found that after 6 months, those on the almond-enriched diet lost 63 percent more weight and 50 percent more body fat while also shrinking their waistlines 55 percent more than those on a high-carb diet.[14] Just beware that almonds are high in calories—a 1-ounce serving (about 28 pieces) has 170 calories, so a little can go a long way toward keeping you satiated. I count them out into a baggie, so I know exactly how many to leave.

● **Avocados:** Creamy avocados aren't just the highlight of a good guacamole. In moderation, they're also a great source of monounsaturated fats, like almonds and other nuts and seeds. Plus, they're high in phytochemicals, especially lutein, which can help keep your eyes healthy. They're also high in vitamin K, potassium, and folate. One study found volunteers who ate avocados every day for a week reduced their total cholesterol by an average of 17 percent, lowering LDL ("bad") cholesterol and triglycerides while improving HDL ("good") cholesterol.[15] Put a few slices on a sandwich in place of mayo; add them to a salad or have a small chunk sprinkled with some lime juice and salt. You can even throw an avocado into a smoothie: It's so mild in flavor you can't even taste it. Just remember that a medium-size avocado has 30 grams of fat, so eat in moderation. A serving size is 2 tablespoons, which has about 55 calories.

● **Apples:** An apple (or two) a day can keep weight gain at bay. Studies have found that subjects who snacked on an apple before each meal lost nearly 40 percent more weight than those who didn't eat the fruit.[16] Another study found those who ate an apple 15 minutes before having an all-you-can-eat lunch ate 15 percent fewer calories than those who had apple juice or applesauce.[17] Apples are high in fiber, so they'll help fill you up and keep you feeling full for several hours. Plus, they're low in calories: A medium-size apple only has about 65 calories.

● **Oatmeal:** A great "stick-to-your-ribs" food, oatmeal offers more than just a good way to lower cholesterol levels. One study found that subjects who ate a reduced-calorie diet that included a high-fiber oatmeal breakfast and walked for 15 to 30 minutes a day lost an average of 10 pounds in 12 weeks, 5 percent body fat, and 2 inches off their waistlines.[18] Oatmeal has a high amount of soluble fiber, which slows down carbohydrate absorption and stabilizes blood sugar levels. I eat mine with walnuts and bananas or blueberries.

● **Peanut butter:** Hurray for PB&J! A little peanut butter or peanuts in your diet can also help stave off the munchies. One study found that subjects who snacked on peanut butter reported feeling fuller and eating less than usual in their regular diet.[19] Peanuts are high in monounsaturated fat (despite the fact that peanuts are actually a legume, and not a nut); they're also high in fiber and protein. Have a small amount (2 tablespoons have about 190 calories) on whole-wheat bread or on apple slices.

MEAL GUIDELINES:

Suggested amounts for each meal

BREAKFAST

2 grains/starchy veggies

1 dairy

1 protein

1 fruit

1 fat

A.M. SNACK

1 dairy

1 fruit

LUNCH

1 grain/starchy veggie

1 protein

2 veggies

1 fat

P.M. SNACK

1 dairy

DINNER

1 grain/starchy veggie

1 protein

2 veggies

1 fat

DAY 9 SUGGESTED MENU

BREAKFAST

1 whole-grain waffle topped with 1 cup mixed berries and 2 tablespoons chopped walnuts. Serve with 3 ounces veggie sausage and 1 cup skim milk.

PER SERVING: 480 calories; 18 g total fat; 2 g sat fat; 51 g carbohydrates; 16 g fiber; 33 g protein; 4 mg cholesterol; 830 mg sodium

NOTE: *This meal is a little high in sodium (you want to aim for no more than 600 to 650 mg per meal), which you should normally avoid, but you'll be sweating a lot throughout the 2-Week Total Body Turnaround, so you can get away with it today.*

SNACK

¹/₂ cup nonfat ricotta cheese topped with ¹/₄ cup raisins and a sprinkle of cinnamon

PER SERVING: 160 calories; 0 g total fat; 0 g sat fat; 34 g carbohydrates; 1 g fiber; 6 g protein; 10 mg cholesterol; 70 mg sodium

LUNCH

Dijon Chicken and Chickpea Salad

PER SERVING: 393 calories; 14 g total fat; 2 g sat fat; 40 g carbohydrates; 10 g fiber; 30 g protein; 52 mg cholesterol; 642 mg sodium

SNACK

1 cup chocolate soymilk

PER SERVING: 90 calories; 2 g total fat; 0 g sat fat; 12 g carbohydrates; 0 g fiber; 7 g protein; 0 mg cholesterol; 180 mg sodium

DINNER

Tofu-Vegetable Marinara with Parmesan

PER SERVING: 352 calories; 16 g total fat; 2 g sat fat; 38 g carbohydrates; 8 g fiber; 18 g protein; 5 mg cholesterol; 603 mg sodium

DIJON CHICKEN AND CHICKPEA SALAD

2 teaspoons olive oil

1 teaspoon Dijon mustard

1 tablespoon cider vinegar

1 tablespoon lemon juice

$^1/_8$ teaspoon black pepper

Pinch of salt

$^1/_2$ cup no-salt-added canned chickpeas

$^1/_2$ cup chopped tomatoes

$^1/_2$ cup sliced red or yellow bell peppers

$^1/_2$ cup shredded carrots

1 cup mixed greens

3 ounces rotisserie skinless chicken breast, sliced

In a small bowl, combine the olive oil, mustard, vinegar, lemon juice, black pepper, and salt, whisking until combined. Set aside. In a medium bowl, toss together the chickpeas, tomatoes, bell peppers, carrots, and mixed greens. Drizzle with the dressing and toss until well coated. Top with the chicken breast slices.

MAKES 1 SERVING (2$^3/_4$ CUPS SALAD MIXTURE)

PER SERVING: 393 calories; 14 g total fat; 2 g sat fat; 40 g carbohydrates; 10 g fiber; 30 g protein; 52 mg cholesterol; 642 mg sodium

TOFU-VEGETABLE MARINARA WITH PARMESAN

3 ounces firm or extra-firm tofu, cubed

1$^1/_2$ teaspoons olive oil

$^1/_2$ cup sliced zucchini

1 cup sliced portobello mushrooms

$^1/_2$ cup marinara sauce

1 tablespoon chopped fresh basil

$^1/_2$ cup cooked whole grain pasta (or brown rice)

1 tablespoon grated Parmesan cheese

In a medium saucepan over medium-high heat, cook the tofu in the olive oil, stirring frequently, for about 5 minutes, or until just browned. Remove from the pan and set aside. Add the zucchini and mushrooms, and cook, stirring frequently, for about 5 minutes, or until tender. Stir in the reserved tofu and the marinara sauce and basil. Cook until warmed through. Spoon over the pasta (or rice), and sprinkle with the cheese before serving.

MAKES 1 SERVING (1$^1/_4$ CUPS MIXTURE OVER $^1/_2$ CUP COOKED PASTA)

PER SERVING: 352 calories; 16 g total fat; 2 g sat fat; 38 g carbohydrates; 8 g fiber; 18 g protein; 5 mg cholesterol; 603 mg sodium

NOTE: *This dish also works well with chicken.*

DAY 10

There are lots of crazy diets out there, and many of you may have actually experimented with a few of them. I recently heard about one called something like the "Ape Diet," and that just hit my funny bone. What has happened to us? There are a million diets out there, and now we have stooped so low that we have to behave as zoo animals to lose weight. But after I got over my giggles, I started listening, and actually it's quite interesting: British researchers asked nine junk-food junkies to follow this diet and actually live in the zoo (oh my goodness!) for 12 days. Participants followed a zoo animal's diet of 11 pounds of fruits and veggies each day. Now that's a heck of a lot of food, but I suppose zoo animals don't dip their veggies in ranch dressing, deep-fry them in trans fats, or drip them with cheese, so therein lies our problem. These self-proclaimed junk-food junkies each lowered their cholesterol and blood pressure and lost 10 pounds in 1 week.

It goes back to what I always say: *Eat clean.* Clean eating means eating more foods that come from a plant, animal, or tree—not a box, bag, or fast-food restaurant. It's food full of information like nutrients, vitamins, and minerals, not just empty calories. I guess the zoo animals are doing it right—although 11 pounds is a lot of food!

But it makes you think. So many foods are stuffed with hidden calories, preservatives, additives, and food colorings that gum up your system and make you feel bloated, sick, and tired. In the last 9 days, you've hopefully started to feel a change in your body for the better, just by eating well and exercising. Maybe you haven't lost 10 pounds, but you've lost the bloat and inflammation caused by junk food. And you didn't even have to live in a zoo.

CARDIO: Pure Power

Today's power walk is a great way to keep building your aerobic endurance while blasting fat. Concentrate on walking at a fast pace for the majority of this workout—as if you were late for a really important appointment! Then take it up a notch for those 30-second mini-intervals. Challenge yourself to see how fast you can keep it up. The half hour will fly by!

INTENSITY	TIME	PACE	RPE	GOAL
Warm up (heart rate: Zone 2)	5 min.	Moderate pace	4-5	You can speak in sentences but are slightly breathless.
Power walk (heart rate: Zone 3)	20 min.	Fast pace	7	Gradually increase intensity until you are walking at the fastest pace you can sustain. You should be mostly breathless, able to speak no more than a few short words at a time.
Cool down (heart rate: Zone 2)	5 min.	Moderate pace	3-4	Slow down until you are walking at a moderate pace. You should be able to speak in full sentences with some breathlessness.

STRENGTH: Total Body

This total body workout will tone your muscles where you want it most—your arms, your butt, your thighs. Try the challenge variations to engage even more of your muscles. Remember to move slowly and take your time with each repetition. Slowing down the movements is going to make a big difference in working the muscles more completely. And building lean muscle is so important, especially as you get older. Starting in our thirties, women will lose about a half-pound of muscle a year. The only way to replace it is by strength training. So get lifting!

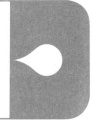

> "Life is 10 percent what you make it, and 90 percent how you take it."
> —Irving Berlin

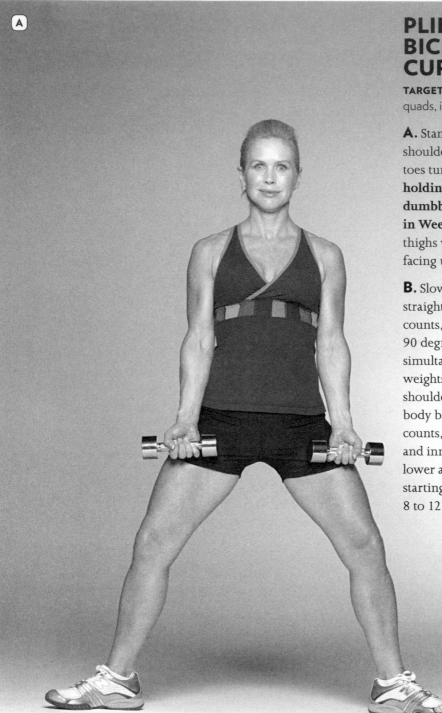

A

PLIÉ WITH BICEPS CURL

TARGETS: Biceps, butt, quads, inner thighs

A. Stand with feet shoulder-width apart, toes turned outward, **holding heavier dumbbells than used in Week 1** in front of thighs with palms facing up.

B. Slowly lower body straight down for 2 counts, bending knees 90 degrees while simultaneously curling weights toward shoulders. Slowly stand body back up for 4 counts, squeezing butt and inner thighs, as you lower arms back to starting position. Repeat 8 to 12 times.

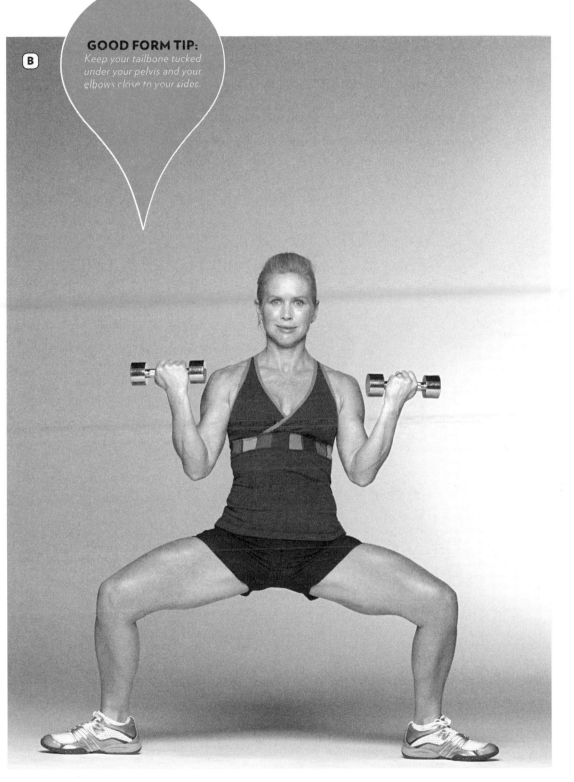

B

GOOD FORM TIP:
Keep your tailbone tucked under your pelvis and your elbows close to your sides.

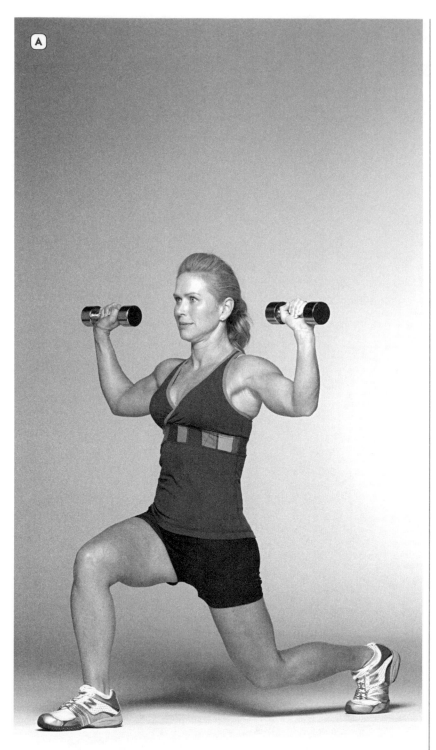

FORWARD LUNGE AND RAISE THE ROOF WITH KNEE-UP

TARGETS: Shoulders, quads, butt, core

A. Stand with feet together, holding dumbbells overhead, palms facing forward. Lunge forward with right foot in 4 counts, bending both knees 90 degrees (keep right knee over right ankle) while lowering weights toward shoulders, bending elbow 90 degrees.

B. Push back to starting position in 2 counts, **lifting left knee to hip height as you straighten arms. Lower to start** and repeat 8 to 12 times; switch sides.

B

GOOD FORM TIP:
Keep your front knee tracking over your shoelaces to avoid putting strain on the kneecap.

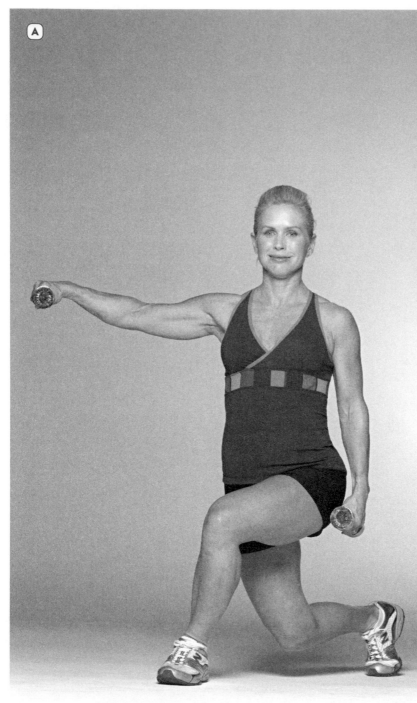

A

CURTSY LAT RAISE WITH FRONT KICK

TARGETS: Shoulders, butt, quads, outer thighs

A. Stand with feet shoulder-width apart, holding dumbbells at sides. Cross right leg 2 to 3 feet behind left, bending knees (keep left knee over left ankle). At the same time, lift right arm out to side at shoulder height. Take 4 counts to perform.

B. Stand up in 2 counts, **kicking right leg out as you lower arm.** Go directly into next curtsy lunge/lat raise. Repeat 8 times. Switch sides and repeat 8 times.

GOOD FORM TIP:
Keep the front knee over the ankle facing forward; don't turn it to the side. Use your shoulder to raise the arm out to the side; don't scrunch up your neck.

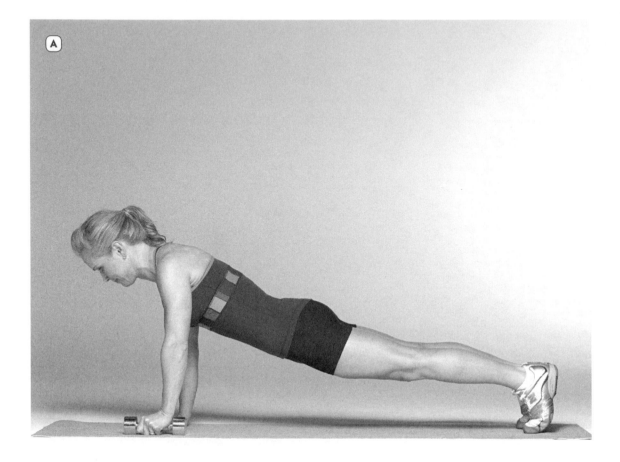

FULL PUSHUP ROW

TARGETS: Chest, back

A. Start in **full pushup position,** legs extended behind you and balancing on toes, holding dumbbell in left hand on floor under shoulders.

B. Slowly bend elbows 90 degrees as you lower chest toward floor for 4 counts, keeping abdominals tight and back straight.

C. Push back to start position for 2 counts, pulling left elbow up toward ribs. Lower weight back toward floor in 4 counts. Repeat the pushup 6 to 8 times. Switch hands and repeat 6 to 8 times, this time holding weight in right hand and lifting right elbow.

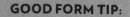

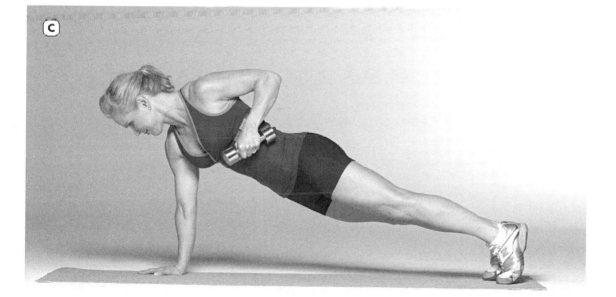

B

GOOD FORM TIP:
Keep abs tight and spine long; don't allow your lower back to sag.

C

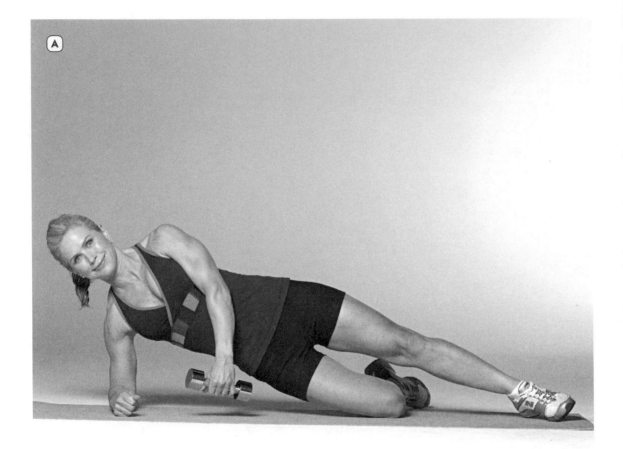

FOREARM SIDE PLANK WITH SHOULDER RAISE AND LEG LIFT

TARGETS: Shoulders, obliques, abs

A. Lie on right side, hips stacked, elbow under shoulder and right forearm on floor with bottom knee on floor and top leg extended. Hold a dumbbell in left hand on floor, just in front of body. Lift hips, forming a straight line from shoulders to heels, keeping abdominals tight.

B. Lift left arm above shoulder for 2 counts; **at the same time, lift left leg as high as you can, keeping abs tight.** Lower both arm and leg slowly for 4 counts. Repeat 8 times each side.

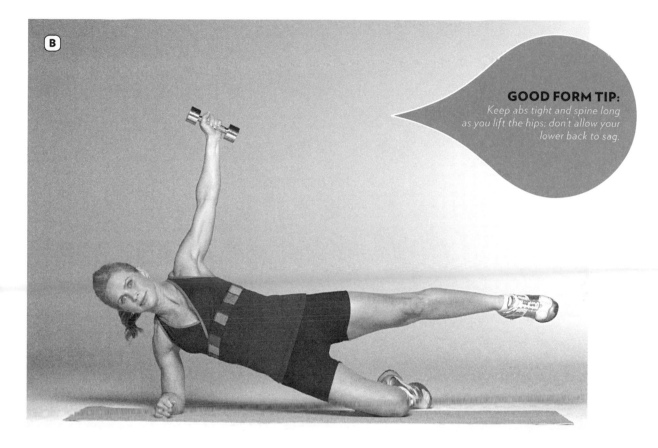

B

GOOD FORM TIP:
Keep abs tight and spine long as you lift the hips; don't allow your lower back to sag.

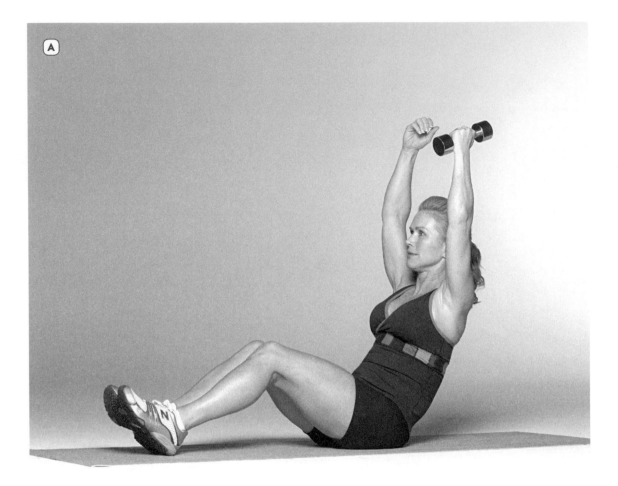

PASS THE BELL

TARGETS: Abs

A. Sit on floor with knees bent and feet on floor in front of you. Raise both arms overhead, holding a dumbbell in left hand. Keep your back slightly rounded and abs engaged.

B. Lean back slightly and lower arms out toward shoulder height in 4 counts, keeping weight in left hand and both elbows slightly bent.

C. Lift arms back overhead in 2 counts, then switch dumbbell to right hand and repeat. Continue to "pass the bell" between hands for 8 to 10 repetitions per side.

B

GOOD FORM TIP:
*Imagine pressing your belly
button into your lower back
to activate your lower abs
and protect your back.*

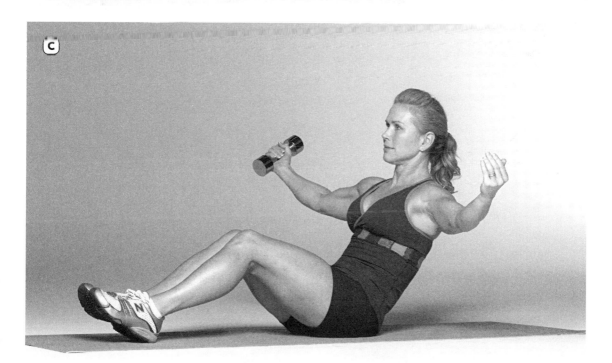

C

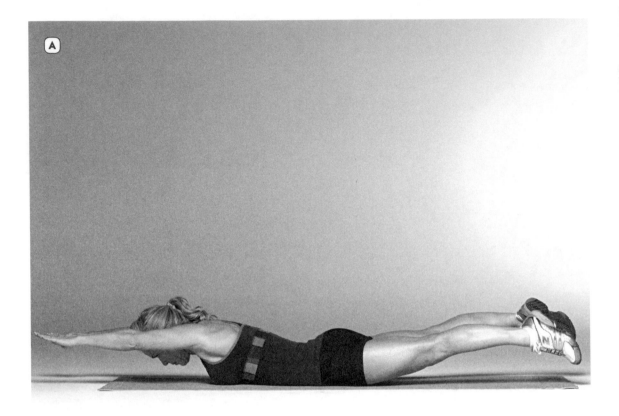

NEW EXERCISE! **CORE CHALLENGE**

SWIMMER

TARGETS: Lower back, abs

A. Lie face down on floor, arms and legs extended. Lift upper body and legs off the floor, keeping arms and legs straight.

B. Pulse arms and legs up and down in a swimming motion, first lifting and lowering right arm and left leg.

C. Then lift and lower left arm and right leg, as if lightly splashing through the water. Try to move only your arms and legs, keeping your torso and hips as still as possible. Do for 30 seconds.

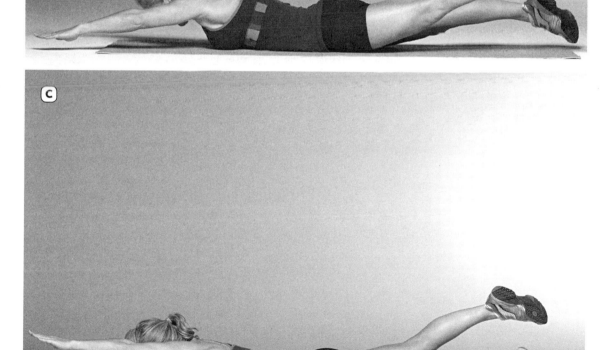

GOOD FORM TIP:
Remember to keep your abs engaged even when you're face down. Move from your shoulders and your hips, not your knees and elbows.

DAY 10 TURNAROUND TIP

Welcome Change

You've taken this 2-Week Total Body Turnaround trip because something about the concept motivated you to try it. You were ready for a change and you thought that this could be the shake-up you need to get on a path to better health.

Well, plateaus and ruts are about as welcome as rainy days. Everyone has a different reason for hitting a plateau or falling into a rut, and the answers aren't the same for everyone, either. But there is one word that applies to all of us—*change*. Something has to change to break that barrier and budge the scale. Shake it up, do something different, eat something different, think different, but *make a change*.

A common question I get from readers on my Web site is: "I'm doing my 30 minutes of cardio every day on the treadmill, but my weight loss is at a standstill. Should I go longer?"

What I tell my readers is that while going longer does burn more calories, that isn't necessarily the only or best fix. Your body has adapted to the typical 30 minutes of walking or jogging or whatever you've been doing. What used to take more effort is now clockwork. Your body has become more efficient, which means it can do the same exercise but expend less energy (read: you'll burn fewer calories doing the same workout).

Instead, do something different during those 30 minutes. Try interval training and vary your intensity, like the intervals we're doing throughout these 2 weeks. Or switch it up entirely—slip in a kickboxing or dance DVD, ride your bike, jump rope, or put on some skates.

Also, remember that doing cardio alone will not boost your resting metabolism. To increase the number of calories your body uses on a daily basis, you need to strength train. But you can still plateau with your strength: Doing the same exercises with the same weights in the same order for the same amount of time will stall your results. Try using a new machine at the gym, or a new accessory, like a medicine ball instead of a dumbbell. Or do a typical strength move like a biceps curl or a chest press on a stability ball instead of a bench. You'll work your abs along with your upper body. By shocking your system, you work harder and burn more calories. If you keep doing what you're doing, you'll keep getting what you're getting.

Change can also play an important role in your diet. My clients will sometimes tell me that they're eating chicken breast and salad greens every day, but the scale has stayed frozen in one place. They'll want to know what's next—only celery and water? My answer: Add some variety and change it up before you go crazy. Change the time you eat, what you eat, and where. Keep eating healthy, but try different foods—ground flax seed or turkey sausage with your breakfast, a wheatberry salad with lunch, or some stir-fried tofu and vegetables (light on the oil!) with dinner. Or take a hard-cooked egg, mix it with some Dijon mustard, add some chopped veggies, and wrap it up! And don't eat the same three squares at the same time—eating several smaller meals throughout the day (as you'll do on this program) can help boost your metabolism because your body has to expend energy to digest the food (just be sure to keep an eye on your portion sizes).

Bottom line: Just do something different than what you are currently doing. It feels safe to always do things the same way, but change will do you good. Step outside your comfort zone and try something new. Without change, one cannot grow—so to bust through a plateau, make adjustments and add variety.

New habits are hard to form because that requires change. This program has forced you to change. You wake up every day and have a choice: How will you embrace today? What will your attitude be? You can't change the past. You can't change the fact that people will act in a certain way. We can't change the inevitable. The only thing you can do is to be in charge of yourself and surround yourself with people who give you love and support. To paraphrase the quote at the start of today's entry, life is 10 percent what happens to us and 90 percent how we react to it. You are in charge of your attitude.

WHAT OUR TEST PANELISTS TOLD US

"I put on a pair of capris today that I couldn't wear last week. Awesome! I've lost a few pounds so far, but most importantly, I have more energy. I'm eating better and I am sleeping like a rock! Life is good."
—Terrie A., 50

AS I'VE DRILLED INTO your heads, strength training is a very important part of your 2-Week Total Body Turnaround. You're working your muscles hard each and every day—especially during the strength workouts on 12 out of the plan's 14 days. So it's important to make sure you're giving your muscles all of the fuel they need to get strong, lean, and sculpted. And that means making sure you're eating an adequate amount of protein.

Protein plays a crucial role in helping muscles repair and get stronger. Most active women should be eating diets made up of at least 15 to 30 percent protein. On a 1,600-calorie diet program, that's about 60 to 120 grams of protein (1,600 calories times 15 to 30 percent, divided by 4 calories per gram). Over the course of a day, that might include a cup of milk (8 grams), a 4-ounce chicken breast (18 grams), some tuna (20 grams), some yogurt (8 grams), and about 14 almonds (3½ grams).

LEARN ABOUT: **POWER FOODS**

That doesn't mean that more protein is better: Eat too much protein and, like everything else, it will be stored as fat. And simply eating a lot of protein won't build muscle—only doing the exercises will. So be careful not to consume protein at the expensive of everything else: You still need to eat enough carbs, because ultimately carbs are used as fuel to power you through your workouts, not to mention the ups and downs of life. For a 1,600-calorie diet, about 55 to 60 percent should come from carbs, or about 220 grams (1,600 x 55 percent, then divided by 4 calories per gram).

If you've ever walked into a supplement store, you'll know that there's an awful lot of hype out there about protein powders and pills. But most of it is backed more by the bottom line than by hard science. Taking extra amino acids will not make your muscles bigger or stronger without strength training. Remember that you don't have to spend a lot of money to eat well—you'll get all of the amino acids you'll need from real food. I personally use plain whey protein in my fruit smoothies when I'm on the go or after a workout, but I use it as a supplement. My supply of protein every day comes from eggs, chicken or fish, nuts, and yogurt. These are some of my favorite foods to power up your workouts:

EGG WHITES: Eggs are a powerhouse food. They're easily digested, easy to prepare, and are packed with protein. If you want to eliminate some of the calories and fat, use just the egg whites. They're almost pure protein: There are about 3½ grams of protein and just 16 calories from the whites of just 1 egg. Scramble them up with some oregano, curry, chives, or pepper for a delicious snack! (I usually add 1 yolk to make it more like an omelet.)

CHICKEN BREAST: I love chicken! It's so mild that you can use it with so many different flavors, and it always tastes delicious! It's incredibly versatile and easy to cook, plus it's a great way to make a low-fat, protein-filled meal (just avoid using lots of butter or oil; bake, don't fry). A 4-ounce serving of chicken breast contains 30 grams of protein. I always cook up extras for snacks and salads the next few days.

TUNA: Easy and portable, tuna is a no-brainer when it comes to finding protein in a pinch! I am a major tuna eater. One 4-ounce can of tuna contains about 40 grams of protein. Plus, tuna is loaded with omega-3 fatty acids, so it's good for your muscles *and* your brain. Just be careful not to overload the mayo: You can still prepare a delicious tuna salad with just a dab of fat-free mayo, or skip it altogether and pile it onto salad greens with some balsamic vinegar. My favorite way to eat it is to mix Dijon mustard with a dash of mayo and toast it open face with a thin slice of Swiss cheese. I also have been known to mix tuna with cottage cheese and toasted almond slices. Note that because of high mercury levels, pregnant women should minimize the amount of tuna they consume.

SOYMILK: You used to only be able to find soymilk in the back of the health-food store, but now this tasty beverage is front and center at most grocery stores. I love it as a great alternative to regular milk for smoothies, but many of my clients who are lactose-intolerant pour it on everything from cereal to coffee. One cup of enriched soymilk has 7 grams of protein, not to mention more than 100 IU of vitamin D and more than 340 milligrams of calcium (amounts vary, so check the label to see what you're getting). Pick a brand that has 130 calories or fewer to keep your weight loss in line. (Many are surprisingly high in sugar. Look carefully: If it says, "vanilla-flavored," it's probably full of sugar.)

PROTEIN SHAKES: Okay, this one is a powder, but there are some advantages to adding some whey powder to your smoothies. For one, whey has been shown to increase satiety, so you'll feel fuller longer. Whey (which makes up 20 percent of the protein found in milk; casein makes up the other 80 percent) is also digested and absorbed much faster than other forms of protein. Plus, it's rich in the branched-chain amino acids (BCAA) leucine, isoleucine, and valine, which go right to the muscles to use in rebuilding tissue, rather than having to first be metabolized by the liver. (Note that casein also contains these three BCAAs.) Of course, you can also stick to good old-fashioned milk and get the same effect for a lot less money than some protein powders. When you're making a smoothie, you need to mix it with frozen fruit and milk or juice to taste sweet. Avoid the powders with lots of sugar already added!

NUTS: I toast almond slices and/or chopped walnuts and keep them in a baggie to sprinkle on everything from my cereal to my smoothie, tuna, or yogurt. Or you can have a light layer of peanut butter on whole-wheat toast for breakfast. Just be careful of portion size, because while they are loaded with protein and "good" fats, nuts also have lots of calories.

WHAT OUR TEST PANELISTS TOLD US

"I am proud to be sticking with the program and not making too many eating mistakes. I have to admit I've made a few. But, I try to make up for it by being really good the next day, and not 'giving in' again. It's hard, but worth it! I enjoy doing my workouts in the a.m. I have young twins, so it makes a difference to get it out of the way early. I can see that my waist is smaller based on how my clothes are fitting, and I feel so much healthier. I love it and really will work to continue on to lose the weight I need to lose to get to my goal weight!"
—JoAnn Q., 42

MEAL GUIDELINES:
Suggested amounts for each meal

BREAKFAST
2 grains/starchy veggies

1 dairy

1 protein

1 fruit

1 fat

A.M. SNACK
1 dairy

1 fruit

LUNCH
1 grain/starchy veggie

1 protein

2 veggies

1 fat

P.M. SNACK
1 dairy

DINNER
1 grain/starchy veggie

1 protein

2 veggies

1 fat

DAY 10 SUGGESTED MENU

BREAKFAST

Apple-Pecan Oatmeal

3 vegetarian sausage links

PER SERVING: 456 calories; 12 g total fat; 1 g sat fat; 62 g carbohydrates; 10 g fiber; 26 g protein; 5 mg cholesterol; 587 mg sodium

SNACK

½ cup fat-free cottage cheese with 2 cups diced cantaloupe

PER SERVING: 170 calories; 1 g total fat; 0 g sat fat; 27 g carbohydrates; 3 g fiber; 15 g protein; 5 mg cholesterol; 340 mg sodium

LUNCH

Salad and sandwich combo: 3 ounces of skinless chicken breast (about ½ cup pulled from a rotisserie chicken) and 2 slices of tomato served on 1 slice of toasted whole-grain bread spread with 1 tablespoon lite mayonnaise. Serve with 1 cup of mixed greens and ¼ cup each diced red bell pepper and shredded carrot, tossed with 1 tablespoon olive oil and a splash of white wine vinegar.

PER SERVING: 400 calories; 23 g total fat; 4 g sat fat; 21 g carbohydrates; 5 g fiber; 27 g protein; 63 mg cholesterol; 350 mg sodium

SNACK

Moroccan Dip with Crudités

PER ¼-CUP SERVING: 37 calories; 1 g total fat; 0.5 g sat fat; 5 g carbohydrates; 0.5 g fiber; 3 g protein; 3 mg cholesterol; 39 mg sodium

DINNER

3 ounces grilled fish of choice served with 2 cups mixed steamed veggies, 10 olives, and ½ whole grain pita

PER SERVING: 310 calories; 15 g total fat; 3 g sat fat; 17 g carbohydrates; 6 g fiber; 23 g protein; 55 mg cholesterol; 620 mg sodium

APPLE-PECAN OATMEAL WITH SAUSAGE

1 cup fat-free milk

$^1/_2$ teaspoon cinnamon

$^1/_4$ cup old-fashioned oats

1 small apple, peeled, seeded, and chopped (about 1 cup)

2 teaspoons brown sugar

$^1/_2$ teaspoon vanilla extract

1 tablespoon chopped pecans

3 vegetarian sausage links

In a small saucepan over medium heat, heat $^1/_2$ cup milk and the cinnamon until boiling. Stir in the oats and cook for 3 to 5 minutes, or until thickened. Stir in the apple, sugar, vanilla, and pecans, and cook for 1 minute longer. Remove from heat.

In a small skillet coated with nonstick cooking spray, cook the sausage until heated through, about 5 minutes. Serve with the oatmeal and the remaining $^1/_2$ cup milk.

MAKES 1 SERVING (1 CUP)

PER SERVING: 456 calories; 12 g total fat, 1 g sat fat; 62 g carbohydrates; 10 g fiber; 26 g protein; 5 mg cholesterol; 587 mg sodium

NOTE: *Look for low-sodium vegetarian sausage.*

MOROCCAN DIP

$^3/_4$ cup plain low-fat yogurt

1 cup peeled, chopped cucumber

$^1/_4$ teaspoon hot sauce (like Tabasco)

$^1/_2$ teaspoon cumin

$^1/_2$ teaspoon garlic powder

1 tablespoon chopped fresh mint

Combine the ingredients and serve with 1 cup sliced veggies, such as carrots, red bell pepper, and cucumber.

MAKES 4 SERVINGS (1 CUP)

PER $^1/_4$-CUP SERVING: 37 calories; 1 g total fat; 0.5 g sat fat; 5 g carbohydrates; 0.5 g fiber; 3 g protein; 3 mg cholesterol; 39 mg sodium

REAL 2-WEEK TURNAROUND SUCCESS STORY

Nancy Haley

AGE:
51

HEIGHT:
5'2¹/₄"

START WEIGHT:
125.4
pounds

AFTER 2 WEEKS:
118.4
pounds

RESULTS:
7 pounds,
7³/₄ inches
lost

(including 2 inches
from waist and
2 inches from hips)

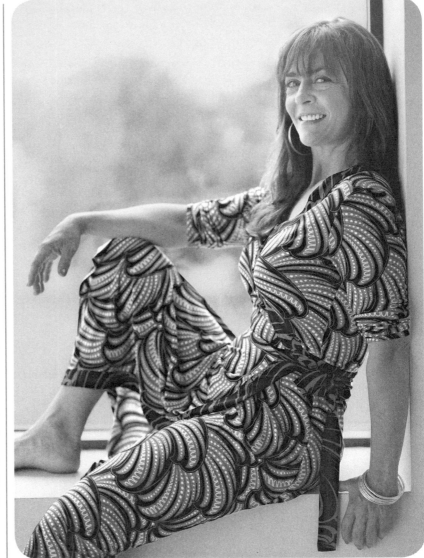

Minnesota winters can be long, cold, and dark, and it's easy to stay holed up inside as much as possible. Factor in working from home—in an office set up just inside the kitchen—and it's not hard to see how Nancy, a marketing consultant, was able to put on more than a dozen pounds by the time spring rolled around. "I spent all winter in my sweats, and my only regular exercise was dashing out to walk my dog," she says. "I was snacking all the time, and I just couldn't get into the flow of a regular workout routine."

Still, as a former aerobics instructor, she says she was surprised to discover that her jeans weren't fitting her anymore. "I never had a weight issue before. But since I hit my fifties, I guess the way I'd always eaten wasn't working for me anymore. I really needed a motivational jumpstart!"

The day before she started her plan, Nancy went to the grocery store and bought almost everything she would need for the next 14 days. "I went online to *Prevention*'s My Health Tracker at prevention.com and planned out what I was going to eat. This way I had everything in the house. Those were my only choices, instead of it being a free-for-all foodfest whenever I wanted."

The first couple of days on her Turnaround were challenging. "I was so used to munching all of the time, and I missed that constant hand-to-mouth feeling," she says. "And I was feeling sore from the weight sessions." By Day 4, though, something clicked. "I'd never really eaten breakfast before, so I made a smoothie in the morning that would carry me for a few hours." Other key treats to keep her satisfied included drinking diet green tea, or water with mint, ginger, and cucumber, as well as munching on vegetables with salsa or a small amount of nuts and raisins.

She also began to feel stronger, both inside and out. "The strength training made a difference for me both physically and emotionally. Seeing my biceps again just made me feel more powerful. That kept me going and gave me even more incentive to eat well." Her dog-walking sessions turned into interval training with multiple speed bursts. By the second week, she noticed a significant improvement in her energy levels and less pain in her back, and her clothes started to fit better. By the time the 2 weeks were up, she'd dropped 7 pounds and more than 7 inches, including 2 inches off her waist.

Nancy has kept her healthy eating habits and regular exercise routine up since then, going so far as to store her weights at a place in the kitchen where she can see them for motivation. "I figure that's where you eat, so it's a good reminder." By the time the Fourth of July came around, Nancy proudly traded her sweats for a pair of white skinny jeans. "I don't even own a scale, so the idea that I could zip these up with ease made me feel like I had really reached my goals!"

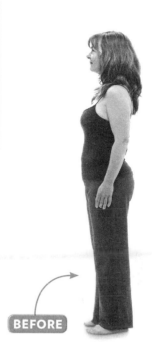

BEFORE

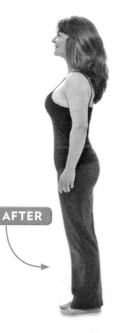

AFTER

DAY 11

Today is your final "active rest" day. Take advantage of this time to regroup and recover, but remember to stress the "active" part over the "rest." This isn't a day off as much as it is a day of activity, albeit less formal activity than you've been doing the rest of the week. It's all about trying to work bursts of activity into your day. Walk to work or get off a stop early on the bus, walk fast while doing errands, stand up when you answer the phone, get up to change the channels instead of using the remote, play with your kids, dance to the radio when you are making dinner. And remember to think "NEAT." Just moving around a little bit can add up to big changes.

One way to get inspired to move around even more is to clip on a pedometer. These handy little devices have been shown to help increase the amount of steps you take over the course of a day. A recent review of several studies on pedometers and walking found walkers lost on average of 1 pound every 10 weeks, or 5 pounds over a year, but

"Nothing great was ever achieved without enthusiasm." —*Ralph Waldo Emerson, American poet*

that's without doing any other formal exercise or dieting.[20] Another review of studies found pedometer wearers increased the number of steps they took each day by more than 2,000 steps (about 1 mile).[21] When you consider that walking 1 mile burns about 75 calories, that's an extra 500-plus calories you're burning each week, outside your regular workouts. Aim to take about 10,000 steps a day, or roughly 5 miles.

You might already come close to that goal, depending on your job. A recent study by the American Council on Exercise (ACE) looked at 10 different occupations, from secretarial work to restaurant servers. Researchers found that mail carriers take the most steps—almost 19,000—while secretaries take the fewest—about 4,300. (FYI, teachers took 4,700, lawyers about 5,000, police officers 5,300, nurses 8,600, construction workers 9,600, factory workers 9,900, restaurant servers 10,000, and custodians almost 13,000.)[22] Moral of the story? If you work in an office environment, move around as much as possible! Walk instead of sending an e-mail to a colleague; go to the restroom on a different floor; take a water walking break and walk to the farther water cooler in your office. Using a pedometer can help you see how much all these extra steps can add up!

Several years ago I gave my kids each a pedometer in their Christmas stockings. My two boys immediately turned it into a contest for the first few days (that's what brothers do), and my little one got so into it, he kept going in the basement to add another 500 steps on the treadmill. ("Mom, don't tell Nick–I'm gonna go do 500 steps.") Of course the novelty wore off on my then-9-year-old, but it proved my point that data and feedback are motivating!

One other quick note about work and activity: As much as possible (or as much as is permitted) wear comfortable clothes. Another study from ACE found that when men and women were allowed to wear "casual" clothes to the office (jeans and comfortable shoes), they had an 8 percent increase in activity levels and burned an extra 25 calories a day.[23] Do that for 50 weeks and it equals 125 calories a week, or 6,250 calories a year— almost 2 pounds! That goes for shoes, too. I always wear comfortable shoes at the airports and breeze right by the high-heel gals painstakingly making it to their gates!

TIP: Remember, if you missed a workout day earlier this week or think you'll miss one over the next 3 days, switch your "rest" day around. Every active day counts when it comes to helping you stay on track and reach your goals!

WHAT OUR TEST PANELISTS TOLD US

"I had a huge 'a-ha' moment last night. When I finished my workout, I turned to the next page and saw it was an 'active rest day.' Instead of feeling what I thought I would (RELIEF, which I did feel in Week 1!), I felt strangely bummed out. This morning as I was planning my day, part of me said, 'Oh good, I don't have to fit in a workout to an already overloaded day,' but another part was trying to figure out when I could at least do a strength-training set or 30 minutes on the bike. For someone who has always HATED exercise, this is an incredible shift. I have chronic pain and fibromyalgia, so the energy boost I've gotten these last 10 days has been amazing."
—Stephanie T., 42

DAY 11 TURNAROUND TIP
Make Every Moment Count

You've been spending a lot of time over the past 11 days working out on a daily basis, and some of you might be thinking that, while you could do this for 2 weeks, there's no way you could keep it up for too much longer. I know it might be hard to find the time to carve out a full hour every day, but if you even keep it up with half that time, you will continue to see results. Don't think you can squeeze it in? Try this exercise:

List the top 10 ways you currently spend your time (#1 being the most important thing you do each day). Now list the top 10 ways you waste time each day: Include things like waiting in store lines, holding on the phone, sitting in traffic, waiting for clients, watching TV, reading the junk mail, etc. Beside each entry, state how much time gets spent, and add up an average daily total. List #1 tells you how you spend your day. List #2 tells you how you waste your time each day.

Take a look at your life and find ways to be active instead of just "wasting time." Get on the treadmill while paging through your latest fashion magazine. Do exercises on the ball while watching TV. If family time is on your list of how you spend time each day, get active together. After work, exercise with your family, whether at home, at the gym, or outdoors.

The truth is, time management is a job, and you have to take ownership of your health. It's all a matter of getting motivated. If you can find the time to deposit your paychecks, fill your gas tank, wait in the fast-food drive-thru, etc., you can find more time to be active. Planning your time more wisely can free up time in other parts of the day. For example, eat at your desk and pay bills or make a grocery list. While waiting in a doctor's office or in the airport, take care of paperwork. You can actually save enough time each day so you will have time to exercise or do something active and fun!

It boils down to "How much do you care?" I hear it every day: "I'm just too busy to exercise." Make your health your priority and get rid of the little time-wasting things that bog your days down. Getting into better shape doesn't happen by accident. It's up to you! Take a look at your lifestyle—are you "active" or just "busy" doing things that don't matter?

If you're not going to do this now, then what are you going to do to take control of your health? There's an Arabian proverb I love: "He who has health has hope; and he who has hope, has everything." Make the time to treat your body right, and your rewards will be immeasurable.

IF YOU'RE LIKE MOST people, there's a pretty good chance you've had some caffeine today. In fact, the average American adult consumes about 3 milligrams per kilogram of body weight (for a 150-pound person, that's about 204 milligrams of caffeine, or 1½ cups of coffee). And caffeine is in more than just your daily morning drip: You'll find it in tea, chocolate, colas—even certain yogurts, ice cream, and orange soda!

Caffeine has no nutritional value, but it's safe to say that it's the world's most consumed drug—one that is both a disease-fighter and an ergogenic aid (science-speak for helping to improve sports performance). A half-dozen studies show people who drink coffee regularly are 80 percent less likely to develop Parkinson's.[24] A recent study from Harvard, which examined 126,000 people for up to 18 years, found having 1 to 3 cups of caffeinated coffee a day significantly reduced diabetes risk.[25] And other research has shown that having at least 2 cups a day will reduce the risk of colon cancer by 25 percent.[26]

LEARN ABOUT: CAFFEINE

Athletes have long known that caffeine also improves performance by stimulating the brain and nervous system to ignore fatigue or recruit extra motor units. Numerous studies have shown that caffeine reduces your level of perceived exertion and blunts pain perception, enabling you to push through your discomfort. It also helps dilate blood vessels and improve lung function, so more oxygen can get to your working muscles. And it's been shown to boost several types of activities, from sprints to endurance runs to strength training.[27]

Of course, as with anything that sounds too good, there's always a catch: Consume too much caffeine and you're left with the jitters—a churning stomach, rapid heartbeat, and trembling hands. Plus, the more you get used to it, the more you need to consume in order to feel the effect. And as anyone who's ever tried to give up their morning mocha knows, there is a withdrawal period as with any drug, usually in the form of pounding headaches, sometimes accompanied by nausea.

Here's my take on coffee or other caffeine-containing beverages: If you like it, sip away. I usually treat myself to a small skim latte a few times a week as a reward after my morning workout. There's no harm—and apparently a lot to gain—by having a moderate caffeine intake. But if coffee is your engine of choice, remember that calories can quickly add up, especially when you're stopping at the local coffee house. A grande latte can have about 220 calories at a major chain; an iced flavored vanilla drink with whipped cream has a whopping 430. Go with fat-free milk and skip the whip; you'll save 90 calories on the latte and 240 calories on the iced drink!

MEAL GUIDELINES:
Suggested amounts for each meal

BREAKFAST
2 grains/starchy veggies

1 dairy

1 protein

1 fruit

1 fat

A.M. SNACK
1 dairy

1 fruit

LUNCH
1 grain/starchy veggie

1 protein

2 veggies

1 fat

P.M. SNACK
1 dairy

DINNER
1 grain/starchy veggie

1 protein

2 veggies

1 fat

DAY 11 SUGGESTED MENU

BREAKFAST

Breakfast sandwich: Toast 2 slices of multigrain bread and fill with 3 ounces Canadian bacon and $1/5$ of a medium avocado. Serve with 1 cup of nonfat or low-fat yogurt mixed with 1 cup of sliced strawberries.

PER SERVING: 490 calories; 11 g total fat; 3 g sat fat; 81 g carbohydrates; 7 g fiber; 22 g protein; 24 mg cholesterol; 760 mg sodium

NOTE: *This meal is a little high in sodium (you want to aim for no more than 600 to 650 mg per meal), which you should normally avoid, but you'll be sweating a lot throughout the 2-Week Total Body Turnaround, so you can get away with it today.*

SNACK

1 part-skim string cheese with 1 cup grapes

PER SERVING: 200 calories; 6 g total fat; 4 g sat fat; 30 g carbohydrates; 1 g fiber; 8 g protein; 15 mg cholesterol; 150 mg sodium

LUNCH

Simple Salad "Niçoise"

PER SERVING: 349 calories; 11 g total fat; 1 g sat fat; 32 g carbohydrates; 6 g fiber; 28 g protein; 53 mg cholesterol; 565 mg sodium

SNACK

1 cup skim milk

PER SERVING: 80 calories; 0 g total fat; 0 g sat fat; 12 g carbohydrates; 0 g fiber; 8 g protein; 0 mg cholesterol; 100 mg sodium

DINNER

Tomato Chicken Thighs with Zucchini and Lentils

PER SERVING: 360 calories; 17 g total fat; 3 g sat fat; 29 g carbohydrates; 11 g fiber; 24 g protein; 55 mg cholesterol; 375 mg sodium

SIMPLE SALAD "NIÇOISE"

$\frac{1}{2}$ cup cooked whole grain pasta

3 ounces chunk light tuna, packed in water, drained

$\frac{1}{2}$ cup chopped tomatoes

$\frac{1}{2}$ cup green beans, steamed and cut into 1" lengths

1 tablespoon chopped Kalamata or niçoise olives

1 clove garlic, chopped

1 tablespoon balsamic vinegar

2 teaspoons olive oil

Pinch of salt and pepper

In a small bowl, combine the pasta with the tuna, tomatoes, green beans, olives, and garlic. Toss with balsamic vinegar, olive oil, and salt and pepper.

MAKES 1 SERVING (2 CUPS)

PER SERVING: 349 calories; 11 g total fat; 1 g sat fat; 32 g carbohydrates; 6 g fiber; 28 g protein; 53 mg cholesterol; 565 mg sodium

NOTE: *If you're a vegetarian, don't worry! Simply substitute $\frac{3}{4}$ cup chickpeas or other white beans for the tuna.*

TOMATO CHICKEN THIGHS WITH ZUCCHINI AND LENTILS

$\frac{1}{8}$ cup dry green or brown lentils

1 bay leaf

1 tablespoon chopped garlic, divided

$\frac{1}{8}$ teaspoon salt

$\frac{1}{8}$ teaspoon black pepper

1 tablespoon olive oil

1 cup chopped tomatoes

1 cup sliced zucchini

1 skinless, boneless chicken thigh (3–3.5 ounces), sliced

1 tablespoon chopped fresh basil

In a medium saucepan, combine the lentils, bay leaf, and 1 teaspoon of the garlic. Cover the lentils with 1 to 2 inches of water, and bring to a boil. Reduce the heat, cover, and simmer for 25 minutes, or until the lentils are tender, draining any liquid if necessary. Discard the bay leaf; stir in the salt and pepper. Meanwhile, heat the oil in a medium skillet over medium-high heat. Add the remaining garlic and cook, stirring frequently, for 30 seconds. Add the tomatoes and zucchini, and cook for about 2 to 3 minutes, or until barely tender. Add the chicken slices and continue cooking with the vegetables for another 5 minutes. Cover, and reduce heat to a simmer for 5 to 10 minutes more, or until the chicken is cooked through. Spoon the chicken and vegetables over the lentils to serve. Sprinkle with the basil.

MAKES 1 SERVING (1$\frac{1}{4}$ CUPS)

PER SERVING: 360 calories; 17 g total fat; 3 g sat fat; 29 g carbohydrates; 11 g fiber; 24 g protein; 55 mg cholesterol; 375 mg sodium

DAY 12

Keep up the good work! You've come so far, you can't give up now. You owe it to yourself. You can follow this program the full 14 days, and hopefully this will propel you to the next 14 days and beyond!

I always revert back to the best advice-givers we all know: our mothers.

You remember what your mother told you, right? Snack on fresh fruit. No dessert until you finish your vegetables. One scoop of ice cream, not the whole pint. Two cookies, not the whole bag. Get a good night's sleep, it will be better in the morning. Even 40-plus years ago, my mom was onto the basic advice. You see, it's not rocket science—it's common sense. Moderation is the key to a healthy lifestyle. I am definitely a high-energy gal, so whenever I start to go off the chart, either up or down, I have trained myself to step back, take a deep breath, and listen to mom!

I know you can do this. I am your biggest fan, and I have seen so many success stories in my past 20 years. I know there is room for you!

> "If you don't know where you are going, you'll end up someplace else."
> —*Yogi Berra, baseball legend*

CARDIO: Pyramid

Pay attention to your form as you do this workout. Stand tall with your head up, chin level. Look a few feet in front of you. Lift your chest and relax your shoulders. The better your posture, the more oxygen you can take into your lungs—so the more efficient your workout will be. Bend your elbows slightly, swinging them from front to back as you walk. If you think about the center of your body being the midline, try not to let your elbows go across your belly button, and don't swing them higher than chest level. Keep your abs tight. When you walk, push off with the balls of your feet, landing on your heels. Then roll through the toe to push off. Try not to take extra-long steps—your natural stride length will keep you walking fastest.

INTENSITY	TIME	RPE	TALK TEST
Warm up (heart rate: Zone 2)	3 min.	4–5	You can speak in full sentences (slightly breathless)
Increase pace (heart rate: Zone 3)	2 min.	6–7	You can speak mostly in short phrases (breathless)
Slow down (heart rate: Zone 2–3)	2 min.	5–6	Somewhat breathless (brisk walk)
Speed up, pump arms (heart rate: Zone 4)	4 min.	8–9	Very breathless
Slow down (heart rate: Zone 2–3)	4 min.	5–6	Somewhat breathless (brisk walk)
Speed up, pump arms (heart rate: Zone 4)	5 min.	8–9	Very breathless
Slow down (heart rate: Zone 2–3)	2 min.	5–6	Somewhat breathless (brisk walk)
Speed up, pump arms (heart rate: Zone 4)	4 min.	8–9	Very breathless
Slow down (heart rate: Zone 2)	4 min.	5	Somewhat breathless (brisk walk; gradually moving into cooldown)

STRENGTH: Upper Body + Core

Today is our final upper-body focus! Remember that adding balance challenges to upper-body moves will work your abs and butt at the same time that you're sculpting your arms, chest, shoulders, and back! Try to hold the balance by looking at a stationary spot a few feet ahead of you. The great thing about improving your balance is the more you do it, the easier it gets!

BALANCING SINGLE-LEG FLY AWAY
(WIDE AND HIGH)

TARGETS: Back, shoulders

A. Stand with right foot in front of left, leaning forward slightly but keeping spine long and abs tight. Hold dumbbells next to right leg, elbows slightly bent and palms facing each other. **Raise left leg behind you, balancing on right leg.** Keep abs tight to help you maintain balance.

B. Lift arms up and back, keeping elbows bent and squeezing shoulder blades together for 2 counts **as you continue to balance on right leg.** Lower back to start position for 4 counts. Repeat 6 times and switch legs, **balancing on left leg for the final 6 reps.**

GOOD FORM TIP: *Pull the weights back and squeeze your shoulder blades together; focus on using your back, not your neck. Press your shoulders away from your ears. Focus on one point to help maintain balance.*

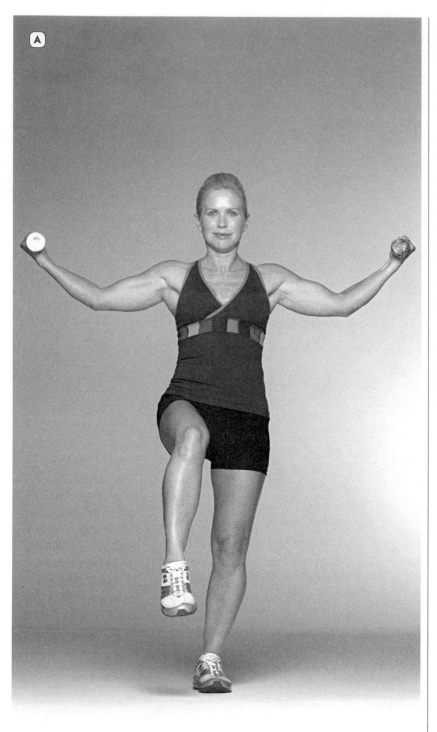

BALANCING SUSPENDED BICEPS CURL

TARGETS: biceps

A. Stand with arms extended out to sides at shoulder height, holding dumbbells with arms extended, palms facing up, elbows slightly bent. **Lift right foot, balancing on left leg.** Curl weights toward shoulders in 2 counts.

B. Reverse the move in 4 counts, lowering arms out to sides. Do 6 reps, **then switch legs** and repeat for 6 more reps.

B

GOOD FORM TIP:
Keep the elbows parallel to the floor. If your elbows do start to fall toward the floor, use a lighter weight. Focus on one point to help maintain balance.

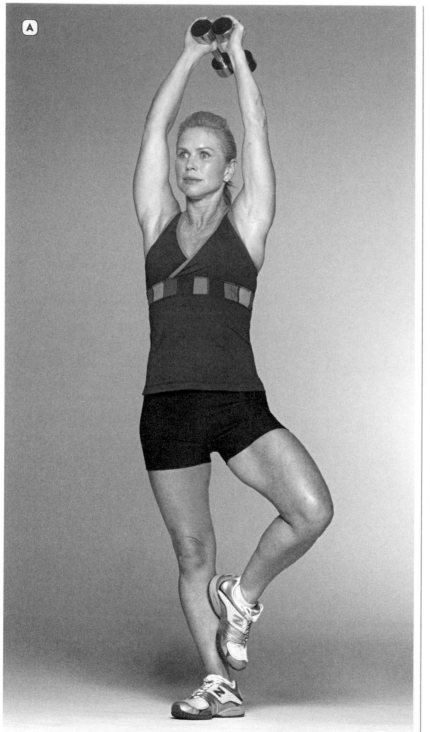

A

TRICEPS TONER WITH TREE POSE

TARGETS: Triceps, core

A. Stand with feet hip-distance apart, arms extended over head, holding one or two dumbbells with both hands. **Bring bottom of left foot to inside of right calf, knee pointing to left side, balancing on right leg.**

B. Slowly bend elbows and lower weight behind head for 4 counts. Lift weight back above head for 2 counts, squeezing triceps and keeping arms next to ears while balancing on right leg. Repeat 6 times; switch legs and repeat for 6 more reps.

GOOD FORM TIP:
Keep your elbows close to your ears; focus on using the back of your arms. Gaze at one point to help maintain balance.

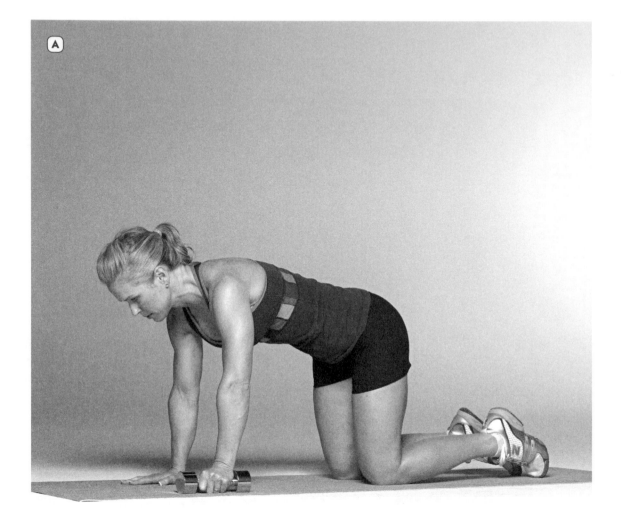

BIRD DOG SHOULDER SHAPER

TARGETS: Shoulders

A. Starting on all fours in kneeling position, hold dumbbell in left hand.

B. Keeping abdominals tight and a slight bend in the left elbow, reach dumbbell out to left side slowly for 2 counts. **At the same time, lift right leg straight behind you.** Lower arm and leg back to start position for 4 counts. Repeat 8 to 12 times, then switch sides and repeat.

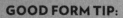

B

GOOD FORM TIP:
Focus on working the top back area of your shoulders as you lift your arm out to the side. Keep your abs tight to help maintain balance.

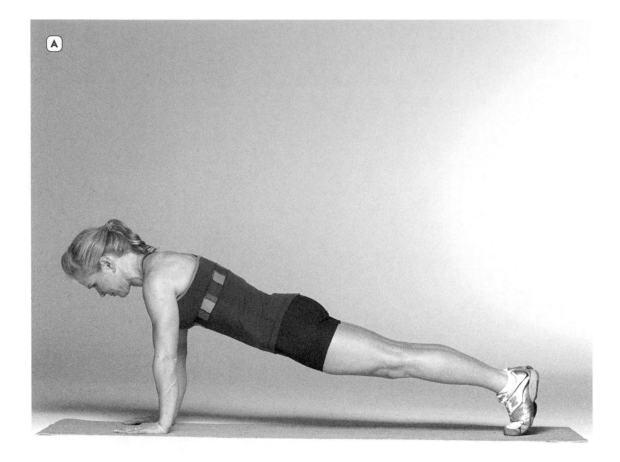

AIRPLANE FULL PUSHUP

TARGETS: Chest, triceps, shoulders, back, abs

A. Start in full pushup position, toes on floor and hands shoulder-distance apart.

B. Bend elbows 90 degrees, lowering chest toward floor in 4 counts; keep abs tight and body in a straight line.

C. Push back up to start position in 2 counts, reaching left arm forward and right leg backward. Balance here for a moment, then repeat, lifting right arm and left leg. Do 6 to 8 repetitions on each side.

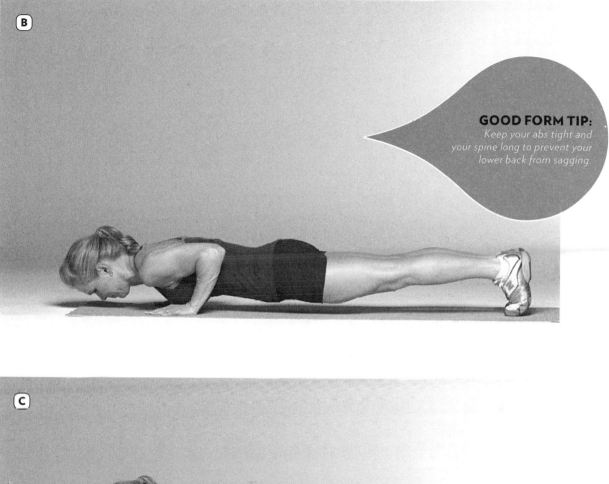

GOOD FORM TIP:
Keep your abs tight and your spine long to prevent your lower back from sagging.

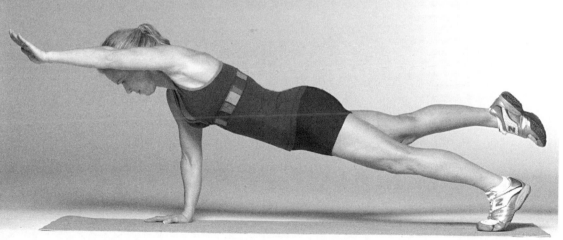

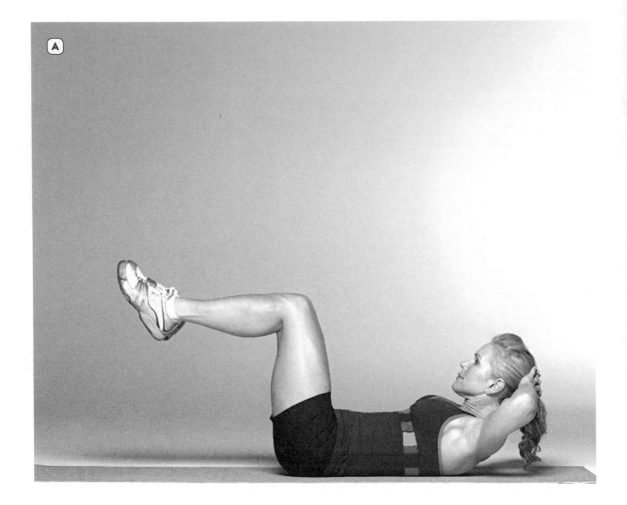

TABLE-TOP CRUNCH WITH REACH

TARGETS: Abs

A. Lie face up on floor with knees bent 90 degrees, feet lifted with shins parallel to floor, and fingers behind head. Curl your upper body up off the floor in 2 counts, using abdominal muscles.

B. Slowly lower upper body back toward floor in 4 counts, straightening left leg toward floor on the 4th count. Bend knee back to start and repeat, this time lowering right leg. Repeat 8 to 10 times per side.

GOOD FORM TIP:
Slightly press your lower back into the mat and think about "sewing" your belly button into your low back.

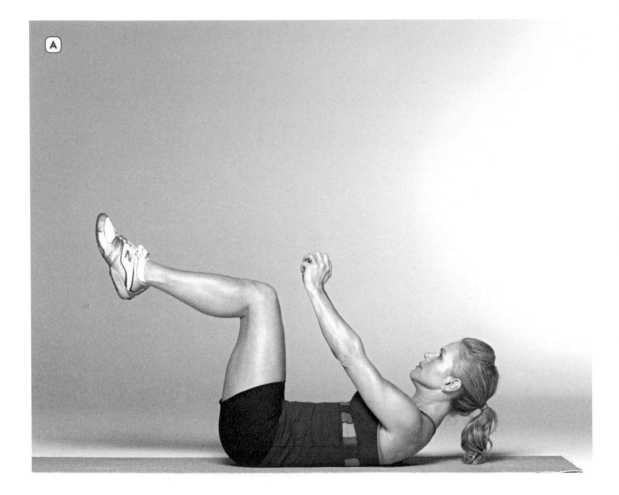

NEW EXERCISE! **CORE CHALLENGE**

DUMBBELL V-OPEN

TARGETS: Abs

A. Lie face up on floor, knees bent 90 degrees above hips. Hold one dumbbell horizontally with both hands, reaching toward legs.

B. Extend arms behind head and straighten legs in 4 counts, until body forms a V-shape. Exhale and lift arms and legs back to start position for 2 counts. Repeat 8 to 10 times.

B

GOOD FORM TIP:
Slightly press your lower back into the mat and "sew" your belly button in toward your low back. If you feel some strain in your neck, put your head on the mat.

DAY 12 TURNAROUND TIP
Work Your Willpower

How strong is your willpower? Do you bypass the doughnuts at a morning meeting? Skip the whip on your latte? Resist the urge to order fries with your sandwich at lunch? You may find that the later you get into your day, the less willpower you have, so that by the time you get home, that hunk of Cheddar in the fridge or the fudge ripple in your freezer can look mighty tempting. Now science is showing that you're not actually being weak when your willpower seems to fail you—you're actually victim to your body's biochemistry.

According to Dr. Roy Baumeister, a researcher at Florida State University who has studied willpower for the past 15 years, willpower isn't a skill or a virtue—it's more like a muscle. Willpower can be strengthened, but it can also be exhausted.

The groundbreaking idea here is that as humans, we have a limited amount of willpower, so if you exert your willpower on one task, whether it's passing on the potato chips or avoiding the urge to buy that cute pair of pumps, you may fail when it comes to exerting willpower on another task. A recent article in the *New York Times* speculated that low consumer confidence levels could actually cause us to gain weight, because we are using up our willpower on financial issues. Exerting willpower in one area, said the article, can lead to backsliding in others.

Researchers have found that there is a biological response to willpower: One study that asked subjects to test their willpower by eating carrots and resisting cookies found the most successful participants showed a temporary increase in heart-rate variability (the beat-to-beat fluctuations of the heart).[28] That's important because heart-rate variability ties into the body's "fight-or-flight" response, as well as the relaxation response, which means that willpower triggers a nervous system response necessary to survival.

But the act of exerting willpower can literally make you fatigued. Another study found subjects who practiced "mental self-control" actually decreased muscular endurance. This also ties into blood sugar levels. Our muscles use glucose for fuel; our brains need it for most tasks. And according to researchers, willpower engages many areas of the brain, and therefore requires high levels of fuel. One study found participants experienced a drop in blood sugar levels immediately after trying to exert self-control. Half the group was then given some lemonade, the other half a sugarless lemonade. When asked to repeat the experiment in exercising self-control, the lemonade drinkers (whose blood sugar levels were replenished) performed equally well in both exercises, while those who had the diet drink had more difficulty the second time around.[29]

Which makes sense: If you skip breakfast, your willpower is impaired, so you're more likely to go for the chocolate croissant. By choosing foods that help to keep blood sugar levels stable, like complex carbs and protein, you can strengthen your willpower for longer periods. That's why I'm always harping on the importance of eating a healthy breakfast to keep your blood sugar stable, as well as eating consistent smaller meals throughout the day. Binge eating at night is a perfect example of what happens to our willpower when our blood sugar levels get too low. We all know the scenario: You've been eating very little all day or skipped meals, and by bedtime you're starving and can't resist the urge to start eating high-fat, high-sugar foods to boost that low blood sugar.

And willpower doesn't have to just revolve around eating fattening foods. Each act of self-control that you exert during the day can add up: Refrain from surfing the Web at work or resist the urge to buy those shoes and you might not want to go to the gym at night. So set priorities: You can only control so much in your life. Don't try to change everything. It's too much stress. Go for progress, not perfection. And allow yourself a little treat now and then—a manicure, a massage, a few more minutes searching online. Giving yourself some breaks from willpower can help you resist temptation down the road.

There are also other things you can do to boost your willpower. With practice, our capacity for willpower can be increased! For one, get enough sleep. Research shows sleep can restore depleted willpower and help you maintain healthy habits. Then take baby steps. Researchers who have tried "willpower training regimens" asked people to control one thing they aren't used to controlling, and do it every day. Just like exercise, the first steps are the hardest. Work your willpower like a muscle. It can feel difficult at first, but after a while you'll find it easier to exert self-control. Make healthy choices in advance, like planning your dinner before you come home hungry or arranging to meet a friend for a walk. By figuring out in advance what obstacles you might have to overcome, you won't have to think about your response: You'll just switch into your strategy. With practice, your ability for willpower can grow! I am sure that you have had to practice willpower in the last 12 days, but hopefully this practice has made you stronger, not just physically, but also mentally. You'll have more willpower to resist life's temptations, and to keep going on the journey to better health.

> ## WHAT OUR TEST PANELISTS TOLD US
>
> "I was talking to a friend about diet and exercise. She's taken the route of 'I'm going to lose 5 pounds, then I'll go on to the next 5, and so on. I've decided that's how I'm going to look at this journey, only instead of 5 pounds, I'm going to approach it 2 weeks at a time."
> —**Barb R., 52**

I'VE BEEN STRESSING THE importance of "clean" eating for the past 12 days. I know you've been working hard, and giving your body the right fuel can help keep it running at its best. But it's also important to eat the right foods *after* a workout. In fact, research has shown that what—and when—you eat can play a big part in helping to reduce injury, improve recovery, and keep you going strong.

Some experts maintain that there is a "glycogen window"—basically a short period (lasting anywhere from 30 minutes to 2 hours) immediately after an intense workout when your muscles are especially responsive to refueling. It's also when you have your best chance at replenishing the glycogen stores that were depleted during a workout.

LEARN ABOUT: **RESTORATIVE FOODS**

And having both protein and carbs together can speed recovery. One study found glycogen levels were 27 percent higher when testers consumed a protein/carb combo (about 75 percent carbs, 25 percent protein) rather than just a high-carb snack.[30] Protein can also play an important role here because your body needs to start repairing the muscle tissue that's been broken down during exercise. Remember, it's this rebuilding process that actually makes you stronger. You don't need expensive (and often highly caloric!) energy bars, protein shakes laced with ice cream, and syrupy fruit. Instead, keep your snack at about 200 calories, and go for healthy protein/carb combos like a yogurt and berries, a half of a turkey sandwich on whole-wheat bread, or some low-fat string cheese and an apple.

Oxidation is a normal process that occurs in your body, but it's a potentially dangerous one: A small percentage of cells can become damaged during oxidation, and become free radicals. These radicals roam your system, harming other cells and potentially causing disease such as heart disease and cancer. When you're exercising aerobically, your body also produces a small number of free radicals. Although recent research shows that this only takes place with extreme levels of exercise, such as running a marathon, it still makes sense to include a diet rich in antioxidants, like fruits and vegetables, to help offset whatever free radical damage might be taking place. Antioxidants help to prevent and repair the stress that comes from oxidation.

Following are a few of my favorite restorative foods:

● **Berries:** Strawberries, blueberries, raspberries, blackberries—all berry good sources of antioxidants! One cup of berries provides all of the anti- oxidants you need in a single day, offering up the most antioxidant bang for the buck. Just 1 cup of wild blueberries has 13,427 total antioxidants, from vitamins A and C to flavonoids like quercetin and anthocyanidin. Berries are a great treat—mix them with some low-fat yogurt for breakfast, add them to a smoothie as a snack, or have a bowl of mixed berries for dessert.

● **Apples:** They're a favorite snack among schoolkids everywhere for good reason. Apples are delicious, tart, crisp, and satisfying. They're also vitamin- and antioxidant-packed. Red Delicious has the highest antioxidant levels— with more than 5,900 a serving—Granny Smith has 5,381, and Gala, 3,903. These varieties are usually available year-round. And don't peel: Most of the antioxidants (as well as the fiber!) are found in the apple skin. I eat an apple almost every day of the year and have one in my bag at all times.

● **Salmon (or herring or mackerel):** These deep-water fish are great sources of omega-3 fatty acids, as well as being high in monounsaturated fats. Omega-3s work to decrease inflammation in the body, suppressing enzymes that erode cartilage. Some researchers speculate that omega-3s might improve performance by increasing bloodflow to the muscles and might reduce muscle inflammation following a strenuous workout. I buy salmon in the foil water packs like you would buy tuna. It's great for quick lunches. Not a fan of fish? Try walnuts, flaxseeds, or eggs that have been fortified with omega-3s.

● **Green tea:** A ton of articles have been written about the benefits of green tea as it relates to lowering cholesterol, inhibiting cancer, and even aid- ing in weight loss. Now add exercise recovery to its credits. A small study out of Brazil found that green tea may counter the effects of resistance exercise by reducing the amount of oxidative stress. They found subjects who drank green tea had a 37 percent increase in levels of a protein called glutathione, which helps protect the body from free radical damage.[31] My favorite smoothie is mango and green tea.

● **Broccoli:** These florets pack a big punch and are a great superfood. Part of the cruciferous family of vegetables (along with cauliflower, cabbage, Brussels sprouts, bok choy, and kale), it contains a phytochemical called sul- foraphane that may block an enzyme that triggers inflammation and joint pain. It doesn't hurt that broccoli is considered a key cancer fighter, linked to the reduction of breast, lung, colon, liver, and cervical cancers in laboratory studies. And the veggie might also help combat heart disease, ulcers, and even the eye disease macular degeneration.

MEAL GUIDELINES:

Suggested amounts for each meal

BREAKFAST

2 grains/starchy veggies

1 dairy

1 protein

1 fruit

1 fat

A.M. SNACK

1 dairy

1 fruit

LUNCH

1 grain/starchy veggie

1 protein

2 veggies

1 fat

P.M. SNACK

1 dairy

DINNER

1 grain/starchy veggie

1 protein

2 veggies

1 fat

DAY 12 SUGGESTED MENU

BREAKFAST

1 whole-wheat English muffin spread with 1 tablespoon peanut butter. Serve with 3 ounces Canadian bacon, 1 apple, and 1 cup skim milk.

PER SERVING: 430 calories; 12 g total fat; 3 g sat fat; 61 g carbohydrates; 9 g fiber; 23 g protein; 19 mg cholesterol; 690 mg sodium

NOTE: *This meal is a little high in sodium (you want to aim for no more than 600 to 650 mg per meal), which you should normally avoid, but you'll be sweating a lot throughout the 2-Week Total Body Turnaround, so you can get away with it today.*

SNACK

1 cup vanilla soymilk with 1 peach

PER SERVING: 140 calories; 3 g total fat; 1 g sat fat; 20 g carbohydrates; 1 g fiber; 7 g protein; 0 mg cholesterol; 170 mg sodium

LUNCH

Open-Faced Mushroom-Onion Veggie Burger

PER SERVING: 310 calories; 16 g total fat; 2 g sat fat; 28 g carbohydrates; 8 g fiber; 17 g protein; 3 mg cholesterol; 567 mg sodium

SNACK

$^{1}/_{2}$ cup nonfat cottage cheese

PER SERVING: 60 calories; 0 g total fat; 0 g sat fat; 1 g carbohydrates; 0 g fiber; 12 g protein; 5 mg cholesterol; 290 mg sodium

DINNER

Seared Chicken Fajita Salad

PER SERVING: 360 calories; 14 g total fat; 2 g sat fat; 30 g carbohydrates; 12 g fiber; 30 g protein; 49 mg cholesterol; 464 mg sodium

OPEN-FACED MUSHROOM-ONION VEGGIE BURGER

1 teaspoon olive oil

¼ cup sliced sweet onion

¼ cup sliced red bell pepper

¼ cup sliced baby portobellos

1 tablespoon balsamic vinegar

1 veggie burger patty (I used Boca Original to analyze)

½ crusty whole-wheat roll or whole-wheat English muffin, toasted

1½ teaspoons mayonnaise

½ teaspoon spicy mustard

¼ cup mixed greens

Heat 1 teaspoon of the olive oil in a medium skillet over medium heat. Add the onion, pepper, and mushrooms and cook, stirring frequently, for about 5 to 7 minutes, or until tender. Remove from the pan, drizzle with the balsamic vinegar, and set aside. Add the veggie burger to the same pan and cook, turning once, for about 8 to 10 minutes, or until heated through. Spread the roll or muffin with the mayonnaise and mustard. Top with the veggie burger, mixed greens, and vegetable mixture.

MAKES 1 SERVING

PER SERVING: 310 calories; 16 g total fat; 2 g sat fat; 28 g carbohydrates; 8 g fiber; 17 g protein; 3 mg cholesterol; 567 mg sodium

SEARED CHICKEN FAJITA SALAD

1 skinless, boneless chicken breast (3 ounces)

½ cup canned no-salt-added black beans, rinsed and drained

¼ cup diced avocado

2 tablespoons minced red onion

1 teaspoon chopped fresh cilantro

2 cups mixed greens

1 tablespoon lime juice

1 clove garlic, chopped

¼ teaspoon cumin

1½ tablespoons red wine vinaigrette dressing

Heat a skillet coated with nonstick cooking spray over medium-high heat. Add the chicken breast and cook, turning once, for about 3 to 5 minutes per side, or until cooked through. Remove from the pan and set on a cutting board. Meanwhile, in a medium bowl, combine the beans, avocado, onion, cilantro, and mixed greens; toss to combine. In a small bowl, whisk the lime juice, garlic, cumin, and vinaigrette dressing. Slice the chicken into thin slices. Toss the salad with the dressing and top with the chicken.

MAKES 1 SERVING

PER SERVING: 360 calories; 14 g total fat; 2 g sat fat; 30 g carbohydrates; 12 g fiber; 30 g protein; 49 mg cholesterol; 464 mg sodium

REAL 2-WEEK TURNAROUND SUCCESS STORY

Linda Madden

AGE:
61

HEIGHT:
4'11"

START WEIGHT:
142 pounds

AFTER 2 WEEKS:
136.8 pounds

RESULTS:
5.2 pounds, 10 inches lost
(including 1¼ inches from waist and 2 inches from hips)

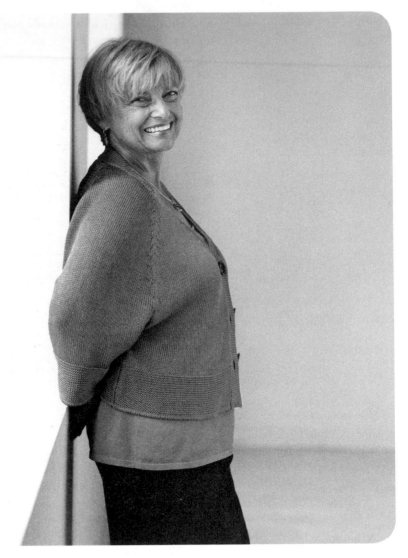

Linda spends about 75 percent of her time traveling as part of her job as a clinical research monitor for a medical device company. With so much time on the road, it's no surprise that her weight has risen steadily along with her frequent-flier miles. And at a little less than 5-feet tall, every extra pound made a big difference on her petite frame. In the past 8 years, she gained at least 25 pounds—about as much as she weighed at the end of her pregnancies 30-something years before.

"I'd skip breakfast, run around all day, then binge with a big steak or pizza for dinner, capped by some candy or popcorn in the room," she says. Even when she was home, she ate out more than she stayed home. "It was just easier to go to a restaurant than keep groceries in the house, since no one was home most of the time to eat them." And while she'd occasionally pack her workout clothes and shoes, more often than not they'd never make it out of her suitcase.

A mere 2 days into her 2-Week Total Body Turnaround, Linda was on the road again—this time for pleasure, with a group of friends. But instead of succumbing to the temptations of travel food, she kept to her program of eating healthy and exercising. "Rather than suffer in silence, I told my friends what I was doing, and they were really encouraging. I realized that there are things on every menu that I can eat without going overboard, and that I can eat real food and still lose weight." And she woke up early enough to finish her workout and shower before her companions were even out of bed.

"Something inside me just clicked," she says. "I started to look forward to going to work out every morning. Now the first place I head in the morning is the gym to do both my cardio and strength. And anywhere I go, my workout gear goes with me." And she finds her energy levels are high even when she's traveling. "I travel across multiple time zones, but I'm not as tired as I used to be."

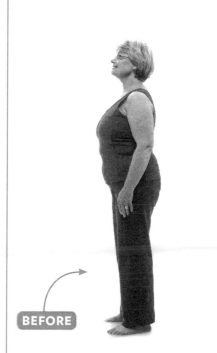

BEFORE

After 2 weeks, she'd lost 5 pounds and an amazing 10 inches; 4 weeks later and still on the plan, she dropped almost 5 more pounds and several more inches. "I'm down at least one clothing size, but I'm only buying two pairs of pants at a time because those numbers are going to continue dropping downward. But when I get to that goal number of 120 pounds, watch out, because I am hitting the stores!"

Key for her is the idea of portion control. "I now know what 3 ounces of protein looks like—it's about the size of a deck of cards. So when I get a dish at a restaurant, I'll cut the portions and set the remaining food aside." Still, she's surprised at what she can eat and still be satisfied. "For breakfast, I'll have two pieces of whole-wheat toast with peanut butter, some fruit, and some scrambled egg substitute. That's a lot of food! And it's all well within my calorie guidelines." Nowadays she'll snack on some string cheese or pop some gum when she's craving food in her hotel room at night. "I don't think of myself as being on a diet, because that makes me think of deprivation. This is about making healthy choices."

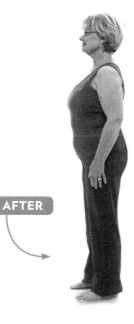

AFTER

At 61, Linda says she looks forward to spending more time with her children and grandchildren, who range in age from 1 to 14. "For a while, my philosophy was, 'I'm older so I don't want to worry about dieting or the way I look. I just want to enjoy life.' But I realized that I'm going to keep getting older, so I might as well be in the best health that I can, both physically and mentally. I just may have added a few years to my life."

DAY 13

■ ■ ■ ■ ■ ■ ■ ■ ■ ■ ■ ■ **13** ◯

As you close in on the end of your 2-Week Total Body Turnaround (time flies!), I want you to think about what you've done over the past 13 days. Despite its short length of time, this plan is all about inspiring long-term change. Think about how far you have come. Are you willing to go back to the way you were before? Or are you ready to try another 2 weeks? Or if not the exact same 2 weeks, at least another 2 weeks of eating less, moving more, and thinking more positively? Then after that, another 2 weeks, 2 months, 2 years? Once you get into the habit of eating clean and moving more, it's hard to go back to doing anything else.

The purpose of the jumpstart was to do just that—SHOCK you into making a change. You were motivated to try it probably for a few reasons: You were ripe for a change, you thought 2 weeks was doable, and it gave you a reason to stay committed. And guess what? You did it.

If you remember on Day 1, I told you that losing weight is a simple math equation: calories in versus calories out. There are really four ways to deficit calories in order to lose weight:

1. Eat less

2. Move more

3. Increase your metabolism by consistently strength training

4. Or, *all of the above* (the best answer!)

You have been eating a controlled amount of calories.

You have been doing cardio and trying to pump up the intensity, and getting into the habit of being more active each and every day.

You have been strength training, which you may not have done before

"Obstacles are those frightful things you see when you take your eyes off your goals." —Sydney Smith, British writer

or for a long time. Not only have you been working every muscle group, you've been doing it slow and controlled to maximize your results.

You have the recipe for losing weight, increasing energy, increasing self-esteem, improving your mood . . . the list goes on. The rest is up to you. When people ask me, "What's the best way to lose weight?" I turn the question around and ask, "How do you think?" Everyone knows the answer: Eat less, move more. It just takes that kick in the seat to get moving. Can you feel my kick?

CARDIO: Speed Ladder

For today's cardio challenge, really focus on your intensity level. I'll bet you can go faster during the speed challenges than you could even just a week ago. In fact, your old "speed" pace may now be what you're using for your warmup or cooldown! Step out of your comfort zone and challenge yourself. Try jogging when the RPE climbs. Your breathing should reflect the higher intensity level. Give yourself time to recover, and try again!

INTENSITY	TIME	RPE	TALK TEST
Warm up (heart rate: Zone 2)	4 min.	4–5	You can speak in full sentences (slightly breathless)
Speed up (heart rate: Zone 2)	5 min.	5	Slightly breathless (brisk walk)
Speed up (heart rate: Zone 3)	4 min.	6	Somewhat more breathless (pace is slightly faster than before)
Slow down (heart rate: Zone 2)	2 min.	5	Somewhat breathless (brisk walk)
Speed up (heart rate: Zone 3)	3 min.	7	Breathless (pace is slightly faster than last speed burst)
Slow down (heart rate: Zone 2)	2 min.	5	Slightly breathless (brisk walk)
Speed up (heart rate: Zone 4)	2 min.	8	Very breathless (pace is slightly faster than last speed burst; you can take this into a slow jog)
Slow down (heart rate: Zone 2)	2 min.	5	Somewhat breathless (brisk walk)
Speed up (heart rate: Zone 4)	1 min.	9	Very breathless (Take this into a jog if you can, or walk as fast as possible)
Cool down (heart rate: Zone 2)	5 min.	4–5	Slightly breathless

STRENGTH: Lower Body + Core

You've gotten through almost 2 straight weeks of strength training nearly every day! This is the time to challenge yourself. Focus on moving slowly through the full range of motion. You should feel stronger and more confident, and perhaps you can even see the change in your muscle definition. Keep it up! This is just the beginning of a more powerful you.

Ⓐ

POWER LUNGE WITH KICK

TARGETS: Quads, butt

A. Stand with feet together, arms at sides holding dumbbells. Step left leg back and lower into lunge position for 4 counts, keeping right knee over ankle as you bend knees 90 degrees.

B. Stand up in 2 counts; **kicking left leg forward to hip height.** Repeat 8 times. Switch legs and repeat.

GOOD FORM TIP:
Step back far enough so your front knee stays in line with your shoelaces (not past your toes) to avoid straining your kneecap.

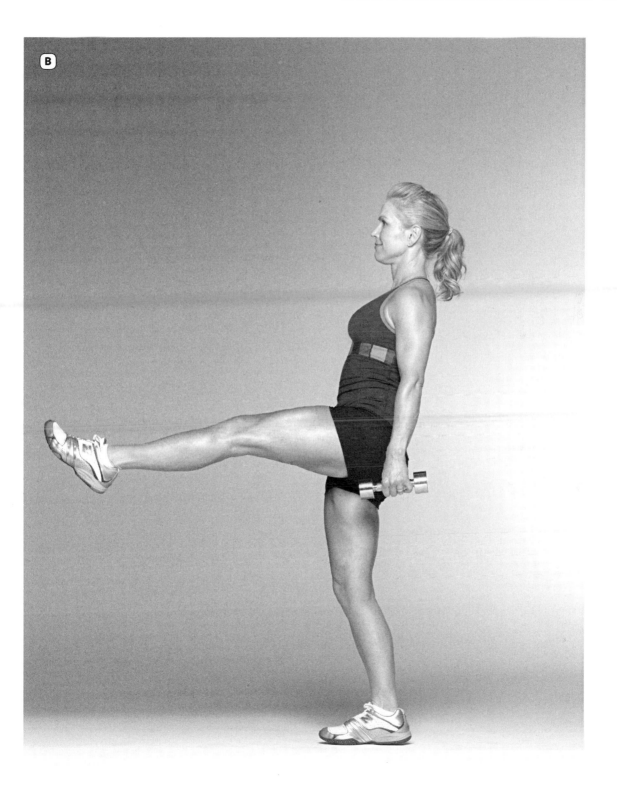

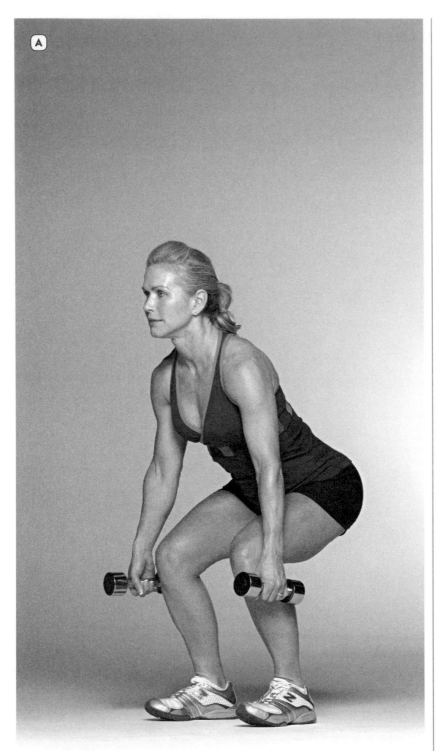

DUMBBELL STILETTO SQUATS

TARGETS: Quads, butt, calves

A. Stand with feet shoulder-width apart, **arms extended next to thighs holding dumbbells.** Squat down, as if sitting in a chair behind you, for 4 counts, lowering dumbbells toward floor.

B. Lift heels, balancing on balls of feet.

C. (not shown) Rise back up to standing for 2 counts, keeping heels lifted. Lower heels to floor. Repeat 8 to 12 times.

B

GOOD FORM TIP:
*When squatting back,
keep your knees tracking over your
shoelaces (not past your toes) to avoid
putting pressure onto kneecaps.
Keep torso lifted, chin
parallel to the floor.*

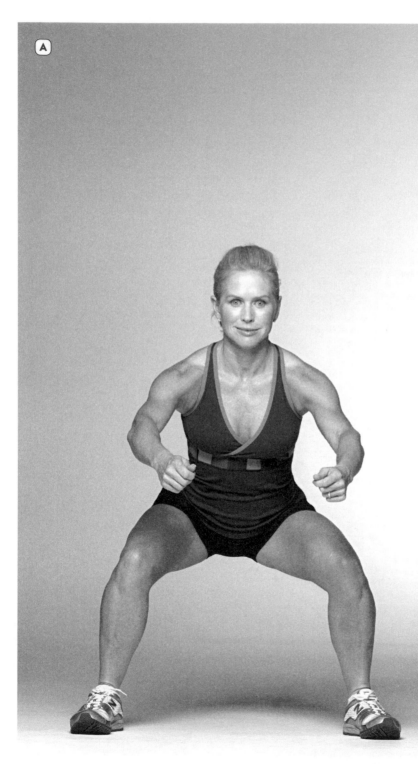

A

JUMPING CLOCK SQUATS

TARGETS: Quads, butt

A. Stand with feet wider than shoulder-width apart. Imagine yourself standing on a big clock, with your right foot on the center and your left foot on the "9." Lower into a squat for 4 counts, keeping weight in heels.

B. Rise up for 2 counts, and **jump with both feet** one-quarter turn to the right (facing "3") on the 2nd count as you stand up.

C. Repeat squat, **jumping with both feet** one-quarter turn to the right or "6" on the 2nd count as you stand up.

D. Repeat squat, **jumping with both feet** one-quarter turn to the right "9" position on the 2nd count as you stand up. Repeat squat, **jumping back to start position** ("12") on 2nd count. Repeat the entire series, this time turning counter-clockwise. Then repeat the entire series 2 more times in each direction.

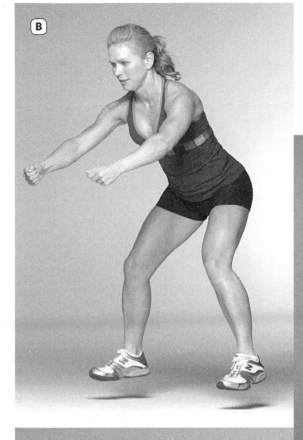

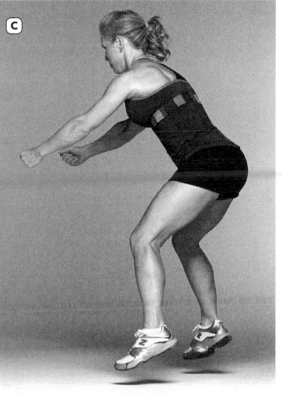

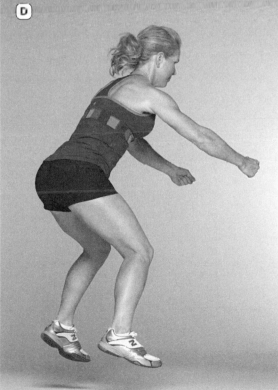

GOOD FORM TIP:
When squatting back, keep your knees tracking over your shoelaces (not past your toes) to avoid putting pressure onto kneecaps. When you jump, land with your knees soft.

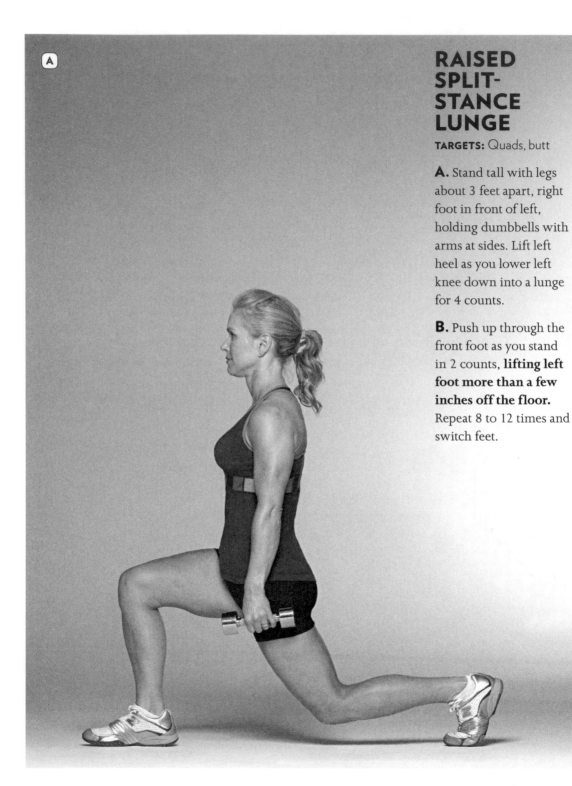

RAISED SPLIT-STANCE LUNGE

TARGETS: Quads, butt

A. Stand tall with legs about 3 feet apart, right foot in front of left, holding dumbbells with arms at sides. Lift left heel as you lower left knee down into a lunge for 4 counts.

B. Push up through the front foot as you stand in 2 counts, **lifting left foot more than a few inches off the floor.** Repeat 8 to 12 times and switch feet.

B

GOOD FORM TIP:
Keep front knee tracking over your shoelaces (not past your toes) to avoid putting pressure onto kneecap.

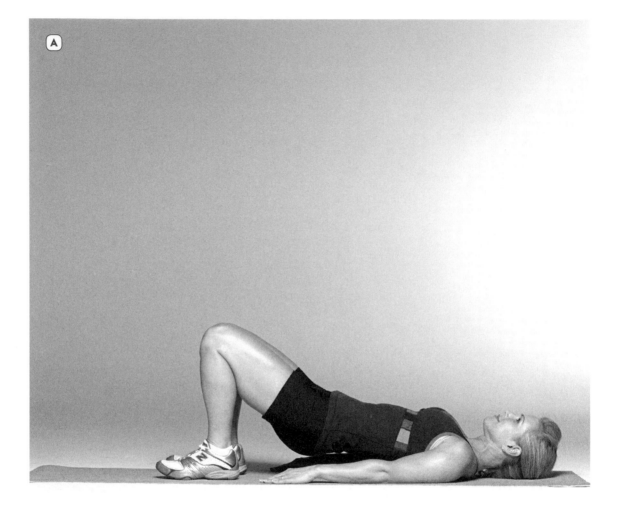

ONE-LEGGED BRIDGE

TARGETS: Hamstrings, butt

A. Lie face up on floor, knees bent, feet flat on floor.

B. Extend left leg, keeping thighs parallel. Pushing right foot into floor, lift hips up for 2 counts, keeping abs tight and body in a straight line **from left heel to chest.** Slowly lower body back to floor for 4 counts. Repeat for 6 reps; switch legs and repeat.

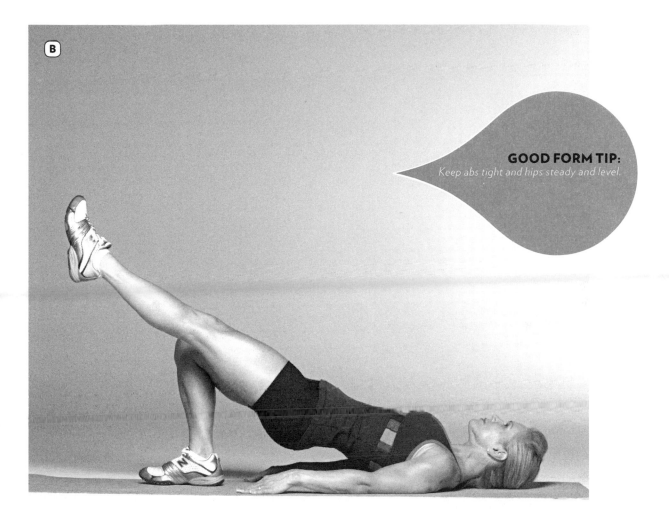

GOOD FORM TIP:
Keep abs tight and hips steady and level.

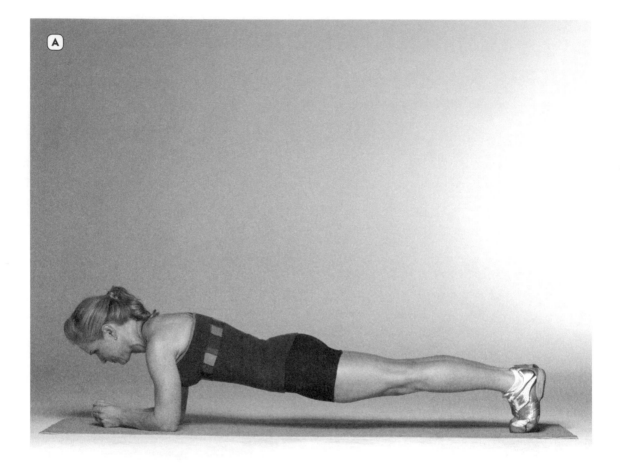

HIP DROP

TARGETS: Abs, obliques

A. Lie face down on floor, legs extended, with elbows and forearms on floor. Lift hips, keeping abs tight while forming a straight line from head to heels.

B. Tip slightly to the right, keeping back straight, as you lower right hip to floor in 4 counts. Slowly return to start position in 2 counts. Tip toward left side for 4 counts. Come back to start in 2 counts. Continue for 8 to 10 repetitions on each side.

GOOD FORM TIP:
Keep abs tight and spine long to avoid sagging through low back, even as you dip from side to side.

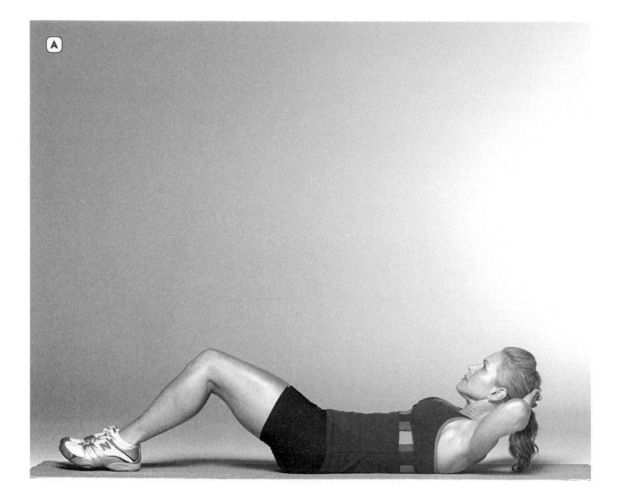

NEW EXERCISE! **CORE CHALLENGE**

GUT CHECK

TARGETS: Abs

A. Lie face up on the floor, hands behind head, knees bent with feet flat on the floor. Lift head, neck, and shoulders off the floor.

B. Crunch up in 2 counts, keeping a fist-size space between your chin and chest. Hold 1 count, then slowly lower in 4 counts. Do 12 reps.

B

GOOD FORM TIP:
Peel up off the mat, engaging your lower abs; lower slowly and with control. Imagine a piece of Velcro beneath you as you peel up and back down.

DAY 13 TURNAROUND TIP
Quash Your Cravings

Cravings can seem to hit out of the blue, although most times they are associated with something specific, like stress or hormonal fluctuations. Indulging yourself once in a while in moderation is okay—that's what today is for!—but if your cravings become regular, you need to find a way to calm them. One tried-and-true way is distraction: Leave the kitchen and do something else. If that's not possible, try some of these craving quenchers.

● **POP SOME PICKLES.** Strong-tasting foods like olives, pickles, and hot peppers overwhelm your tastebuds, which experts say cuts cravings off at the pass.

● **GUM UP THE WORKS.** I chew bubble gum when I feel like I cannot stop eating. It keeps my jaw going and it's sweet!

● **SATISFY YOUR HUNGER.** When cravings strike, ask yourself if you are really hungry. If so, make a deal with yourself to first satisfy your hunger with some healthy food, and then you can have a taste of whatever you're craving if you still want it.

● **BRUSH YOUR TEETH.** Ever notice how nothing tastes very good after some toothpaste? Next time you're trying to avoid the box of chocolate bars you bought from a school fundraiser, give your pearly whites a quick cleaning. A swish of mouthwash or popping a mint can have the same effect.

What if these strategies don't work and you find yourself slipping? Remember that we all blow it sometimes and that a single episode of overeating does not have to turn into 3 days of dietary havoc. No one ever got fat from a single overindulgence. Don't beat yourself up about it. Remember, it's what you do most of the time—not those few occasions you fall off the wagon—that determines your success!

THERE'S NO DENYING THAT we all have cravings for certain types of foods. Maybe it's a throwback to the time when you came home from school and your mom served you some milk and cookies to hold you over until dinner; maybe it's the desire to munch while watching TV. Whatever the case, nothing can weaken your willpower like a midafternoon or after-dinner snack attack. And if a well-stocked cookie jar or open bag of chips is within reach—watch out.

Rule #1, of course, is to junk food proof your house. (It's the idea of childproofing when your kids are little: If you don't want your kid to break something, you remove it!) Keep the chips, cookies, and ice cream out of there entirely. But when your body is yearning for certain sweet or salty snacks, it can be a big mistake to deny it entirely. Hold out on

LEARN ABOUT: **SATISFYING FOODS**

cravings too long, and you risk going overboard the second you see some cookies, cake, or chips. For these 2 weeks, we'd like you to stick with our snacking guidelines if at all possible—with one 200-calorie snack (including one serving of dairy and one serving of fruit) in the morning, and another 200-calorie snack (including one dairy serving) in the afternoon or evening. But if you are finding it difficult to stay on track with these restrictions, make some smart, nutritious, and low-calorie substitutions that will satisfy your cravings without sabotaging all of your hard work. See page 355 for some deliciously satisfying low-calorie ideas.

MEAL GUIDELINES:
Suggested amounts for each meal

BREAKFAST
2 grains/starchy veggies

1 dairy

1 protein

1 fruit

1 fat

A.M. SNACK
1 dairy

1 fruit

LUNCH
1 grain/starchy veggie

1 protein

2 veggies

1 fat

P.M. SNACK
1 dairy

DINNER
1 grain/starchy veggie

1 protein

2 veggies

1 fat

DAY 13 SUGGESTED MENU

BREAKFAST

1 whole-grain pita filled with 5 scrambled egg whites and ¼ cup shredded colby. Serve with 1 banana and 1 cup nonfat or low-fat yogurt.

PER SERVING: 510 calories; 3 g total fat; 2 g sat fat; 75 g carbohydrates; 7 g fiber; 46 g protein; 10 mg cholesterol; 650 mg sodium

SNACK

1 apple with 1 slice reduced-fat Cheddar

PER SERVING: 160 calories; 6 g total fat; 4 g sat fat; 20 g carbohydrates; 3 g fiber; 6 g protein; 20 mg cholesterol; 240 mg sodium

LUNCH

Beef Tostadas

PER SERVING: 325 calories; 18 g total fat; 4 g sat fat; 20 g carbohydrates; 4 g fiber; 22 g protein; 53 mg cholesterol; 645 mg sodium

SNACK

1 cup skim milk

PER SERVING: 80 calories; 0 g total fat; 0 g sat fat; 12 g carbohydrates; 0 g fiber; 8 g protein; 0 mg cholesterol; 100 mg sodium

DINNER

Tofu Stir-Fry with Peanut Sauce

PER SERVING: 387 calories; 13 g total fat; 2 g sat fat; 50 g carbohydrates; 12 g fiber; 23 g protein; 0 mg cholesterol; 689 mg sodium

BEEF TOSTADAS

3 ounces 95% lean
ground beef

2 teaspoons taco
seasoning

1 tablespoon olive oil

$^1/_2$ cup chopped onion

$^1/_2$ cup chopped green or
red bell pepper

$^1/_2$ cup sliced mushrooms

$^1/_2$ cup broccoli florets

2 small (4") corn tortillas,
warmed

$^1/_4$ cup fat-free sour
cream (optional)

In a nonstick skillet, combine the beef and taco seasoning and cook, stirring frequently, until crumbled and cooked through. Drain any fat; remove from the skillet and set aside.

Heat the olive oil over medium-high heat in the same skillet. Add the onion and pepper, and cook 2 minutes. Stir in the mushrooms and broccoli and sauté about 5 minutes, or until tender. Return the beef to the pan; cook until heated through, stirring occasionally. Top the warmed tortillas with the beef-veggie mixture and top with sour cream, if desired.

MAKES 1 SERVING

PER SERVING: 325 calories; 18 g total fat; 4 g sat fat; 20 g carbohydrates; 4 g fiber; 22 g protein; 53 mg cholesterol; 645 mg sodium

TOFU STIR-FRY WITH PEANUT SAUCE

3 ounces firm tofu, cubed

$^3/_4$ cup sugar snap peas

$^1/_2$ cup asparagus, sliced
on the diagonal

$^1/_4$ cup sliced mushrooms

1 tablespoon creamy
peanut butter

2 tablespoons vegetable
broth

$^1/_2$ teaspoon brown sugar

1 teaspoon white wine
vinegar

2 teaspoons lite soy sauce

Pinch of red-pepper flakes

$^1/_2$ cup julienned
(matchsticks) carrots

$^1/_2$ cup cooked whole-
grain spaghetti

In a medium nonstick skillet coated with cooking spray, cook the tofu over medium heat, stirring frequently, for about 5 minutes, or until browned. Remove from the pan and set aside. Add the peas, asparagus, and mushrooms, and cook, stirring frequently, for about 3 to 5 minutes, or until crisp-tender. In a small bowl, combine the peanut butter, broth, sugar, vinegar, soy sauce, and pepper flakes, stirring to combine. Pour the sauce over the vegetables and simmer for 1 minute. Add the tofu, carrots, and pasta, stirring to coat, and cook until heated through.

MAKES 1 SERVING ($1^3/_4$ CUPS VEGETABLES AND $^1/_2$ CUP PASTA)

PER SERVING: 387 calories; 13 g total fat; 2 g sat fat; 50 g carbohydrates; 12 g fiber; 23 g protein; 0 mg cholesterol; 689 mg sodium

NOTE: *This recipe is a little high in sodium (you want to aim for no more than 600 to 650 mg per meal), which you should normally avoid, but you'll be sweating a lot throughout the 2-Week Total Body Turnaround, so you can get away with it today.*

DAY 14
FINAL
DAY!!!

■ ■ ■ ■ ■ ■ ■ ■ ■ ■ ■ ■ ■ **14**

You've done it! You've made it through the 2-Week Total Body Turn-around—and more importantly, you've proven to yourself that you can do this. You've achieved something great. Now it's time to keep it up. Momentum is a force. It gathers speed as it keeps going. You've got your speed, so start the next race.

You've found success because you've taken this challenge on for just 2 weeks. Moving in small increments is key to long-term success, so think about how you will treat your body for the next 2 weeks, and then the 2 weeks after that. Before you know it, eating right and exercising is a way of life!

"The surest way not to fail is to determine to succeed."
—Richard B. Sheridan, British playwright

And remember that you can use this jumpstart anytime your engine needs it. I am personally proud of each and every one of you who made it through the 2-Week Total Body Turnaround. Now is your time to keep the momentum going and create a healthy and happy life. There's a Gatorade commercial that I love and that perfectly sums up this feeling:

"It's not where you're from; it's where you're going. It's not what you drive; it's what drives you. It's not what's on you; it's what's in you. It's not what you think; it's what you know."

CARDIO: Mini-Bursts

Power through the final cardio workout of your 2-Week Total Body Turnaround with this steady-paced walk. Remember to keep your intensity level as high as you can sustain for the full 25 to 30 minutes. If you have time, challenge yourself to go even longer! For every 5 minutes you add on, you'll burn about 30 extra calories!

INTENSITY	TIME	PACE	RPE	GOAL
Warm up (heart rate: Zone 1–2)	5 min.	Moderate pace	2–4	You can have a conversation but are starting to get breathless.
Power walk (heart rate: Zone 3) with mini-bursts (heart rate: Zone 4)	20 min.	Fast pace	7 (8–9 for mini bursts)	Gradually increase intensity until you are walking at the fastest pace you can sustain. Every few minutes, try jogging or walking as fast as you can for 30 seconds, then return to fast walking pace. Try to do at least 5–7 of these mini speed bursts.
Cool down (heart rate: Zone 1–2)	5 min.	Moderate pace	3–4	Slow down until you are walking at a moderate pace. You should be able to speak in full sentences with some breathlessness.

STRENGTH: Total Body

It's your final strength day of the 2 weeks, and we're going to put every major muscle to work! By now you're a little more familiar with what's involved, so try to do at least 2 sets of each exercise. Do them as a circuit, moving from one to the next, and take as little rest as possible between each move.

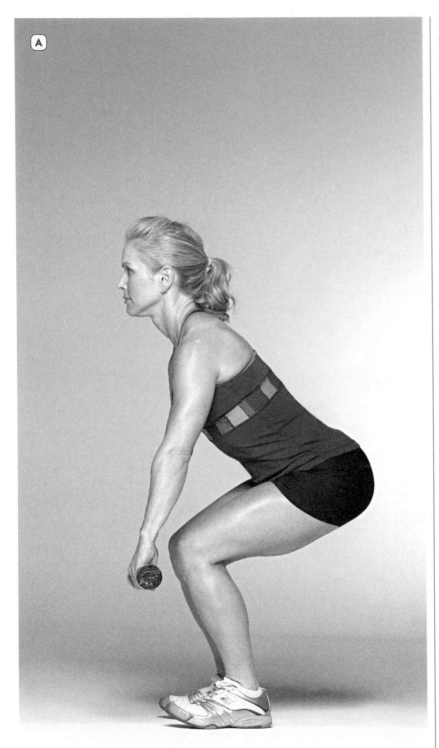

SQUAT WITH STRAIGHT ARM PRESS AND LEG LIFT

TARGETS: Shoulders, arms, quads, butt

A. Stand with feet about 4 inches apart, holding dumbbells at sides with palms facing behind you. Slowly lower into squat position for 4 counts, keeping weight over heels as arms move forward.

B. Stand back up in 2 counts **lifting left leg behind you, squeezing butt** while simultaneously pressing palms behind you. Repeat 6 times; switch legs and do 6 more reps.

B

GOOD FORM TIP:
*Keep abs tight and spine long.
Use backs of shoulders to press,
keeping arms straight.*

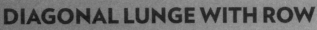

DIAGONAL LUNGE WITH ROW

TARGETS: Quads, butt, back

A. Stand with feet shoulder-width apart, left foot turned out 45 degrees, **holding heavier dumbbells than in Week 1 with arms extended at sides.** Slowly bend left knee, sitting back into left butt in 4 counts while straightening right leg, reaching right dumbbell toward left ankle. (Keep knee in line with shoelaces.)

B. Push back up to start position in 2 counts, keeping left knee slightly bent, and squeezing through left butt while pulling right elbow across body and behind you in a row; keep elbow close to sides (you'll feel this in the middle of your back). Repeat 8 times. Switch to the other side and repeat 8 times.

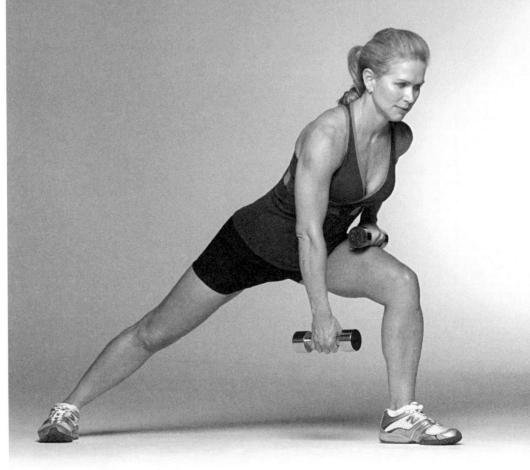

GOOD FORM TIP:
Keep your shoulders pressed down, away from your ears. Focus on using the muscles in your back, not your neck.

HAMMER TIME WITH KNEE LIFT

TARGETS: Arms, quads, butt

A. Stand with feet 2 to 3 inches apart, holding dumbbells at sides. Lunge back with left foot in 2 counts, bending both knees 90 degrees (keep right knee over right ankle) while curling weights toward shoulders with thumbs facing up.

B. Slowly lower arms as you rise back up in 4 counts; **on the 4th count, lift left knee in front of hips,** then step back into lunge with left foot. Repeat 8 times. Switch sides and repeat 8 times.

B

GOOD FORM TIP:
Keep your elbows close to your sides; avoid swinging from your shoulders as you lunge back.

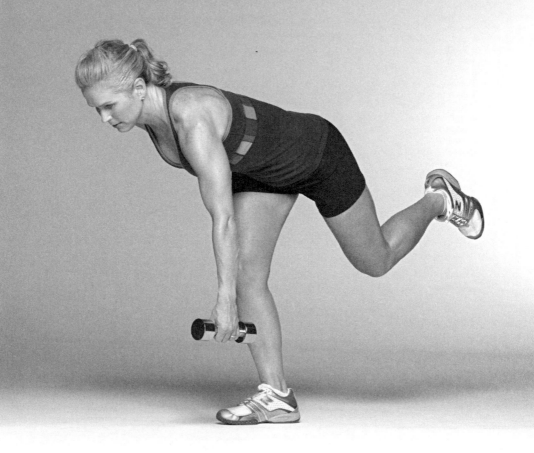

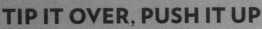

TIP IT OVER, PUSH IT UP

TARGETS: Arms, shoulders, hamstrings, butt

A. Start with feet staggered, right foot in front of left, holding a **heavier dumbbell than in Week 1** in your left hand, **right hand on hip (rather than holding chair)**. Keeping spine straight and abs tight, lean forward in 4 counts, reaching left arm toward floor while lifting left leg behind you, slightly softening knee.

B. Return to start in 2 counts, curling weight toward shoulder in a biceps curl while lifting left knee to hip height.

C. Slowly press weight up toward ceiling in 2 counts and lower it in 4 counts. Repeat 8 times and switch sides.

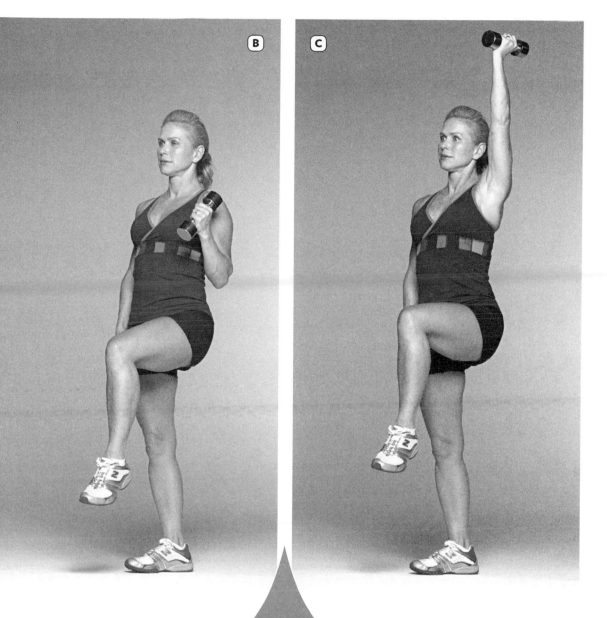

GOOD FORM TIP:
Keep your abs tight and your spine long so your lower back doesn't sag. Stand by pulling up through your hamstrings and butt, not your lower back.

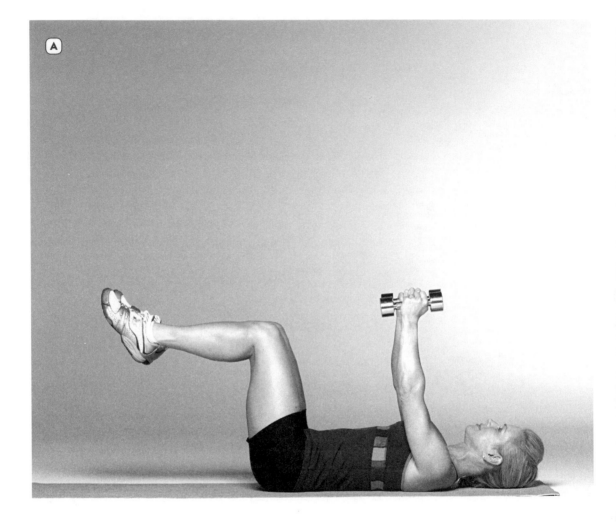

TABLETOP BEACH BALL HUG

TARGETS: Chest, abs, hips

A. Lie face up on floor, **knees bent 90 degrees and feet lifted, shins parallel to floor.** Hold dumbbells above chest with arms extended, elbows slightly bent, palms facing each other.

B. Slowly lower arms out to sides in 4 counts, keeping elbows slightly bent while simultaneously straightening legs 45 degrees to floor. Pull knees back to start in 2 counts while lifting arms back above chest, squeezing your chest muscles as if you're hugging a beach ball. Do 10 to 12 reps.

B

GOOD FORM TIP:
Slightly press your lower back into the mat and "sew" your belly button in toward your lower back.

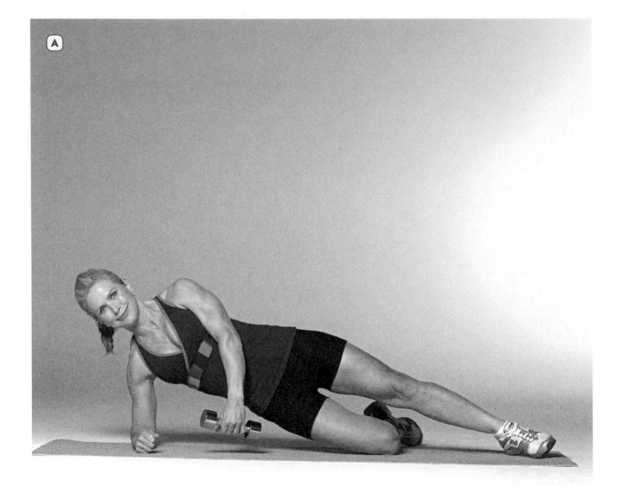

FOREARM SIDE PLANK WITH SHOULDER RAISE AND LEG LIFT

TARGETS: Shoulders, abs, obliques
This move should be familiar to you from Day 10.

A. Lie on right side, hips stacked, elbow under shoulder and right forearm on floor with bottom knee on floor and top leg extended straight. Hold a dumbbell in left hand on floor, just in front of body. Lift hips, forming a straight line from shoulders to heels, keeping abs tight.

B. Lift left arm above shoulder for 2 counts; **at the same time, lift left leg as high as you can, keeping abs tight.** Lower arm and leg slowly for 4 counts, keeping hips still. Repeat 8 times. Switch sides and repeat another 8 times.

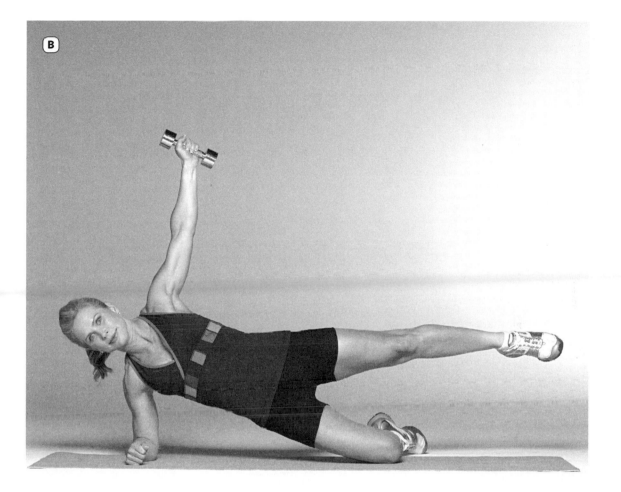

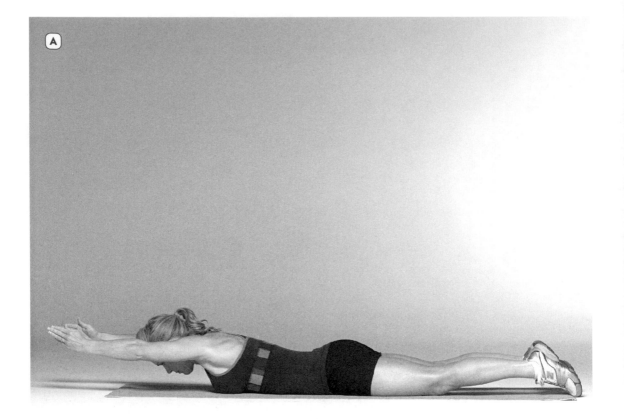

NEW EXERCISE! **CORE CHALLENGE**

BREAST STROKE

TARGETS: Upper and middle back

A. Lie face down on floor, arms extended overhead with palms facing each other. Lift head and arms off the floor, keeping abs tight and head in line with spine. Hold here for 2 counts.

B. Lift chest a few inches off the floor and "swim" your arms down in 2 counts, sweeping them out in semicircles toward the middle of your back (finish with your thumbs pointing down), using the middle back muscles to keep you up. Be sure to keep your abs tight and your feet on the floor. As you lower chest, draw arms in toward body, bending elbows, then "swim" them back overhead to start position in 4 counts. Do 8 to 10 reps.

B

GOOD FORM TIP:
Keep your lower abs engaged even when face down. Imagine there's a rod or a ruler behind your neck to help keep your head in line with your neck.

DAY 14 TURNAROUND TIP
Go for Your Goals

Here we are: Day 14 of your 2-Week Total Body Turnaround. You made it! But this isn't the end: These 2 weeks were only the start of something great.

Now that you've succeeded in getting through these 2 weeks, it's time to establish your next goal. Will you keep this up for 2 more weeks? Will you embark on a new journey, and this time bring along your family and friends? The key is to have a specific plan, and then figure out the best way to implement it.

Start by picking your destination. If it's weight loss, figure out a number that's realistic. Focus on short-term goals, from day to day or week to week.

Then map out your route. Set up what I call my "SMART" goals:

SPECIFIC: What kind of exercise will I do? When will I do it? Be as specific as possible: "I want to lose 5 pounds by June 1" or "I want to zip up my favorite skinny jeans."

MEASURABLE: Determine how many minutes you will spend on exercise each day, and at what intensity level. That might mean a 45-minute power walk, a 30-minute interval routine, or a 20-minute strength circuit.

ATTAINABLE: Is my body up to these challenges? You've made it through the past 2 weeks, so give yourself credit for what you can do. You may surprise yourself!

REALISTIC: Have I created a schedule I can stick to? If you found it hard to squeeze in every minute of the 2-Week Total Body Turnaround workout, you may have to scale back your exercise plan to doing just 30 minutes a day rather than 60.

TIME FRAME: What will I do each day/week/month? I encourage you to use the routines in this book as a guide. There are lots of great workouts to choose from, and you don't have to do them the same way every time: Do the interval routine on an elliptical machine or stationary bike instead of the treadmill; change up the order of the strength moves.

Finally, try to steer clear of distractions. You might hit the occasional rough spots, but keep moving.

Don't forget to reward yourself for the small successes.

WHEN YOU'RE FEELING ANXIOUS, upset, or stressed, certain foods can immediately calm you down. Unfortunately, many of us tend to pick up a box of cookies or tear into a bagel or muffin when stress and anxiety levels rise. Your body has the right idea: High-carb foods raise levels of the brain chemical serotonin, which makes us feel calm and happy. Fortunately, you don't have to swallow hundreds of calories to raise serotonin levels. There are many smart, healthy choices that can give you the same sense of peace without having you pig out.

Let's back up a second and look at what happens to your brain chemistry when you eat. Both protein and carbs are very important in the manufacturing and transport of neurotransmitters, the chemicals in your brain (including serotonin) that transmit thought.

LEARN ABOUT: **CALMING FOODS**

As I mentioned on Day 1, protein is made up of different amino acids. One of these amino acids—tryptophan—is involved in helping to create serotonin. Tryptophan helps the body produce the B-vitamin niacin, which in turn helps the body produce serotonin. You may have heard of tryptophan around Thanksgiving time—people often blame their post-feast feelings of sleepiness on the turkey, which does contain high levels of tryptophan.

Carbs stimulate the release of insulin, which helps more tryptophan get to the brain. So to get the greatest amount of this natural calm, you need to consume both protein and carbohydrates. Ideally, these carbs are complex and high in fiber, such as whole grains. The fiber will slow absorption of the carbs into the bloodstream, so you have a more measured response. Eat too much low-fiber food (like those with white flours or refined sugars) without the accompanying protein and you'll get not just calm, but sleepy and lethargic. Other foods that contain high levels of tryptophan include eggs, milk, bananas, chickpeas, sunflower seeds, and beef.

So if you want to feel calm and alert—not comatose—have a small meal or snack with a combo of protein and carbs. That might include some grilled chicken on whole-grain bread, hummus with whole-wheat pita, fish and rice, or low-fat milk and bran flakes (throw in half a banana for good measure!).

Some people also like a cup of tea when they want to calm down. Remember that all non-herbal tea, whether green or black, does contain caffeine, which can be a stimulant. Still, there's evidence that a spot of tea can soothe your nerves: A study from University College London found subjects who drank tea and were exposed to a stressful situation recovered their pre-stress levels of calm more quickly and felt more relaxed afterward than those who drank a bogus tea drink. Subjects also had lower levels of the stress hormone cortisol in their blood.[32] On the herbal tea side, chamomile has been prized for generations for its ability to help calm stressed-out nerves.

MEAL GUIDELINES:

Suggested amounts for each meal

BREAKFAST

2 grains/starchy veggies

1 dairy

1 protein

1 fruit

1 fat

A.M. SNACK

1 dairy

1 fruit

LUNCH

1 grain/starchy veggie

1 protein

2 veggies

1 fat

P.M. SNACK

1 dairy

DINNER

1 grain/starchy veggie

1 protein

2 veggies

1 fat

DAY 14 SUGGESTED MENU

BREAKFAST

Broccoli-Cheddar Scramble

PER SERVING: 430 calories; 10 g total fat; 5 g sat fat; 54 g carbohydrates; 10 g fiber; 37 g protein; 28 mg cholesterol; 784 mg sodium

SNACK

Slices from 1 orange dipped in 1 cup nonfat or low-fat yogurt

PER SERVING: 200 calories; 1 g total fat; 0 g sat fat; 34 g carbohydrates; 3 g fiber; 15 g protein; 5 mg cholesterol; 190 mg sodium

LUNCH

Chicken salad: Combine 1 cup mixed greens, 3 ounces diced grilled chicken breast, $1/2$ cup halved grape tomatoes, $1/2$ cup sliced cucumber, 1 tablespoon pine nuts, 1 tablespoon olive oil, and a splash of balsamic vinegar.

PER SERVING: 350 calories; 23 g total fat; 3 g sat fat; 9 g carbohydrates; 3 g fiber; 29 g protein; 75 mg cholesterol; 90 mg sodium

SNACK

1 part-skim string cheese

PER SERVING: 80 calories; 6 g total fat; 4 g sat fat; 1 g carbohydrates; 0 g fiber; 7 g protein; 15 mg cholesterol; 150 mg sodium

DINNER

Spiced Salmon with Spinach-Feta Couscous

PER SERVING: 366 calories; 17 g total fat; 3 g sat fat; 32 g carbohydrates; 7 g fiber; 24 g protein; 52 mg cholesterol; 498 mg sodium

BROCCOLI-CHEDDAR SCRAMBLE

$^1/_2$ cup chopped broccoli (fresh or frozen)

$^1/_2$ cup chopped mushrooms

$^1/_3$ cup chopped red or green bell peppers

$^3/_4$ cup egg whites

$^1/_4$ cup shredded reduced-fat Cheddar cheese

$^1/_2$ whole-wheat English muffin, toasted

1 tablespoon low-fat cream cheese

$1^1/_4$ cups strawberries

$^1/_2$ cup freshly squeezed orange juice

In a nonstick skillet coated with cooking spray, cook the broccoli, mushrooms, and peppers, stirring frequently, for about 5 minutes, or until tender. Add the egg whites and cook for 2 to 3 minutes, or until set. Sprinkle the cheese on top of the eggs to melt. Cover for a few seconds. Spread the English muffin with the cream cheese. Serve with strawberries and orange juice.

MAKES 1 SERVING

PER SERVING: 430 calories; 10 g total fat; 5 g sat fat; 54 g carbohydrates; 10 g fiber; 37 g protein; 28 mg cholesterol; 784 mg sodium

NOTE: *This recipe is a little high in sodium (you want to aim for no more than 600 to 650 mg per meal), which you should normally avoid, but you'll be sweating a lot throughout the 2-Week Total Body Turnaround, so you can get away with it today.*

SPICED SALMON WITH SPINACH-FETA COUSCOUS

$^1/_2$ teaspoon brown sugar

$^1/_4$ teaspoon cumin

$^1/_4$ teaspoon coriander

$^1/_4$ teaspoon garlic powder

$^1/_8$ teaspoon cinnamon

$^1/_8$ teaspoon salt

1 salmon fillet (3 ounces), skinned

1 teaspoon olive oil

2 cups fresh baby spinach

1 teaspoon pine nuts, chopped

2 teaspoons crumbled reduced-fat feta cheese

$^1/_2$ cup cooked whole-wheat couscous

Preheat the oven to 375°F. Combine the first 6 ingredients in a small bowl. Rub over both sides of the salmon. Place the salmon on a baking sheet coated with cooking spray and bake for 15 minutes, or until cooked through and fish flakes easily when tested with a fork. Meanwhile, heat the olive oil in a nonstick skillet over medium heat. Add the spinach and cook for about 2 to 3 minutes, or until wilted. Toss the spinach, pine nuts, and feta cheese with the couscous until combined. Serve the salmon with the couscous.

MAKES 1 SERVING

PER SERVING: 366 calories; 17 g total fat; 3 g sat fat; 32 g carbohydrates; 7 g fiber; 24 g protein; 52 mg cholesterol; 498 mg sodium

REAL 2-WEEK TURNAROUND SUCCESS STORY

Kim Regenhard

AGE:
51

HEIGHT:
5'5"

START WEIGHT:
147.4 pounds

AFTER 2 WEEKS:
140.8 pounds

RESULTS:
6.6 pounds, 7³⁄₄ inches lost
(including 2 inches from waist and ¹⁄₂ inch from hips)

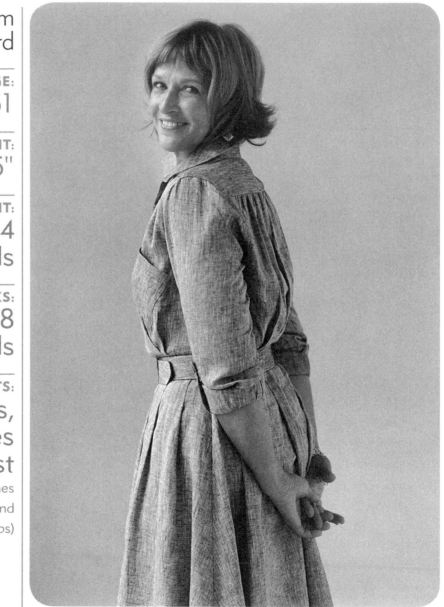

When Kim Regenhard looks at pictures of herself from over the past few years, she's hard-pressed to find one that shows her body from the waist down. "I trained my husband and son well!" she laughs. "Almost all of my photos were just head shots."

Two weeks and counting after her 2-Week Total Body Turnaround plan, and Kim was not only proud to model in front of the camera, she was flaunting her stuff in a white bathing suit. "One of my friends told me I looked awesome, and it made me feel so good—after all, nobody looks good in a white swimsuit!"

A frequent runner, Kim found that since she hit 50, it still wasn't enough to keep the extra weight off. "I've exercised my whole life and I enjoy it, but whatever I was doing wasn't working."

What did make the difference: adding the strength moves to her routine. "I've lifted weights before but very infrequently. When I added the strength part into my workout, it made a big difference." Within 4 days, Kim says, her pants were looser; more than halfway into the program, she started to see more muscle tone in her arms, shoulders, and thighs. After 2 weeks, she'd lost nearly 7 pounds and more than 7 inches.

Since being diagnosed with breast cancer about 10 years ago, Kim has made an effort to eat more healthfully, including having more organic foods in her diet. A bigger challenge for her was keeping track of everything she was eating. "I decided I would write down everything I put in my mouth to see what 1,600 calories looked like and to make sure I was getting a good balance of nutrients. I was really surprised that I could eat so much and still feel satisfied!" Favorite foods included peanut butter on rice cakes, nuts, and fresh fruits and vegetables.

After the 2 weeks were up, she stayed on the plan, albeit modifying the diet a bit to allow her to enjoy her Friday night glass of wine (which she's turned into a white-wine spritzer to save calories). She's also become a dedicated fan of putting the dressing on the side for her salads. "I find myself using just half of the normal serving, and I don't even miss it."

But her favorite thing about the Turnaround is its simplicity. "It's all about eating less and moving more. There are no pills, powders, gimmicks, or hype," Kim says. "Most plans are either a fitness boot camp or a calorie-monitoring approach. This really addresses both sides of the equation, calories in and calories out."

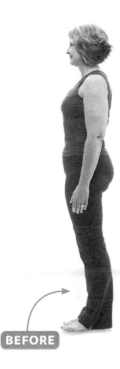

BEFORE

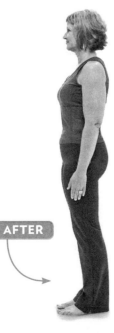

AFTER

Your 2-Week Total Body Turnaround Plan at a Glance

Your 2-Week Total Body Turnaround Plan at a Glance
WEEK 1

DAY	CARDIO	STRENGTH	MENU
1	**SPEED BURSTS** (30 min.)	**UPPER BODY/CORE** (30 min.) Tank Top Toner Single-Arm Row Standing Biceps Curl Pushup Shoulder Tap Triceps Kickback Full Body Rollup	**BREAKFAST:** Whole-Grain Cereal **SNACK:** Yogurt **LUNCH:** Turkey Meatball Pocket **SNACK:** Pear **DINNER:** Garlic Lemon Shrimp
2	**HILLS** (30 min.)	**LOWER BODY/CORE** (30 min.) Floating Lunge Deadlift Plié Heel Taps Scissor Squat Calf Attack Bridge Double Leg Stretch	**BREAKFAST:** Whole-Grain Waffle **SNACK:** Ricotta Cheese with Raisins **LUNCH:** Dijon Chicken and Chickpea Salad **SNACK:** Chocolate Soymilk **DINNER:** Tofu -Vegetable Marinara with Parmesan
3	**PURE POWER** (30 min.)	**TOTAL BODY** (30 min.) Plié with Biceps Curl Forward Lunge and Raise the Roof Curtsy Lat Raise Pushup Row Forearm Side Plank with Shoulder Raise Pass the Bell	**BREAKFAST:** Apple-Pecan Oatmeal **SNACK:** Cottage Cheese with Cantaloupe **LUNCH:** Salad and Chicken Sandwich **SNACK:** Moroccan Dip with Crudités **DINNER:** Grilled Fish
4	**PYRAMID** (30 min.)	**UPPER BODY/CORE** (30 min.) Fly Away Suspended Biceps Curl Standing Triceps Toner Kneeling Shoulder Shaper Airplane Pushup Table-Top Crunch with Reach	**BREAKFAST:** Breakfast Sandwich **SNACK:** String Cheese with Grapes **LUNCH:** Simple Salad "Niçoise" **SNACK:** Skim milk **DINNER:** Tomato Chicken Thighs with Zucchini and Lentils

DAY	CARDIO	STRENGTH	MENU
5	**SPEED LADDER** (30 min.)	**LOWER BODY/CORE** (30 min.) Power Lunge Stiletto Squats Clock Squats Split-Stance Lunge Bridge Hip Drop	**BREAKFAST:** Whole-Wheat English Muffin with Peanut Butter **SNACK:** Vanilla Soymilk with Peach **LUNCH:** Open-Faced Mushroom-Onion Veggie Burger **SNACK:** Cottage Cheese **DINNER:** Seared Chicken Fajita Salad
6	**MINI-BURSTS** (30 min.)	**TOTAL BODY** (30 min.) Squat with Straight Arm Pressback Diagonal Lunge with Row Hammer Time Tip It Over, Push It Up Beach Ball Hug Forearm Side Plank with Shoulder Raise	**BREAKFAST:** Whole-Grain Pita with Egg Whites **SNACK:** Apple with Cheddar **LUNCH:** Beef Tostadas **SNACK:** Skim milk **DINNER:** Tofu Stir-Fry with Peanut Sauce
7	**ACTIVE REST**	None	**BREAKFAST.** Broccoli-Cheddar Scramble **SNACK:** Orange with Yogurt **LUNCH:** Chicken Salad **SNACK:** String Cheese **DINNER:** Spiced Salmon with Spinach-Feta Couscous

Your 2-Week Total Body Turnaround Plan at a Glance
WEEK 2

DAY	CARDIO	STRENGTH	MENU
8	**SPEED BURSTS** (30 min.)	**UPPER BODY/CORE** (30 min.) Balancing Tank Top Toner Single-Arm Row Balancing Biceps Curl Full Pushup Shoulder Tap Balancing Triceps Kickback Full Body Rollup Dumbbell Oblique Twist	**BREAKFAST:** Whole-Grain Cereal **SNACK:** Yogurt **LUNCH:** Turkey Meatball Pocket **SNACK:** Pear **DINNER:** Garlic Lemon Shrimp
9	**HILLS** (30 min.)	**LOWER BODY/CORE** (30 min.) Knee Lift Floating Lunge Single-Leg Deadlift Dumbbell Plié Heel Taps Hands Up Scissor Squat Calf and Inner Thigh Attack Bridge Double Leg Stretch Read the Paper	**BREAKFAST:** Whole-Grain Waffle **SNACK:** Ricotta Cheese **LUNCH:** Dijon Chicken and Chickpea Salad **SNACK:** Chocolate Soymilk **LUNCH:** Tofu-Vegetable Marinara with Parmesan
10	**PURE POWER** (30 min.)	**TOTAL BODY** (30 min.) Plié with Biceps Curl Forward Lunge and Raise the Roof with Knee-Up Curtsy Lat Raise with Front Kick Full Pushup Row Forearm Side Plank with Shoulder Raise and Leg Lift Pass the Bell, Swimmer	**BREAKFAST:** Apple-Pecan Oatmeal **SNACK:** Cottage Cheese with Cantaloupe **LUNCH:** Salad and Chicken Sandwich **SNACK:** Moroccan Dip with Crudités **DINNER:** Grilled Fish
11	**ACTIVE REST**	None	**BREAKFAST:** Breakfast Sandwich **SNACK:** String Cheese with Grapes **LUNCH:** Simple Salad "Niçoise" **SNACK:** Skim Milk **DINNER:** Tomato Chicken Thighs with Zucchini and Lentils

DAY	CARDIO	STRENGTH	MENU
12	**PYRAMID** (30 min.)	**UPPER BODY/CORE** (30 min.) Balancing Single-Leg Fly Away Balancing Suspended Biceps Curl Triceps Toner with Tree Pose Bird Dog Shoulder Shaper Airplane Full Pushup Table-Top Crunch with Reach Dumbbell V-Open	**BREAKFAST:** Whole-Wheat English Muffin with Peanut Butter **SNACK:** Vanilla Soymilk with Peach **LUNCH:** Open-Faced Mushroom-Onion Veggie Burger **SNACK:** Cottage Cheese **DINNER:** Seared Chicken Fajita Salad
13	**SPEED LADDER** (30 min.)	**LOWER BODY/CORE** (30 min.) Power Lunge with Kick Dumbbell Stiletto Squats Jumping Clock Squats Raised Split-Stance Lunge One-Legged Bridge Hip Drop, Gut Check	**BREAKFAST:** Whole-Grain Pita with Egg Whites **SNACK:** Apple with Cheddar **LUNCH:** Beef Tostadas **SNACK:** Skim Milk **DINNER:** Tofu Stir-Fry with Peanut Sauce
14	**MINI-BURSTS** (30 min.)	**TOTAL BODY** (30 min.) Squat with Straight Arm Press and Leg Lift Diagonal Lunge with Row Hammer Time with Knee Lift Tip It Over, Push It Up Tabletop Beach Ball Hug Forearm Side Plank with Shoulder Raise Breast Stroke	**BREAKFAST:** Broccoli-Cheddar Scramble **SNACK:** Orange with Yogurt **LUNCH:** Chicken Salad **SNACK:** String Cheese **DINNER:** Spiced Salmon with Spinach-Feta Couscous

MAINTAIN

"A man too busy to take care of his health is like a mechanic too busy to take care of his tools."—*Spanish Proverb*

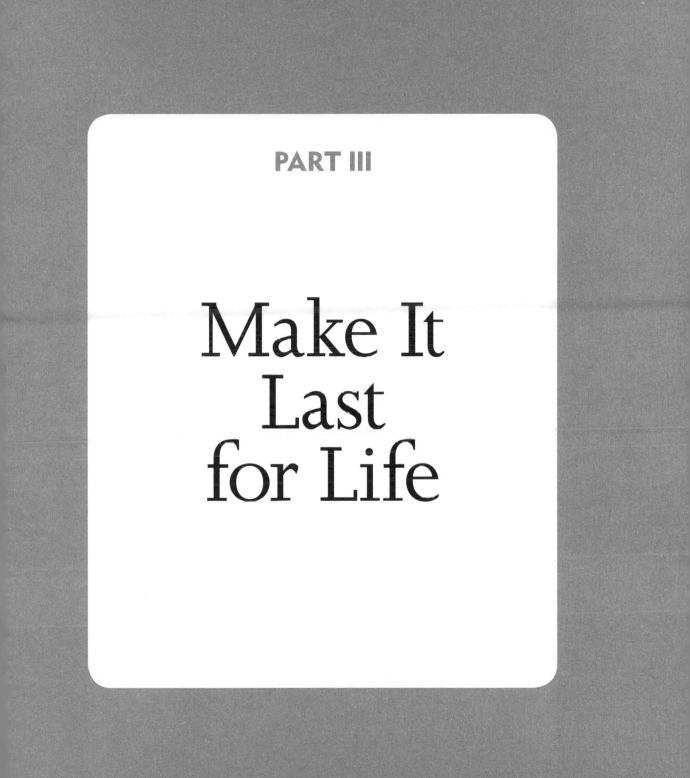

PART III

Make It Last for Life

Staying the Course

Over the course of the 2-Week Total Body Turnaround, you will experience many changes: More energy. Increased stamina. Better sleep. Soaring confidence. Stares of envy from your friends. Motivation that keeps you craving more and more. You may also find your muscles are a bit sore, especially after some of the strength workouts, but remember: That's a sign that your body is getting stronger! In this chapter, you'll find ways to keep feeling healthy and fired up each and every day of your 2-week plan—and well beyond.

Reaching the Highs

You've probably heard about the "runner's high," or the feeling of euphoria you get during exercise. Of course, you don't have to be a runner to experience this sensation. Doing any prolonged activity, whether you're walking, jogging, skating, cycling, skiing, swimming, or so on, can give you this feel-good sense that all is right in the world.

For years, scientists have speculated that this sensation is caused by endorphins, a group of naturally occurring opiates associated with positive mood changes that flood the brain during exercise. Recently, researchers in Germany studied runners before and after a long run, then used PET scans to see if endorphins were being produced. They found that the chemicals were, in fact, present in the area of the brain closely associated with emotions, giving credence to the long-held claim that exercise does affect your brain chemistry.[1] And the more endorphins you produce, the greater the effect. I call it the body's natural "happy drug!"

Rest and Recovery: How to Maximize Your Results

There's no doubt that you are working your body hard over these 2 weeks. And if you haven't been active for a while, or if you're simply not used to getting up and moving around on a regular basis, you might find yourself feeling a bit sore.

There are really two main types of muscle soreness. The first is the soreness you might experience during or immediately after exercise. It usually goes away very quickly and can be blamed on the by-products of muscle metabolism, which involves getting enough oxygen to your cells so they can do their job.

The second type of pain is called delayed onset muscle soreness (DOMS), because it usually comes on about 24 to 48 hours after exercise, then decreases after about 72 hours. I talked about it briefly in Part I. DOMS is a natural body process that's due to microscopic tears in the muscles and surrounding connective tissues. It's when your muscles rebuild that you get stronger and start to see some of that sculpted, sexy muscle tone in your arms, abs, shoulders, and thighs. This soreness is a sign that your workout is working! If you don't challenge your muscles, they won't get stronger, so if you're not feeling at all sore after your workouts, you need to increase your intensity a bit by using heavier weights, slowing down the movements, or doing some combination of both. Remember that women simply do not have the hormonal makeup to get big and bulky, especially if you're spending just 30 minutes a day lifting weights. Bottom line: Strength training will help you get sculpted, sexy muscles that will boost your metabolism.

1. **ICE IS NICE**

If you find the soreness is so bad that it's affecting your daily activities, you can treat it a number of ways. One of the easiest is to simply apply some ice to the affected area. I like using bags of frozen vegetables, like peas, because they conform to your body and are more comfortable than a hard block of ice.

If you've got a strong disposition, you might want to consider taking an ice bath after a workout. Sounds painful, I know, but many athletes swear that gritting your teeth and getting into some very cold water for a few minutes after an intense workout significantly helps to relieve next-day muscle soreness. The theory: The cold water causes your blood vessels to constrict. This slows bloodflow to the sore areas, which decreases swelling. And after about 5 minutes, your blood vessels will relax and return to normal, which results in a pumping action that helps get rid of by-products like lactic acid. Here's how to do it: Fill your bathtub with about 6 inches of water, then dump in a couple of trays of ice cubes. The water should cover your heels, calves, hamstrings, and butt. Try to stay in for 5 to 10 minutes. The first couple of minutes are the most painful, but biting into a towel can help!

Even if you don't want to do your best polar bear imitation, try to avoid the urge to take a long, hot bath or get into a hot tub or sauna immediately after a workout. In addition to being dehydrating, heat can increase inflammation, and since your muscles and joints may already be somewhat inflamed after exercise, the heat will only exacerbate the effect. However, some coaching pros I know recommend taking a shower alternating hot and cold temperatures to increase the bloodflow throughout your body.

2. STAY ACTIVE

Despite the urge you might have to plant yourself on the couch after a workout, remember that the more you move, the less sore you will be (and, by the way, the more calories you will burn throughout the day!). I talked a little bit about this on Day 7, your first "active rest" day of the plan.

Research has shown that active recovery—some low-intensity exercise, like walking casually or playing with your kids—can help reduce muscle soreness. This holds true whether it's immediately after a workout or the next day. One study, for example, tested two groups of exercisers doing hard intervals. The first group rested completely after each interval; the second exercised at just 30 percent of their effort level. When the researchers measured the lactate levels in the blood (the by-product of lactic acid, which your body makes during intense exercise), they found the low-intensity exercise group's levels were 25 percent lower than those from the group who rested completely. And the low-exercise group even had a comparatively greater power output during each interval following the recovery period.[2]

Being a bit more active also helps you recover after your workouts, probably because it helps encourage the removal of lactic acid from the bloodstream. Whether you're walking around the neighborhood or cycling around town to run some errands, you're increasing the blood circulation, which in turn helps remove lactic acid.

3. EAT SMART

Remember what I told you on Day 12 of your 2-Week Total Body Turnaround: The right foods can make a difference in helping your body recover faster. This holds true both for that immediate period after exercise (the "glycogen window"), when your muscles are most receptive to replenishment, and for several hours following it. Exercise makes your muscles more responsive to insulin, which in turn increases glycogen uptake. In other words, your muscles are better able to absorb glucose (in the form of carbs) for a short time after exercising. Adding some protein to the mix spurs even more of the insulin response, so your muscles can store even more glycogen. That'll come in handy the next time you exercise. Remember, too, that your body needs adequate amounts of protein to help your muscles rebuild and get stronger. So, ideally, you'll choose a protein/carb combo like peanut butter on an apple or some low-fat yogurt and fruit to help your muscles recover faster.

One other tasty way to get both carbs and protein in quickly post exercise: Pour yourself a tall glass of fat-free chocolate milk. One recent study found the classic childhood refreshment was as good as sports drinks like Gatorade in helping athletes recover from strenuous exercise. Cyclists who drank low-fat chocolate milk after exercise were able to bike 50 percent longer than those who had a sports drink during their next workout session.[3] Plus, chocolate milk is loaded with calcium and vitamin D. Just watch the amount of powder or syrup you're using: Two tablespoons of the sweet stuff pack in more than 100 calories, so go for the "lite" variety when you can and stir it into fat-free milk.

4. RUB RIGHT

Ahhh . . . There's nothing better than a nice massage, especially when your muscles are feeling achy. It's no small wonder that if you attend a local road race or watch a big sports event on TV that there are always massage therapists on hand, waiting to give athletes a rubdown where they need it most. Massaging helps to increase bloodflow to your muscles, bringing with it oxygen and the nutrients necessary to speed recovery. And let's face it—a good massage just feels good!

There is some science behind the idea of getting a massage to reduce soreness. One study from the University of Iowa found subjects who were given a deep-tissue massage after experiencing muscle soreness had their symptoms of pain reduced by up to 50 percent.[4] An Australian study found subjects who had a brief massage after exercising reduced their muscle soreness by about 30 percent and also reduced swelling.[5]

Of course, most of us can't afford to hit the spa each time we log in a workout. So while treating yourself to a professional massage is a nice idea, it's not always the most practical thing we can do for ourselves. But you can

> ### WHAT OUR TEST PANELISTS TOLD US
>
> "I was drying my daughter's hair this morning and she said, 'Mom! Look at how your pants and shirt are fitting. What a difference!' And she was right. I used to unwind with a glass of wine and was bummed to have to give that up for a couple of weeks. But I haven't missed it at all! The exercise is doing the de-stressing and making me feel great."
> —Stephanie T., 42

do yourself some good with self-massage. With a little practice, rubbing tender areas for just a few minutes can make you feel as relaxed as if you had just stepped off the masseuse's table. (Mind you, a dark room, some pleasant background music, and no interruptions can help enormously.)

Here's my quick and easy massage technique: Begin with your body part that feels the most sore. For me, that's typically my quads, hamstrings, and glutes. Use a little lotion or, better yet, some massage oil to reduce skin friction, and apply just some gentle pressure—don't rub too hard. If it's just a small sore spot, like an area on your neck, press your thumb or a finger into the area (go only as hard as is comfortable), hold for about 30 seconds, and release. For larger muscles, knead the muscles gently with your hands. Keep it up for a few minutes, breathing normally (don't hold your breath) and keeping your muscles relaxed. You can also try the "squeeze" method, especially for your upper body: Start at the base of your neck and give it a gentle squeeze with your opposite hand. Then inch your way down your neck and toward your hand, giving little squeezes down past the shoulders and arm, all the way to the hand until you reach your fingers, giving each of them a little squeeze as well. This will help increase circulation and "wake up" your muscles.

Another option is to focus on one particularly sore area with a foam roller. I try to use one to "roll out" every day! These long, dense foam tubes resemble an oversized pool noodle and have been used for many years in physical therapy to help break up deep scar tissue. More recently, they've migrated into the fitness world, popping up at gyms and for home use. They're fairly inexpensive—anywhere from $15 to $35 (try www.optp.com)—and a great way to work out tight hips or glutes when you feel sore. Use them often enough and you'll also improve your flexibility and range of motion.

Rollers are designed to act as a sort of self-myofascial release, breaking up the scar tissue that can form in the ligaments and connective tissue around your muscles. They can be a little uncomfortable at first, because they act like a "trigger point" as you use your body weight to provide pressure to one small area of your body. Roll out a tight area for just a couple of minutes a day and you'll see real benefits almost immediately. And here's a bonus: You can also use rollers for balance exercises, similar to the way you might use a stability ball. Simply standing on one without holding onto anything can be a big challenge, or even try doing squats. To work your abs, lie on top of it the long way and do crunches; flip over and place both hands on it for a more intense variation of plank pose.

You can also try using a tennis ball to deepen your massage or to target a particularly hard-to-reach spot, especially for the hips and glutes. I'll often bring one with me when I'm traveling, To help relieve sore feet, stand on top of a ball and gently roll it with the bottom of your foot, using your body weight to increase the intensity where it feels sore. Or stand against a wall with a tennis ball behind your back, and roll the ball along your back, stopping when you get to a tender area and rolling just an inch or two back and forth to help release tension. For a bigger release, put two balls in a sock, tie the ends together, and use that as your massage tool.

5. RELIEF IN A BOTTLE—AND BEYOND

Many people find that taking an anti-inflammatory medicine like aspirin, ibuprofen (like Advil or Motrin), acetaminophen (like Tylenol), or naproxen (Aleve) when they have some muscle soreness can help ease the pain. As a group, these medications are known as non-steroidal anti-inflammatory drugs, or NSAIDs, and generally do a good job at helping you feel better fairly quickly by reducing some of the inflammation in your muscles, joints, and connective tissue.

Further, some new research shows a daily dose of anti-inflammatories may actually help boost your training benefits. Researchers at Ball State University studied 36 men and women ages 60 to 78 and gave them daily standard dosages of ibuprofen, acetaminophen, or a placebo while having them complete a 3-month weight-training program. All the participants gained strength, but those in both the ibuprofen and acetaminophen groups had even better gains. The researchers speculate that the medications somehow induce a change in the muscle tissue that makes it more responsive to the exercises.[6] But be careful of taking too many of these pills at once: Chronic use can lead to stomach, liver, or kidney problems, in some cases to a very serious degree.

Not all pain relief comes in a pill. Certain foods are considered natural anti-inflammatories. Omega-3 fatty acids, for one, like those found in salmon and other cold-water fish, walnuts, and flax seeds, have been shown to help reduce inflammation in the body. (If you're not a fan of fish, you can also try taking fish-oil supplements. I keep them in the freezer to eliminate burping up that fishy taste.) Soy-based protein like tofu, soymilk, and soybeans may also reduce the pain. Fruits and vegetables can also help. Studies have shown that quercetin, a phytochemical found in apples and red onions, among other foods, has strong anti-inflammatory properties. And be sure you're drinking plenty of fluids to help flush the waste products out of your body: Water is best, but if you're not a fan of plain water, try flavoring it with lemon, orange, lime, or even cucumber slices.

Finally, you can also experiment with some natural anti-inflammatory medicines. Natural health experts often recommend arnica for treating soreness and swelling. This plant can be used in several forms, including creams, salves, ointments, gels, and tinctures. My family includes a ballerina and two hockey players, so this is a staple in my home! Massage the medicine into your muscles for a soothing rubdown. Note that arnica is considered toxic if you ingest it, so don't apply it to broken skin or an open wound. Some people also try the homeopathic version of the herb, which are tiny white pills that contain extremely small amounts of arnica. Finally, you can also try rubbing with some witch hazel—a distillation of leaves, bark, and twigs that is available at most drugstores—as a gentle way to soothe sore muscles.

6. SLEEP TIGHT

You may find yourself sleeping more soundly in the 14 days that you are on the 2-Week Total Body Turnaround than you have in months. Our test panelists unanimously reported they all experienced much deeper, restful sleep when they started the program. "I not only found that I fell asleep more easily, I also slept through the night and woke up feeling far more refreshed in the morning!" notes tester Diane V. "I slept like a rock!" agrees Terrie A.

And getting a good night's sleep is important for many reasons, not the least of which is that it makes you healthier. Like food and water, your body needs sleep to survive: Rats deprived of sleep die within 2 to 3 weeks. Most experts recommend adults get an average of 7 or 8 hours of sleep a night. But even an hour's less sleep can have your body develop a sleep debt. Accumulate too much of this debt and it can interfere with your daily routine, having a negative effect on your performance, reaction time, and concentration, leading to accidents, injuries, and memory lapses. Not to mention, it puts you in a heck of a bad mood.

Even worse, too little sleep can lead to high blood pressure and increased stress hormones, as well as an irregular heartbeat. In addition, it may alter your immune system's ability to function, including the activity of your natural killer cells, which play a key role in fighting disease.

Finally, don't forget that sleep and weight gain seem to go hand in hand. Scientists speculate that chronic sleep deprivation can lead to weight gain by altering levels of hormones that affect the appetite and the way we process and store carbs. One recent study found that too little or too much sleep can have an effect on your waistline: Canadian researchers found those who got an average of just 5 or 6 hours of sleep a night were 35 percent more likely to gain 11 pounds than those who slept an average of 7 to 8 hours. They also gained 58 percent more fat around their waists and 124 percent more body fat than the 7-to-8 hour sleepers. Surprisingly, those who slept 9 or 10 hours were 25 percent more likely to gain weight.[7]

And here's another bonus of sleeping well: It may improve your exercise performance. A recent study from Stanford University found athletes who slept more swam faster and had better reaction times. Other studies showed basketball players had faster sprint times and better free-throw shooting after getting some extra sleep, and also felt more alert and in a better mood.[8]

In addition to exercising regularly, like you're doing on the 2-Week Total Body Turnaround, try to establish a healthy bedtime routine. Go to bed at approximately the same time every night, and don't go to bed too hungry or full. Exercising right before bedtime can also be problematic, so try to do your workouts earlier in the day. Keep your bedroom quiet, dark, and a little cool. Finally, try to wake up about the same time each morning, rather than cramming in your late mornings on the weekends.

7. MANAGE YOUR HUNGER

With the increased level of exercise and daily activity that you are doing on the 2-Week Total Body Turnaround, you may find yourself being a little hungrier than usual. Many of my clients report that when they're active, they want to eat more.

To stay in control, ask yourself if you are truly hungry, or just bored. If you've recently eaten and are just looking for something to do, put a wad of bubble gum in your mouth and start to do something else—usually the urge to munch goes away when your body realizes it's not hungry. Or make a low-calorie slushie. One of my favorites is to blend together some frozen fruit blended with sugar-free green tea or lightly flavored water. Or when you're really in doubt of hunger, eat an apple! It's a high-fiber snack that only has about 65 calories, and it's a great way to fill up.

You might actually find you are less hungry now than before. One new study has found that aerobic exercise, such as walking, can increase a protein in the blood that suppresses appetite, so you're less likely to overeat![9] Researchers from Chile found that overweight and obese people on a 3-month aerobic exercise program not only decreased their body fat, but also their calorie intake. They speculate the reduced desire to munch is due to an increase in a protein called brain-derived neurotrophic factor, or BDNF, which may act as an appetite suppressant. The more BDNF the subjects had in their blood, the fewer calories they took in, and the greater the weight loss.

> ## WHAT OUR TEST PANELISTS TOLD US
>
> "Normally, I'd go to the store two or three times a week to pick up fresh produce . . . and I'd always get myself some high-calorie treat. I had only been to the store once in the last 10 days. When I went last night in search of more soymilk for my smoothies, it seemed like every packaged product I eyeballed screamed of junk food. Last night, I not only wasn't tempted, but I was a little disgusted by the plethora of high-quantity, low-quality foods out there."
> —Nancy H., 51

REAL TURNAROUND SUCCESS STORY
"I'm finally getting a good night's sleep."
MARIA SLAVENS, 45

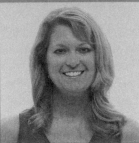

AN UNPLANNED 3 A.M. wake-up call became an unfortunate nightly habit for Maria, age 45. "I'd wake up with a start and toss and turn with a lot of difficulty getting back to sleep," she says, noting that she had to resort to the occasional dose of Tylenol PM. A busy working mom with three kids whose schedule kept her busy from dawn until dusk, Maria found her energy levels had reached an all-time low—and her frequent pillow-pounding sessions weren't helping matters. "Between work, homework, activities, etc., I didn't have any time for myself until I fell into bed at night—I rarely had enough energy to read a book."

But just a few days into her 2-Week Total Body Turnaround, Maria noticed a dramatic shift in her energy. "At the end of the day, I just had so much more to give," she says. "I found I could rev up for my workouts and take the time to eat the right food, instead of just grabbing what was easiest." Moreover, she found she was sleeping far more solidly and through the night. "I sleep so much better than I ever used to!"

Making time for herself was key to her success. "I forced myself to get out of bed and walk in the morning at 5:30 a.m., and I grew to love this time outside, without any interruptions—just me and my dog." In the evenings, her weight workouts gave her more "me-time." "I had to tell my kids that they needed to let me get my workout done, and then we could talk. They were caught a little off guard, but they understood that I needed to occasionally put myself first."

Her efforts paid off on the scale, as well, when she dropped nearly 6½ pounds and 7 inches in 2 weeks, including 2 from her waist. But it's her vigor that is keeping her going. "I will not give up my newfound energy!" she maintains. "This has been the best part of the whole plan!"

Maintaining Motivation

I'm so proud of you for keeping your motivation on high through each day of the 2-Week Total Body Turnaround. But hey—we're human. It's natural to need a little extra oomph in order to get us moving. I have a few favorite strategies that I tell my clients to try whenever motivation starts to lag.

➤ **Press Play.** Numerous studies have shown that listening to music while you exercise can improve your performance. Some researchers say it helps to lower your rate of perceived exertion, so the exercise simply doesn't feel as hard, and you can go stronger and longer. One study, for example, found subjects who listened to upbeat music while exercising went 11 percent farther, and at a significantly higher speed (so they burned more calories).[10] I know that's the case for me—if one of my favorite songs comes on while I'm in a Spinning class or running, I automatically kick it into a higher gear. Music may even help during your strength workouts: One recent study asked men and women to do some leg-toning exercises either with or without music. Those who listened to the beat gained 50 percent more strength than those who exercised in silence.[11]

I really believe that when you exercise to music that keeps a steady pumping beat, you keep moving at that pace. I find that when the music speeds up, or slows down, that's exactly what I do. So if you're doing an interval workout, try to time it so your songs keep pace with you. You can find lots of pre-mixed workout tunes that help you stay on pace. (My own workout mixes are sold on isweatmusic.com.)

● **Write down your workouts.** Keeping a log that details your exercise routine can be incredibly motivating. It's a great check-in with yourself to see how hard you worked and for how long, and also a good way to track your progress. If you were only able to walk at 3.5 miles per hour one week and then stepped it up to 3.8 the next, then 4.0 the week after that, you can see in black and white how you are moving forward. And seeing how far you have gone is incredibly rewarding. You can also use it to track how many miles you've walked this week or how much weight you've lifted.

Journaling is also a good way to get some clarity, helping you determine just how long you've been using those 5-pound weights and maybe helping you decide to step it up to the 8-pound ones. After all, the best way to know where you want to go is to figure out where you are, and keeping a log can help you stay on track and reach your goals. And I don't know about you, but I can't remember exactly what I ate or did yesterday, much less last week. So to be truer to yourself, write it down!

You don't need a fancy hard-covered book: Even a simple binder or pad will do, although having calendar dates can help you stay on track and easily flip back to a previous week's or month's workout. If you're more comfortable on the computer, keep a spreadsheet, or try one of the free online workout logs that you can keep up with and that even send you daily or weekly reminders about your exercise plans.

● **Buddy up.** Working out with a friend or family member is one of the best ways to keep your motivation going. Knowing someone is waiting on a corner for you at 6:00 a.m. means you're a lot less likely to hit the "snooze" on your alarm. A fitness buddy keeps you accountable, and also more consistent. Plus, chatting with a friend makes the time go by much more quickly. And having a friend at the gym is a great way to try out new moves and to help you watch each other's form.

When choosing your workout partner, try to find someone who has fitness goals similar to yours. If you like to walk but your best friend would rather jog, you're probably not going to stick together for too long on a 3-mile jaunt. It's also helpful if your schedules match up—someone who can't squeeze in a workout until the early evening may not be too helpful if you have to be home to make dinner for your family. I always say "I play the field" when it comes to workout buddies. I have a friend I run with on Fridays, another I run with on Saturdays and Mondays, my husband is usually my Sunday date, and Tuesday through Thursday, I exercise with my classes!

● **Reward yourself.** Promising yourself a treat after a particularly hard workout or, even better, after doing a week's worth of them can be just the carrot you need to keep going. Get a mani/pedi, take a long, hot bubble bath, or treat yourself to a movie with a friend. Or take yourself shopping and get a new pair of shoes or a workout outfit or something else that makes you feel good about yourself. Just don't reward yourself with food. It's easy to think you might deserve that sundae after getting up early on Sunday for a morning workout, but don't negate the effects of your hard work with a few spoonfuls of mint chocolate chip!

● **Outsmart the elements.** If you like to exercise outside, it's easy to use the weather as an excuse the moment the skies seem to threaten, or the temperature rises or falls below a comfortable level. Those perfect blue-sky days are usually rarer than we'd like, so take some precautions to deal with variations in the weather. Manufacturers have made great strides in performance activewear, to the point where there's pretty much an outfit for every season and climate. Water-resistant jackets and hats can keep raindrops at bay without making too big of a dent in your wallet. And sometimes what seems like what will be a big storm is merely a threat, so head out early, tie a jacket around your waist, and wear a hat. After all, it's only water!

On cooler days, dress in layers to help you stay comfortable, because as you exercise, your body will start to heat up. A moisture-wicking base layer will keep sweat off your skin. Stay away from cotton, since that will absorb the moisture, leaving you feeling cold and clammy. If it's very cold, include an insulating layer, like a light fleece jacket. And on top, wear a windproof shell to keep you comfortable. Some companies also combine these two benefits into a windproof fleece fabric. Don't forget a hat to keep your temperature regulated, warm socks (again, go with a moisture-wicking fabric so your feet don't get wet or cold), and gloves. A small waistpack will come in handy if you want to store any of these items. I love my SPIbelt (you can find them at www.SPIbelt.com). It stays on your hips and can hold an iPod or BlackBerry, keys, and lots more!

On very warm days, dress in light, cool clothing. Moisture-wicking fabrics work best here, too, to keep the sweat off your skin so your body can continue to cool itself. Don't forget a mesh hat to protect your skin, and put on sweatproof sunscreen before you leave the house.

REAL TURNAROUND SUCCESS STORY
"I wanted to be fit by age 50."
ROXANN MCCAIN, 49

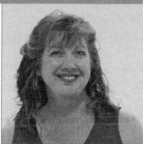

AT AGE 49, ROXANN considered herself an active person—walking regularly, going horseback riding, even using the push mower instead of the rider to mow her lawn. But with the big 5-0 on the horizon (not to mention an upcoming cruise to Alaska), she wanted to be stronger, leaner, and healthier. "I realized that even though I walked a lot, it was always at the same pace, so I wasn't really challenging my body. And adding the strength moves really ramped things up!"

Two weeks also seemed the perfect length of time to focus on. "Going on a diet or exercise program and not having a goal until 9 or 12 months away was just too daunting," she notes. "I knew I wasn't going to lose 25 pounds in 2 weeks, but in the past I haven't even been able to lose 2 pounds in 10 months." But after just 2 weeks on this plan, she lost almost 3 pounds, plus almost 12 inches, including 3 1/2 from her waist. "It's as if my body has shifted, and it's not so focused around my stomach. My clothes are fitting much more nicely." Having this success in just 14 days spurned her to do another 2 weeks, and then 2 after that, and so on.

Her energy levels also got a big boost. "If there was no other difference, that would have been enough to keep me going!" she says. She recalls a recent walk where she was trying to get home before a storm hit. "I even jogged up 'heartbreak hill' near my house and just made it in the door when the sky opened and it started to pour. I was so thrilled that I didn't want to sit down for the rest of the day."

She also had another surprising benefit: A history of incontinence has disappeared. "I was having a bit of a problem making it to the bathroom in the morning, because it's a bit of a walk from the cottage where I sleep to the main house, so I started wearing pads. Sometime in the middle of the second week, I suddenly realized I no longer had a problem holding it until I made it to the house!"

By the time she was on board for her Alaskan cruise, Roxann was fully committed to integrating strength and interval workouts into her routine. "I did a lot of walking on the deck of the ship and hit the fitness room almost every day to do my weight workouts. By the end of the cruise, I hadn't gained a pound!"

● **Find a mantra.** I'm a big believer in positive phrases. It's incredibly empowering to have a phrase that you believe in and that makes you feel motivated to do more whenever you say it in your head (or even out loud!). Your mantra can be whatever moves you, whether that's a phrase you've heard, a poignant poem or quote, even an advertising slogan. Find at least two that you can repeat when the going gets tough.

One of my favorite new mantras is "Strive for Progress, not Perfection." As a trainer and a mom, I have come to find out that perfection *always* leads to disappointment. I'm not telling you to lower your standards; I'm just suggesting you set realistic and worthwhile goals. We all have room for progress. Here are a few other great mantras to consider, courtesy of one of my favorite yoga and athletic apparel companies, lululemon.

"Move your body and your heart will follow."

"Do it now, do it now, do it now!"

"Your outlook on life is a direct reflection of how much you like yourself."

"Do one thing a day that scares you."

"That which matters the least should never give way to that which matters the most."

"Breathe deeply and appreciate the moment. Living in the moment could be the meaning of life."

"Wake up and realize that you are surrounded by amazing friends."

"Choose a positive thought. The conscious brain can only hold one thought at a time."

What If It's Too Much?

Your mind can be a funny thing sometimes. Just when you think you can't take one more minute in your walk at a brisk pace or eke out one more weight repetition, a switch clicks and all of a sudden you're ready to do more. I once heard a doctor say, "You are always capable of doing more than you are doing." The key is to find a safe way to trick your brain into pushing yourself a little harder. It works the other way, as well. How many times while exercising have you started thinking about all of the things you have to do or places you could be—and all of a sudden you feel tired and want to quit? Your brain can most definitely play tricks on your body, and conquering the mental aspect of exercise is just as important as the physical part.

When things do get tough, try practicing "dissociation": Instead of thinking about how hard you are working, focus on something positive. Try out one of those mantras we just talked about. I had a friend who used to go through all the names of her children over and over when she got to that tough "I-don't-think-I-can-finish" point of a 10K race. I personally sing the words to motivating songs in my head over and over when I get to that last mile of a long run. And, when I teach my classes, as we are reaching the last few reps of an exercise, I make them chant, "I think I can, I know I can, I like it, I love it . . ."

Of course, you also want to focus on your technique so you don't get hurt: You don't want to trick your body into ignoring pain, so don't push through an excruciating ache where something might really be wrong. Instead, take your primary focus off how many reps or steps you have left by using your breath, words, or music to keep your mind in the game.

Finally, invite the whole family to join you. Often the best motivation comes from those who surround you. This seems to be especially true with our children. Getting your kids involved in your activity—whether it's having them join you on a walk or bike ride or asking them to keep you company when you do your strength training (or try it for themselves, if they're big enough!)—is more than just motivating, it's essential to help pass along the desire to be fit and healthy to the next generation. One of my best "talk" times is a walk to a local coffeehouse with my kids. If you're ever not into exercising, ask your kids—they'll often call your bluff and remind you of your promises!

Several of our test panelists told me that their children were the ones who helped them get out the door. Barb, for example, asked her teenage son to go with her on her walk. A high-school football player, he not only coached her all the way through it, he also stuck around to help her with her strength workouts. "If it hadn't been for him, I know I wouldn't have done as much, or as well!" she reports.

My Favorite Healthy Eating Tips

Now that you know what to eat, here are a few ways to help you maximize your results and keep on track for a lifetime of good nutritional habits.

Write It Down (or Just Log On!)

Keeping a food diary is one of the best ways to make sure you are staying on track with your healthy eating plan. Most of us can't remember what we did last week, let alone what we ate for breakfast. Plus, logging what you've eaten keeps you honest and accountable. Seeing in black and white (or data bits) can be a reality check when it comes to logging three slices of pepperoni pizza. A recent study from Kaiser Permanente of more than 1,700 participants found keeping a food diary can double a person's weight loss. The more food records a person kept, the more weight they lost; those who kept a daily food record lost twice as much weight as those who didn't keep track at all.[12]

Choose the method that works for you. Many of our test panelists found they really enjoyed using *Prevention*'s free My Health Trackers (www. prevention.com/healthtracker) to keep track of their food choices and automatically see how many calories they'd consumed, as well as the nutrient breakdown. But putting a pen to paper is still a good low-tech option. Here's what to include when writing it down:

- **What kind:** Write down the type of food you ate, being as specific as possible. Include sauces and gravies, plus "extras" like ketchup, mayo, butter, sugar, or salad dressing, and beverages like soda, water, milk, or juice.

- **How much:** Estimate the size, volume or weight, or amount.

- **Time:** Remember the time you had the food or drink.

Try to keep your log with you and be sure to write down or log everything that you eat or drink. Doing it at the time can help prevent memory lapses at the end of the day! Estimate portion size to the best of your ability, using my "handy" measurements (see page 53) or real ones.

Track Your Progress with *Prevention*'s My Health Trackers

AS I'VE MENTIONED, *Prevention* magazine features a fantastic interactive program called My Health Trackers on its Web site, www. prevention.com/healthtracker.

On it, you can create a personal food journal to track calories, fat, protein, fiber, vitamins, and more. You can also log your daily workouts and activities to see how many calories you have burned, as well as track your mood, stress, and energy levels. Plus, you'll find detailed nutritional information on thousands of foods, as well as the ability to keep tabs on individualized concerns such as blood pressure, blood sugar levels, sleep habits, caffeine intake, and more. The graphics are pretty cool, too—and there's nothing more rewarding than literally seeing your waist, hip, and thigh measurements and overall weight dip before your eyes. Best of all, it's totally free!

On the "Foods Eaten" page, you can register your daily calorie intake, your calorie balance, and the amount of carbs, fat, protein, and fiber you've consumed, plus the percentage of recommended daily allowance of vitamins and minerals.

On the exercise side of things, My Health Trackers allows you to track how many calories you've burned by entering the type of exercise you've done and for how long. In addition, you can calculate your daily activity level. Logging in this info makes it incredibly simple to stay on track.

WHAT OUR TEST PANELISTS TOLD US

"I love *Prevention*'s My Health Trackers. It's so easy to use, and it helps me realize just how many calories I'm consuming and where I'm getting (or not getting) nutritional value. I work at home, and it's conducive to snacking. Being a far cry from a nutritionist, I had no idea of the quality and quantity of my daily intake!"
—**Nancy H., 51**

REAL TURNAROUND SUCCESS STORY

"I've gotten my diabetes under control."
DEE RASMUSSON, 63

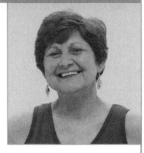

THE PAST FEW YEARS have been challenging for Dee. Three years ago, she was diagnosed with type 1 diabetes. Shortly thereafter, she lost her husband after a long illness and turned, in part, to food for comfort. She put about 20 pounds onto her 5-foot-3 frame, and struggled to find the motivation to eat well and exercise, spending her evenings on the couch instead of doing things around the house.

Dee, now 63, started her 2-Week Total Body Turnaround by writing down 15 things about her body she was thankful for. "It helped me to think positive about the effort needed to stay healthy and in shape," she says.

The first thing Dee noticed after she began the program was that her legs and abs started to firm up and her energy levels began to perk up. "I was a real couch potato at night, but found myself having more energy to do the things I love—even if it's just staying awake to read more."

But the most dramatic change, she says, was for her health. "I very quickly realized that I could keep my glucose level under better control and needed less insulin to do so once I started exercising and eating more healthfully." As a diabetic, she says she frequently studied food labels to see the amount of carbohydrates and sugars. Now, she notes, she looks at the calorie counts as well, and she chooses more fruits and vegetables and fewer packaged goods. "I'm spending a lot more time in the produce section and less in the snack aisle!" she maintains.

Dee lost more than 4 pounds on the plan and 6½ inches, including more than an inch off her hips. Although she wasn't a big fan of strength training in the past, she says she followed through each move one at a time, and before she knew it, she was done with the workout. Seeing her arms and waistline get more toned also motivated her to continue. She's kept up with the program, walking or strength training at least 30 minutes a day. "Having a set plan has made it much easier to accomplish my goals," she says. "It's all about being consistent and having a commitment to stick to the program."

Drink Up

The first thing I reach for when I am thirsty is a cold glass or bottle of water. Water keeps you energized, improves your workouts, helps you feel fuller, and may even boost your metabolism. One recent study from the University of Utah found that students who drank the recommended eight glasses of water a day had more energy, were more inclined to study, and had better concentration. And since previous studies have linked dehydration with a reduced metabolism, the researchers speculate that being fully hydrated will help you burn calories more efficiently.[13] Best of all, water is clean, refreshing, and calorie free!

There are many tempting types of flavored water and energy drinks on the market. Although some brands tout their vitamin and mineral content or herbal ingredients and other "healthy" extracts, many are full of sugar and have high calorie counts—in some cases more than regular soda. Plus, their nutrient levels are often remarkably low—far too low to give you the health benefits they claim. My best advice is to get your nutrients from real foods, and keep your beverages simple. And if you're really thirsty for a nutritious drink, try a smoothie (more on that later!) or a lightly flavored water, like Propel Fitness Water (only 10 calories per serving and about 2 grams of sugar).

Smart Supplements

If you're eating a healthy, well-rounded diet, you don't need to spend a lot of money on supplements. The one daily pill most of us could benefit from is a simple multivitamin that includes minerals to ensure you're getting all of the 40-plus nutrients we need each day. Here's a look at some of the key ones:

B VITAMINS: Thiamin, riboflavin, niacin, and other B vitamins are all involved in helping to break down food for energy. The more active you are, the more your body burns through them, so make sure your multivitamin contains adequate levels of these, even though many of our favorite foods (breads, cereals) are also fortified with these vitamins. Keep in mind that folate is among the B vitamins crucial for prenatal health, so if you're pregnant or planning on becoming pregnant, be sure you're getting enough of this important nutrient.

VITAMIN C: This important vitamin may help keep your immune system healthy, prevent cardiovascular disease, and even minimize wrinkles. And it may also play a role in weight loss: One study found individuals who had healthy levels of vitamin C oxidized 30 percent more fat during moderate exercise than those who had low levels of the vitamin. In addition, those whose low levels were boosted had a better workout and were more energy efficient.[14]

VITAMIN D: Your body needs vitamin D to absorb calcium and promote bone health, but it's also crucial for a number of other reasons. Low levels of vitamin D have been linked to certain cancers (including breast, colon, and prostate), heart disease, depression, and weight gain. Your body does make vitamin D after skin exposure to sunlight, but if you live in a northern climate or always slather on the sunscreen, you may not be getting all the levels you need. Five to 30 minutes of sun exposure to the face, legs, or back at least twice a week should give you enough vitamin D to keep you healthy. (If you get more than that, be sure to wear sunscreen.) Because

GOOD TO KNOW

Another very important healthy-eating tip to keep in mind: It's not just what you are eating, it's how you prepare it. Think about chicken breast: You can grill it with just a little bit of cooking spray or olive oil for about 140 calories, or bread it and fry it for 220 calories (and 9 grams of fat). That's 57 percent more calories for the same basic food! I try to prepare my own food at home, where I am in control. It tastes better, there are fewer preservatives, it's more nutritious, and it's often much cheaper than what you will find in the store. At the end of the day, your prep time will be similar, and your food fresher. My kids would rather eat a piece of seasoned, grilled chicken, some fresh-cut watermelon, and a few baby carrots than a chicken pot pie. Good habits start young!

GOOD TO KNOW

Many of my clients are completely addicted to diet soda. After all, with zero calories, how bad can it really be? Surprisingly, research is showing that artificial sweeteners may actually promote weight gain. Researchers theorize that artificial sweeteners can interfere with your metabolism and your body's ability to count calories, causing you to overeat later on. Plus, research has shown that drinking too much diet soda can have an adverse effect on bone health.[15]

Bottom line: The occasional diet drink won't do you any harm, but don't go overboard. When it comes to artificial sugars and their safety, I refer to my favorite food watchdog, the Center for Science in the Public Interest (www.cspinet.org). So far, only sucralose has earned their "safe" grade, but keep checking for the most up-to-date information on foods and additives.

vitamin D is a fat-soluble vitamin—meaning it is stored in the body instead of excreted out—getting too much of this nutrient through food or supplements can be toxic. The safe upper limit—consumed from food and supplements combined—is 2,000 IU.

CALCIUM: I talked about this important nutrient in Part II, but in addition to being vital for strong, healthy bones (especially for women), calcium also helps to control high blood pressure, reduce PMS symptoms, and may even play a role in improving weight loss. Women over the age of 18 need to get at least 1,000 milligrams of calcium a day (girls ages 9 to 18 should strive for 1,300 because they're in the key bone-building stage).

Breakfast: Start Your Day Right

I am a big believer in eating a healthy breakfast—it really is the most important meal of the day. I always have a good breakfast, which keeps me satisfied until lunch. One of my favorites is a simple fruit smoothie (frozen strawberries, protein powder, and skim milk) with a side of turkey sausage. For about 350 calories, that starts my day right!

Many people skip breakfast in the hopes of saving calories, but research has shown that skipping breakfast is actually linked to obesity, whereas eating a healthy morning meal can help successful dieters stay on track. When you don't eat breakfast, you tend to make up for it later in the day, either by eating more food at lunch or nibbling on high-calorie snacks. And other studies have shown that by eating fewer, larger meals (for example, a big lunch to make up for skipping breakfast), you'll accumulate more body fat than by eating smaller, more frequent meals. If you have kids, it's especially important to not only feed them a good breakfast, but to set a good example by eating a healthy meal yourself. Research has shown children who eat breakfast have better attention spans, recall, and happier moods the rest of the day. A study from the University of Minnesota of more than 2,000 adolescents found the more often a person ate breakfast, the less likely he or she was to be overweight or obese.[16]

The ideal breakfast follows my three-food rule: It contains a fruit or vegetable (loaded with vitamins and carbs necessary for energy), whole grains (more good carbs plus vitamin E, folate, and fiber), and protein (to keep you satisfied and aid muscle growth).

I hear lots of excuses from my clients about why they don't eat breakfast. "There isn't enough time." "Food makes me sick that early in the morning." "I don't like breakfast foods." But you might just need to rethink your traditional breakfast choices. It doesn't always have to be a bowl of cereal or eggs and toast. Think a bit outside of the box. At home, do one-half whole-wheat bagel or bread with peanut butter and jelly, or a grilled cheese sandwich with some fruit. Or have some low-fat yogurt with berries and a bit of high-fiber cereal.

If you and your family are always on the go in the morning, mix up some low-fat trail mix—cold cereal, a handful of nuts, and dried fruit—and throw it into a baggie. Or make a "breakfast taco" of low-fat melted cheese on a whole-wheat tortilla with some salsa, and roll it up. Or just grab some low-fat string cheese and a piece of fruit.

REAL TURNAROUND SUCCESS STORY
"I'm getting my body back after having twins!"
JOANN QUACKENBUSH, 42

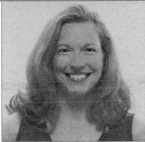

THANKS TO A STEADY exercise program through her pregnancy, JoAnn, 42, didn't have much trouble losing the baby weight after having twin boys. In fact, just a week after giving birth, she was fitting back into her non-maternity pants. The trouble, she says, came shortly thereafter. "I was so sleep deprived dealing with all of the feedings and with raising my 3-year-old daughter, plus a 16-year-old, that I just didn't have the energy to work out." Seven months later, she'd gained close to 20 pounds. "I was so proud that I had gotten through the pregnancy in such great shape, but then I just couldn't stick with it afterward."

She decided that what she needed was more structure and accountability, which she found in the 2-Week Total Body Turnaround. "I knew how to eat right and exercise, but I had trouble putting that into practice. Having everything spelled out in front of me—how much to eat, what exercises to do and for how long—made it so much easier to put those ideas into practice."

When her boys woke up at 5:00 a.m., she'd feed them, then do her strength workouts while they were awake, and later she'd get on the treadmill while they napped and her daughter played. She soon found her energy levels starting to rise. "I used to be simply exhausted by the end of the day, but now I'm still going strong until at least 10:00 p.m."

She lost almost $3\frac{1}{2}$ pounds in her first 2 weeks and a total of $6\frac{3}{4}$ inches ($1\frac{1}{2}$ inches off her waist). Since then, she's lost more weight and dropped a full size. The strength exercises have also helped reduce the pain of an old back injury. Most important, she says, is that she's discovered the necessity of putting herself first. "It's hard to get up and down off the floor with the kids when you're 20 pounds heavier! And I have a lot more energy right now to take care of my family. I've realized that I need to take care of myself in order to take care of everyone else."

Smoothies: My Quick-Fix Option

I love smoothies! You can tailor them to your own preferences and change them up depending on what you feel like that day. They make great grab-and-go breakfasts and snacks, but can also be used as a well-balanced meal replacement at any time of the day by adding some protein powder. (Kids love smoothies, too, since they look and taste like milkshakes—smoothies are also a great way to sneak more fruit into kids' diets!)

Just remember that the smoothies you make at home are a lot more nutritious (and less fattening!) than the ones you'll find at fast-food restaurants, juice bars, and coffee shops. Some of those contain the same number of calories as a Big Mac! It all goes back to the idea that "It's not what you eat, it's how it's prepared." Use fresh or frozen fruit, without any sugary syrups, to keep it low-cal—add in low-fat milk and yogurt, and you've got a delicious and nutritious treat! Kids love to slurp it through a straw.

Here's a trick: I often make up to four smoothies at once, then stick them in my freezer. And if I'm in a hurry in the morning, I'll just grab one and it will dethaw in my car within the hour.

Here are a few of my favorites:

CRAZY FOR COFFEE

1 cup brewed coffee

3 ounces vanilla fat-free yogurt

1 scoop (1 ounce) protein powder (chocolate)

9 ice cubes

1 tablespoon sugar-free hazelnut syrup

SERVINGS: 1 (3 CUPS)

PER SERVING: 184 calories, 0% calories from fat, 1 g total fat, 1 mg cholesterol, 73 mg sodium, 310 mg potassium, 21 g carbohydrates, 0 g fiber, 15 g sugar, 21 g net carbs, 25 g protein

TEA BERRY

$^1/_2$ cup frozen cherries

$^1/_2$ cup frozen strawberries

$^1/_2$ banana

1 cup green tea, brewed and chilled or bottled diet green tea

3 ounces vanilla fat-free yogurt

5 ice cubes

SERVINGS: 1 (3 CUPS)

PER SERVING: 196 calories, 3% calories from fat, 1 g total fat, 2 mg cholesterol, 71 mg sodium, 439 mg potassium, 44 g carbohydrates, 4 g fiber, 32 g sugar, 39 g net carbs, 6 g protein

CHOCOLATE-COVERED CHERRIES

$^3/_4$ cup frozen cherries

6 ounces vanilla fat-free yogurt

1 scoop (1 ounce) whey protein powder (chocolate)

$^3/_4$ cup soymilk or fat-free milk

$^1/_2$ teaspoon almond extract

6 ice cubes

1 tablespoon sliced almonds

SERVINGS: 1

PER SERVING: 352 calories, 12% calories from fat, 5 g total fat, 3 mg cholesterol, 206 mg sodium, 578 mg potassium, 44 g carbohydrates, 1 g fiber, 35 g sugar, 44 g net carbs, 33 g protein

---

WHAT OUR TEST PANELISTS TOLD US

"I didn't realize how much bad stuff I was eating until I used *Prevention*'s My Health Tracker. I always thought I ate healthy with lots of fruits and veggies. But I also ate lots of bad stuff as well without realizing how much it was adding up!"
—Maria S., 45

FEELIN' PEACHY

$1/2$ cup frozen peaches

$1/2$ cup frozen strawberries

$1/2$ banana

3 ounces vanilla fat-free yogurt

$3/4$ **cup** soymilk or fat-free milk

1 tablespoon wheat germ

$1/8$ **teaspoon** almond extract (optional)

SERVINGS: 1 (2 CUPS)

PER SERVING: 288 calories, 12% calories from fat, 4 g total fat, 1 mg cholesterol, 132 mg sodium, 792 mg potassium, 53 g carbohydrates, 5 g fiber, 37 g sugar, 49 g net carbs, 12 g protein

NUTTY BUDDY

2 tablespoons natural peanut butter

1 tablespoon slivered toasted almonds

1 tablespoon ground flaxseeds

$3/4$ **cup** frozen vanilla yogurt

$1/2$ **cup** soymilk or fat-free milk

SERVINGS: 1 ($1^{1}/_{2}$ CUPS)

PER SERVING: 545 calories, 38% calories from fat, 23 g total fat, 98 mg cholesterol, 205 mg sodium, 192 mg potassium, 61 g carbohydrates, 4 g fiber, 38 g sugar, 57 g net carbs, 24 g protein

I Love Chicken!

Chicken breasts are a great source of lean protein. They're low in fat and usually easy on the wallet. And they're like a blank canvas—you can cook them any way you want (grill, broil, sauté, poach) and add almost any spices and sauce you choose to come up with for a different flavor every time, whether Asian-inspired or Southwestern in feel. But eating the same thing day in and day out can get boring, which means you have to be a little creative in your cooking. Here are a few of my favorite ways to jazz up chicken for my family:

➤ **POUR ON THE MARINADE.** The right marinade will make your chicken tender and tasty. Experiment with different sauces you find in your local market or use low-fat salad dressings to find your favorites— Asian, Tex-Mex, lemon pepper, curried, fruity. Just watch out for marinades that are high in fat, sodium, and calories. Always be safe in the kitchen and toss any leftover marinade you already used on the raw chicken to prevent food-borne illnesses.

- **SOUTHWEST EXPRESS.** Shred a cooked chicken breast and mix with black-bean and corn salsa (you can find a commercial version of this in most supermarkets). Spread the mixture on a whole-grain tortilla and top with low-fat cheese, lettuce, and tomato.

- **CHICKEN AND THE EGG.** Making chicken for dinner? Cook an extra breast or two and refrigerate overnight, then slice up with your eggs in the morning for a double dose of protein.

- **SWORD SMART.** Thread chicken strips onto a skewer, throw them on the grill, and serve with (a little!) Thai peanut dipping sauce for chicken satay. (Kids love this!)

- **ROMAN HOLIDAY.** Cube up a cooked chicken breast and toss with some fresh cherry tomatoes, basil, and whole-wheat noodles for a healthy Italian twist.

- **SERVE UP THE SALAD.** Chicken is a great centerpiece for a healthy, protein-rich salad. Sliced, cooked chicken breasts can be mixed with any number of veggies on top of any kind of greens for a nutritious meal. Play around with different combinations. Some of my favorite add-ins include artichokes in water, shredded carrots, cherry tomatoes, mushrooms, red pepper, chickpeas, edamame, and sliced almonds.

Snack Attack

Who doesn't like to snack? We certainly have become a snack-food nation, as witnessed by the hundreds of chips, candies, and snack cakes that fill grocery store aisles. But snacks can be a dieter's best friend, provided you make some healthy choices. A good snack will satisfy a midafternoon hunger attack and keep you from feeling ravenous by the time you eat your next meal. Research has shown that eating both regular meals and snacks keeps blood sugar and insulin levels steady, so you're less like to have cravings. Plus, snacking regularly will keep you more mentally alert and prevent that midday blood sugar dip that can make you feel tired and moody.

To keep you feeling satisfied, be as smart in your snack choices as in your meals. Avoid high-sugar, processed foods and stick with clean, natural ones. High-fiber foods are generally good choices to help you feel fuller, longer. That may require a little more planning on your part, since it's hard to find fresh veggies or other healthy choices at the vending machine, so stock up on some of these new staples and enjoy!

GOOD TO KNOW

Researchers at the University of Liverpool gave 60 young adults lunches and snacks on 4 separate days. On half of their visits, the subjects chewed two sticks of gum after lunch. The subjects said they felt less hungry after chewing gum, and when they were offered treats like cookies, chips, or candy 3 hours after lunch, they ate an average of 36 fewer calories than when they didn't have the gum.[17]

Following are a few of my favorite snack ideas, most of which are about 200 calories or fewer. You'll be amazed at how satisfying they can be!

ON THE SAVORY SIDE

VEGGIES AND DIP: Cut one large cucumber, one large carrot, and a celery stalk into sticks. Mix a pouch of dry onion soup mix into a container of fat-free sour cream. Dip your veggies into ½ cup of dip, or use Dijon mustard, salsa, or hummus.

SEASONED POPCORN: This is one of my favorite snacks when I'm seeking something salty. Sprinkle 1 tablespoon of garlic salt, chili powder, or Lawry's seasoning salt over 3 cups of air-popped popcorn.

NACHOS: Sprinkle 1 tablespoon of shredded Cheddar cheese over a dozen baked tortilla chips and melt under the broiler. Add 2 tablespoons of salsa.

PITA AND HUMMUS: Cut a piece of whole-wheat pita bread into wedges and toast. Top with 1 tablespoon of garlic or red-pepper hummus.

TUNA MELT: Put ¼ cup of canned tuna and a slice of low-fat cheese on a slice of whole-wheat bread. Broil and top with chopped tomato.

CHICKPEA SALAD: Combine ½ cup of chickpeas with a chopped tomato, ½ tablespoon of olive oil, the juice of ½ lemon, and a pinch of salt and pepper.

CRACKERS AND VEGETABLE JUICE: Enjoy approximately 7 whole-wheat crackers with 1 cup of vegetable juice cocktail.

MINI BAGEL MELT: Spread 1 tablespoon of low-fat ricotta cheese over a whole-wheat mini bagel and broil. Sprinkle with fresh chives.

SWEET TREATS

RICE CAKES AND PB: Spread a thin layer (about 1 teaspoon) of peanut butter over two caramel-flavored rice cakes.

TRAIL MIX: Mix 1 tablespoon of golden raisins with ½ cup of Cheerios and 1 tablespoon of almond slivers.

MELON "SUNDAE": Combine ½ cup each of cantaloupe and honeydew melon slices. Mix in a small container of low-fat yogurt.

PEANUT BUTTER AND FRUIT: Cut an apple into 4 wedges and spread ¼ teaspoon of low-fat peanut butter over each wedge.

SMOOTHIE: Blend 1 cup of vanilla soymilk with ½ frozen banana and ½ cup of frozen strawberries. (Add a scoop of protein powder if you like.)

GRANOLA PARFAIT: Sprinkle ¼ cup of Fiber One cereal into low-fat yogurt; add a few berries.

FROZEN FRUIT: Pluck some fresh grapes off the stem and freeze. Store them in a freezer bag for up to 2 months. Or peel a banana, cut into "coins," and cover them in plastic wrap and freeze. Then eat and enjoy!

CINNAMON-BAKED APPLE: Core an apple and fill with 1 tablespoon of raisins; sprinkle with cinnamon and a touch of brown sugar. Microwave for 3 minutes or until apple is tender.

Our Test Panelists' Favorite Foods

Our test panelists loved their new, healthy food choices! Here are some of the favorite things they enjoyed while on the 2-Week Total Body Turnaround:

- Edamame
- Scrambled egg whites with salsa
- Low-fat breakfast sausage made with chicken and apples
- Popcorn
- Whole-wheat crackers
- Whole-wheat toast with peanut butter
- Fruit smoothies made with fruit, protein, milk, flax seeds, and yogurt
- Cut-up fruits and veggies
- Frozen blueberries and blackberries for smoothies
- Salads with balsamic vinegar and lots of fresh veggies
- Baked pita chips
- Organic almond and peanut butter
- Chocolate banana smoothies with skim milk and whey protein
- Spreadable light cheese (like Laughing Cow)
- Tuna salad made with light mayo and lots of chopped celery on double-fiber whole-wheat bread
- Grilled chicken or salmon and grilled asparagus
- Mashed sweet potato with cinnamon
- Veggie burgers

The FAST Track Routine

One thing you might expect over your 2 weeks is the unexpected. I know that you are committed to doing this plan in its entirety. That means fitting in both the full strength and cardio workouts each of the given days, and also keeping on track with healthy eating. But there are times for all of us when we just can't do what we set out to do. Maybe you've gotten called home to take care of a sick child, or had an unexpected deadline pop up at work. You might have hit heavy traffic on the way home, or felt a little under the weather. Whatever the case, you simply cannot squeeze in your workout plan.

With the idea that something is better than nothing, consider my FAST Track Routine your emergency workout for days when you absolutely, positively cannot make time for anything else. FAST stands for *Fitness and Strength Together*. It's only 15 minutes, but it will work all of your major muscles and get your heart rate going; plus it burns about 135 calories (based on a 150-pound person). I know you can find 15 minutes in your day to do at least a little bit of exercise. And while you will not get the same results by doing just this quickie routine, it is definitely better than nothing!

THE FAST TRACK ROUTINE

1-MINUTE WARMUP:
POWER MARCH

Walk in place, lifting knees and using arms for momentum.

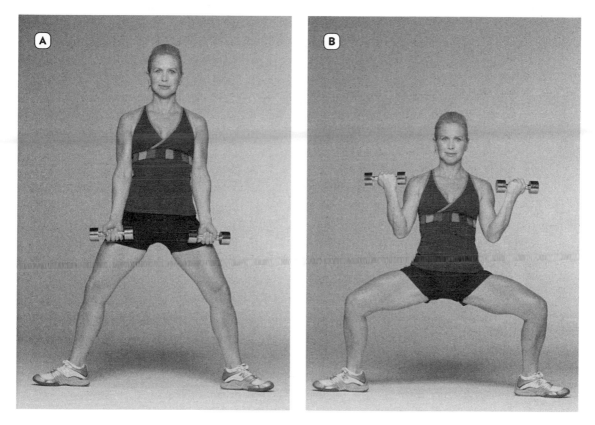

2-MINUTE STRENGTH:
PLIÉ WITH BICEPS CURL

TARGETS: Biceps, butt, quads, inner thighs

A. Stand with feet shoulder-width apart, toes turned outward, holding dumbbells in front of thighs with palms facing up.

B. Slowly lower body straight down for 2 counts, bending knees 90 degrees while simultaneously curling weights toward shoulders. Slowly stand body back up for 4 counts, squeezing butt and inner thighs as you lower arms back to starting position. Do 12 to 15 reps.

2-MINUTE CARDIO BURST:
INVISIBLE JUMP ROPE

Stand with feet hip-distance apart, arms at sides. Pretend that you are holding a jump rope with one end in each hand (of course, if you have the real thing, that will work, too!). Skip over the "rope," keeping arms close to sides and feet close to floor. Repeat for 2 minutes.

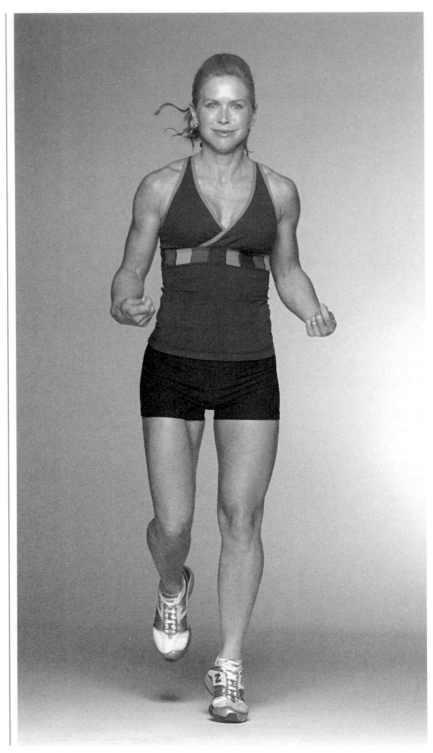

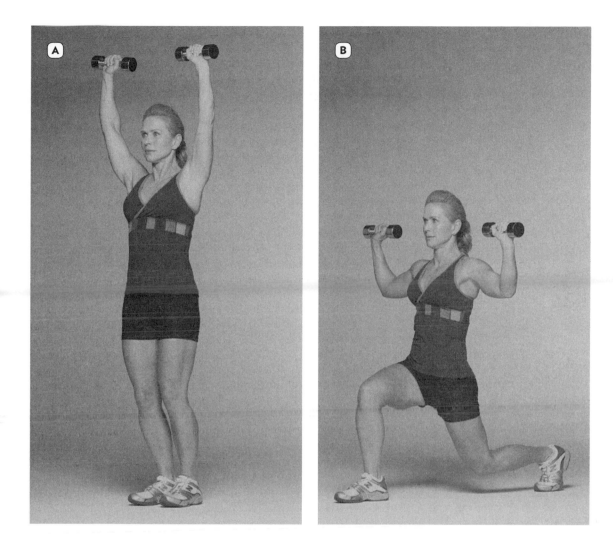

2-MINUTE STRENGTH:
FORWARD LUNGE
AND RAISE THE ROOF

TARGETS: Shoulders, quads, butt, core

A. Stand with feet together, holding dumbbells overhead, palms facing forward.

B. Lunge forward with right foot in 4 counts, bending both knees 90 degrees while lowering weights toward shoulders, bending elbows 90 degrees. Push back to starting position and straighten arms in 2 counts. Repeat 8 to 12 times; switch sides.

2-MINUTE CARDIO BURST:
JUMPING JACKS

Stand with feet together, arms at sides. Step or jump legs apart while raising arms overhead. Step or jump legs together and lower arms back down to sides. Continue for 2 minutes.

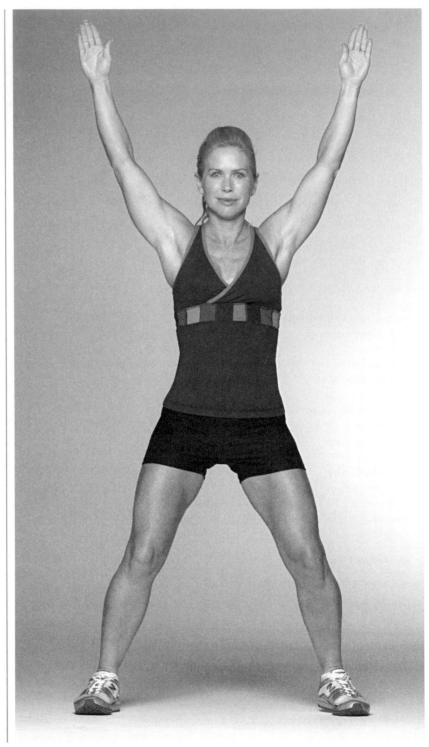

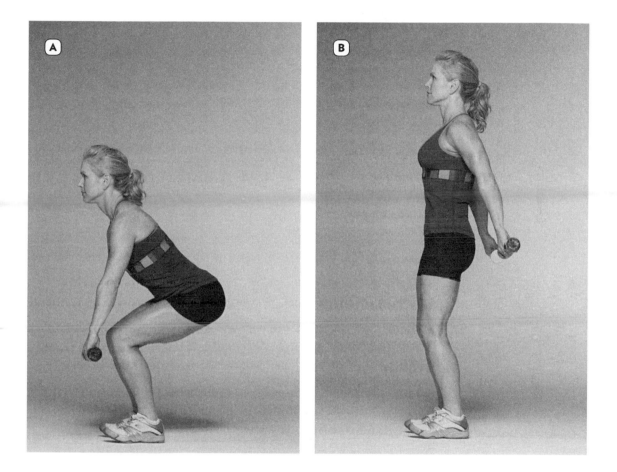

2-MINUTE STRENGTH:
SQUAT WITH
STRAIGHT ARM PRESS BACK

TARGETS: Shoulders, arms, quads, butt

A. Stand with feet about 4 inches apart, holding dumbbells at sides with palms facing behind you. Slowly lower into squat position for 4 counts, keeping weight over heels as arms move forward.

B. Stand back up in 2 counts while pressing palms behind you. Repeat 8 to 12 times.

2-MINUTE
CARDIO BURST:
STAIR
STEPPER

Stand in front of a flight of stairs or a step bench. Step up onto the first step with your right foot and then your left. Step down with your right foot, followed by your left. Switch, stepping up and down with your left foot first. Continue for 2 minutes, alternating your lead foot.

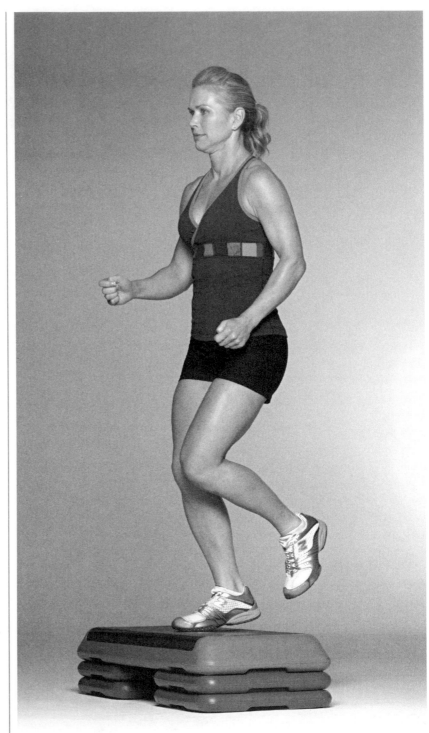

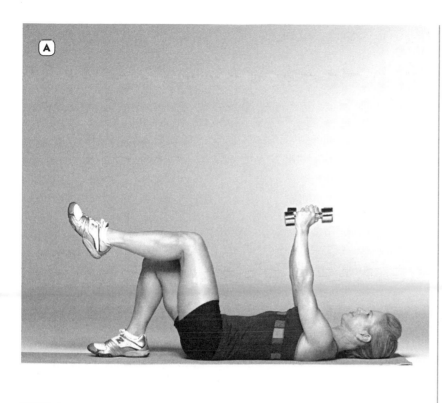

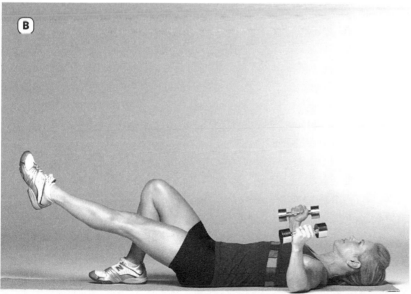

2-MINUTE STRENGTH:
BEACH BALL HUG

TARGETS: Chest, abs, hips

A. Lie face up on floor, knees bent and feet flat on floor, holding dumbbells above chest with arms extended, elbows slightly bent, palms facing each other. Lift left leg, keeping knee bent 90 degrees, shin parallel to floor.

B. Slowly lower arms out to sides in 4 counts, keeping elbows slightly bent while simultaneously "reaching" left foot out to straighten leg.

C. Pull knee back to start in 2 counts while lifting arms back above chest, squeezing your chest muscles as if you're hugging a beach ball. Repeat 8 times with left leg, then do the exercise 8 times with right leg.

NOTE: *You can do my FAST routine with any of your favorite strength moves. Just mix and match 4 moves and do a cardio burst for 2 minutes between each one. Be sure to pick exercises that target your upper body, lower body, and core.*

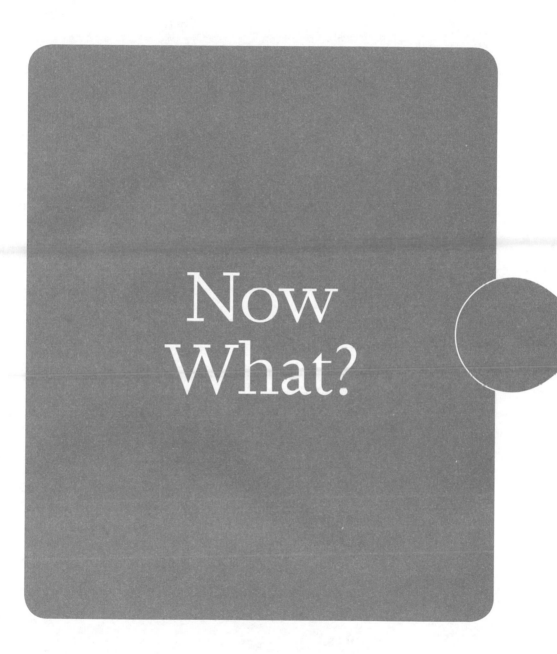

Now
What?

Shelly J., one of our testers, told us, "This 2-Week Total Body Turnaround was just the start that I needed. The single most important thing that it has taught me is that I can overcome all of the mental obstacles that block my way:

"As a mom, it's selfish to work out and take time away from the kids."

"I don't have time to do this."

"I can't get to the store, so I might as well eat the candy in the house."

"It's just one more cookie." "I worked hard today—let's eat a whole cake!"

But here's what I tell myself now:

"It's only 2 weeks. I can do anything for 2 weeks. (And then I start over every 2 weeks.)"

"Every Monday starts a new week. Start fresh."

"Weight loss is a very simple concept: It's all about calories in versus calories out."

"I need to be a leader for my family in making healthy choices."

"I work out regularly. I eat more healthfully. I watch my calories. I think more positively. I keep losing inches and weight. Hooray! Thank you!"

Take a moment, like Shelly, to think about how far you've come in a mere 14 days. Hopefully, you—like the women on our tester panel—have really changed your attitude and your lifestyle. You've helped your body get stronger and leaner. You've fueled up with smart choices and eaten "clean," getting rid of the junk that slows you down and makes you feel bloated. You've boosted your energy, lost inches and pounds, and revved your metabolism. But most importantly, you've gained confidence in yourself. You *can* do this—you've proven it to yourself in a mere 2 weeks. And here's the good news: This is just the beginning of a whole new you.

The 2-Week Total Body Turnaround was meant to be intense—a kick in the butt, a mental challenge, a contest to keep you going for 14 days. It was designed to give you the skills and tools to move forward. For the past 2 weeks, we've focused on establishing a solid base upon which to build. You've learned how to make healthy choices when it comes to buying and preparing foods. You've discovered the importance of building lean muscle, and how essential that is to keeping your body strong, healthy, and revved up. You've challenged your body aerobically and trained yourself to push through plateaus and past limits that you might not have thought possible. You've found out how important it is to move, stretch, and grow—even outside of a formal "workout."

Now that those 14 days are up, what's next?

First off, let's reflect on the past 2 weeks. What did you find out about yourself? How did you squeeze in your workouts? What food substitutions did you make? How did you find motivation when you needed it most? Take some of the lessons that you've learned over the course of the 2-Week Total Body Turnaround and make them a fundamental part of your approach to healthy living.

Here are a few things our test panelists told us they learned from doing the 2-Week Total Body Turnaround:

● **EXERCISE IN THE A.M.** Even on their crazy-busiest days, our testers say they managed to find time to exercise largely by getting up a little earlier than usual. "I found that if I don't get up early and go to the gym before work, I won't go later in the day. And it sets the right tone for me: I feel like I'm accomplishing something right away!" notes Colleen O.

● **ENLIST A PARTNER.** It's definitely easier when you have someone doing the plan right along with you. For Michele Ke., that was her husband, Joe. "He kept me going when I was tired, and I kept him going when he didn't want to exercise. We really motivated each other." Or get your kids involved. (It's a great way to teach them to be physically active and committed to a lifetime of health—a lesson you're never too young to learn!)

WHAT OUR TEST PANELISTS TOLD US

"These were my 3 Cs. Commitment: I promised myself that I would do this. Consistency: I did something every day. Convenience: I did it when I wanted to. And it worked!"
—Sue P., 57

- **GIVE IT A FEW MINUTES.** An hour a day can seem intimidating, so start small and build from there. You'll be surprised at how quickly the time will go—and often you'll naturally want to do more. "The key for me was to remind myself that I was only going for a half hour. I typically did a little more just by being out there!" says Michelle Kn.

- **TUNE INTO YOUR INTENSITY LEVELS.** "The kind of high-intensity walking workouts that were in this plan were not the kind of walking I was doing before!" says Kim R. "If you can carry on a conversation, you probably aren't walking fast enough. I used to try and read a magazine while I was on the treadmill, but I realized that if you are able to do that, it's probably not doing anything for you!"

Other testers discovered the power of using a heart-rate monitor for feedback. "It allowed me to follow the program exactly," says Maria S. "If I didn't have it on, I would have thought I was exerting myself, when in reality I wasn't hitting the higher zones. I could push myself more."

- **TRACK YOUR PROGRESS.** Almost all of our test panelists who tried *Prevention's* My Health Trackers (online at www.prevention.com/health-tracker) gave the tool a thumbs-up. "I really liked and appreciated My Health Trackers. I don't like to journal or write down what I eat, but doing it on-line with this tool made it easy and interesting," reported Barb R. Logging in what you are eating and seeing the nutritional breakdown and calorie count can make it incredibly simple to ensure you are staying on track for your eating goals.

- **EXPLORE NEW OPTIONS.** Whether it's your workout (getting on a new machine at the gym or walking on trails instead of the same neighborhood path) or your shopping list, mix things up to stay motivated. "I became an investigator at the grocery store," says Linda A. "I found myself at the meat counter, buying fresh fish, shrimp, and chicken. And I read labels: I wasn't just studying to see what I could eat for the rest of the program, but for the rest of my life."

- **EAT SMART, EVEN WHEN YOU'RE EATING OUT.** We all enjoy eating out, but a restaurant meal doesn't have to be a diet killer. "I tried to look at the menu ahead of time, and that helped me stick to healthier choices," says Colleen O. "It really surprised me how high the fat levels were on some restaurant foods," notes Maria S. "I had to make some adjustments." The same be-prepared motto also works for social engagements. "I ate plenty of fruits and vegetables before going to a party so I'd fill up, and then once I was there, I avoided the bread and chips and chose salads," reports Jane S. But most importantly, remember you're there to have a good time. "I realized that you don't have to eat to have fun at a social gathering. I could go and drink bottled water without eating the cake. No one else cared, and we all had fun!" says Sue P.

● **FORGIVE YOURSELF AND MOVE ON.** If you skip a day (or 2 or 3) of exercise, don't let it snowball. Same goes for your diet: One bad snack, or meal, or day, does not signal the beginning of the end. Remember how far you've come, and that every day is an opportunity to start fresh. "I realized that you don't have to deprive yourself completely of a 'cheat' food—just have a small amount. And if you fall off, get back on the next day!" says Tammy M.

Make Your Own Rules

I've given you a very structured program to follow for the past 2 weeks. That was the point—I wanted you to have all of the tools that you need to jumpstart your path to a healthier lifestyle. And this plan will always be here for you should you need it. But I know that eventually "real life" will interfere and that you will need to come up with your own program to keep feeling strong and healthy. So I want you to keep a few "rules" in mind.

RULE #1: YOU DON'T ALWAYS HAVE TO FOLLOW THE RULES. I've been a rule-follower my whole life. But when I first started personal training, I quickly learned that human beings don't always conform to the rules of exercise and that trying to force them into it was like trying to get my kids to make their beds every day! I've learned to get to know my clients' lifestyles and then suggest things that will work for them. And everyone is a little different.

Too often, we force ourselves to follow the rules for diet and exercise, even if they don't work in our lives. The truth is, rules don't matter if we aren't following them in the first place. If that's the case, we may be better off making our own rules. There are plenty of rules for exercise that we follow because they make sense and they keep us healthy and safe. We have heart-rate training zones to guide us so we burn fat and don't overdo it. We have strength-training rules that tell us how often to lift, how much to lift, and how to do the moves safely. We have guidelines for stretching to reduce injury and muscle soreness. But every so often, when we read exercise rules and guidelines in the media, we get overwhelmed and confused. We end up feeling defeated if they don't exactly fit in with our lives, needs, and goals. We all know that person who collects information on every diet and exercise program but follows none of them. We're all guilty of being influenced by what we read or hear without even realizing it. So do what's right for you, just as long as you do it.

RULE #2: EXERCISE WHEN IT WORKS FOR YOU. I recently got an e-mail from a woman who was desperate to lose weight. She mentioned she'd been trying for years to get up early and exercise and she'd never managed to do it. When I suggested that morning exercise wasn't right for her, she was surprised. She mentioned how I always advocate morning exercise as my favorite way to stay consistent and be more successful at weight loss. My question to her was this: "If you're not exercising in the morning now, how much weight are you losing anyway?" A calorie burned at 6:00 a.m. is the same calorie burned at 6:00 p.m. I believe in morning exercise, but when I find a client who absolutely won't go for it, then I suggest another time of day that works for them. And I must be honest, when my kids were infants, morning exercise just didn't work! I was either too tired, or feeding a baby! But then my "rules" changed as

---

REAL TURNAROUND SUCCESS STORY
"I want to avoid my family history of diabetes."
SELETA RANDLE, 45

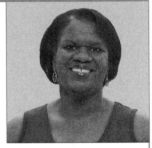

WHEN SELETA RANDLE VISITED her doctor for her annual checkup, her blood glucose levels revealed that she was on the borderline of having pre-diabetes. She knew firsthand what this devastating disease could bring: Almost all of her paternal family members had been diagnosed with diabetes. She'd lost her father to a stroke that was likely diabetes-related, and all of her father's six siblings had died from some form of the disease. And she watched a close cousin with kidney failure undergo dialysis 4 days a week.

"The day I decided to do the 2-Week Total Body Turnaround, I heard the doctor's words 'You need to lose weight' echoing in my ears," says Seleta, age 45. "At this point in my life, I still have control over what will happen, and I knew I needed to do something to make a change."

Seleta started the plan hoping to jumpstart her way to a healthier lifestyle, and perhaps drop 5 pounds in 2 weeks. After 14 days, she'd doubled that goal, losing more than 10 pounds and almost 11 inches, including more than 2 from her waist. "The first thing I noticed were that my clothes felt looser, and my face looks slimmer. I actually have some dimples in my cheeks!"

Since then, she's kept up with her exercises but modified them slightly, doing her cardio or strength sessions at least 5 days a week. She's also made changes to her diet. "I'm paying more attention to what I'm eating and trying to space things out so I never get too hungry." She's also subbing in healthier choices, like an apple instead of a cookie, when she gets the urge for sweets.

"By having the structure and variety of 2 weeks, I was able to get myself into a steady routine," she says. Having some discipline over her schedule has spilled over into other areas of her life, as well. "I'll get up earlier and do some Bible study, or do things around the house. This is the beginning of my continued life change."

my kids got older. Be wise and insightful and make changes as your life changes.

You see, what you may find is that what works for you is a little different than what you read or heard on TV. Set your schedule to work out when it is easiest for you, whether that's before the sun comes up, on your lunch hour, or right after work—or a combination of all three! Just try to set aside specific days and times for exercise, making it just as much a regular part of your schedule as everything else.

RULE #3: MIX IT UP. I've given you a structured program for exercise and eating, but there's no rule that says you can't try new things. Mix up the order of your strength and cardio. Do both moderate and vigorous intensity levels, like walking twice a week and jogging twice a week. Try new exercises—there are lots and lots out there to choose from. Experiment with using a new workout tool like a stability ball to work your core or a BOSU ball to test your balance. Swap your dumbbells for some resistance bands and see how it feels to work against that type of resistance, or if you go to a gym, ask one of the trainers who work the floor to show you how to use a machine you've never tried before. Try a new class—belly dancing, kickboxing, Latin dance, boot camp, even cardio striptease! And remember the gym itself isn't a necessity—you can get just as good a workout on your own. If you want to get the feel for a new group exercise class, try exploring a new workout DVD. Try one of our many Prevention Fitness Systems DVDs and work out with me! Or maybe enter a race to get motivated: There are thousands of races in almost every community in the country, from local 5Ks to half or full marathons everywhere from big cities like New York, Chicago, and LA to scenic locales like Big Sur, California, or Moab, Utah, to fun ones like Las Vegas and Disney World.

RULE #4: DON'T DEPRIVE YOURSELF. Cravings are completely normal. Everyone has them. And there's no more guaranteed way to have a big binge than to ignore your cravings entirely. Research from Tufts University has shown that 94 percent of dieters still have cravings, even after 6 months of being on a diet. Among the most desired: calorie-dense foods like chocolate, chips, and fries.[18] It's how often that you give into these cravings that makes a difference. Those dieters who gave into their cravings on occasion were the most successful at maintaining weight loss. So, if you must, split a small order of fries with your friend, or have a few squares of dark chocolate. Just don't go overboard, or do it too often. One of my favorite sayings: "Divide, don't deprive."

RULE #5: EVEN A LITTLE BIT COUNTS. I've advocated working out for 30 to 60 minutes on most days, but I know that just isn't practical for many of us. Just remember that no matter how busy you are, you can still

WHAT OUR TEST PANELISTS TOLD US

"The scale is my friend, and I am still heading to the gym on a daily basis when I'm home. My workout gear goes with me on business trips now and actually gets used! I want to thank you for introducing me to healthy living! I certainly don't get tired of hearing 'Boy, you really can tell you've lost weight— you look great!'"
—Linda M., 61

GOOD TO KNOW

If you enjoy working out with DVDs, visit pvtwoweekturnaround. com/TR and pick up a copy of the 2-Week Turnaround DVD series, which includes a Strength and a Cardio DVD, both featuring me. As you know, the 2-Week Total Body Turnaround program includes 30 minutes of strength training and 30 minutes of cardio every day for 6 days per week for 2 weeks. Use each DVD every day for 6 days per week while you are following the program. The exercises on the DVDs and in the book are not exactly the same but are very similar and can be used interchangeably. You can even mix it up by using both the book and the DVDs as long as you get in 30 minutes of cardio and 30 minutes of strength daily.

find little gaps of time in your day to be active. It only takes three or four 10-minute windows of time in your day to have an impact on your health. And research shows that three bouts of moderate-intensity activity accumulating in 10-minute bouts are just as effective as exercising for 30 minutes straight. So forget that all-or-nothing attitude: It doesn't work when dieting and it doesn't work when it comes to promoting activity in your life.

We all have 10-minute slots when we can be more active. For example, instead of turning on the television to catch the last 10 minutes of a show, walk around the block. Instead of waiting for a crowded elevator, take the stairs. There are always little opportunities to squeeze in some activity—you just have to be open to finding them! Wake up 10 minutes earlier and do some yoga stretches instead of hitting snooze. Speed-walk around the playground or soccer field or do some lunges while you watch your kids instead of sitting on the park bench or your lawn chair. Ideally, you'll find a 10-minute slot in the morning, another in the afternoon, and a third in the evening to keep your metabolism revved up all day. Or try to get in 20 minutes in the morning and 10 more after dinner. It can make a big difference!

Moving On: The 2-Week Total Body Turnaround Maintenance Plan

Millions of people with the best intentions try some of the craziest workouts out there, only to find they're impractical, too hard to follow, and sometimes unsafe. Inevitably, they'll drop out and feel like failures—which leads to unhealthy eating and weight gain until another gimmick comes along.

I don't want that to happen to you. You have come so far in the past 2 weeks, and you've started to build a firm foundation for the rest of your life. I know these 14 days have been hard and have involved some sacrifice and struggle on your part. But it's also been a launching point to help propel you forward into a lifestyle that works. Whether you realize it or not, you have been learning how to make changes on a behavioral level. Reading some tips on a Web site or in a newspaper can be helpful, but it's often not enough to enforce healthy habits. What you have done for the past 14 days has been to dig into your inner layers of behaviors and psyche in order to elicit long-term change. Constantly reminding yourself about eating right and exercising can help cement those healthy habits for good!

And remember, this book is here for you anytime you need it. If weight loss is a continued goal, you might want to opt in completely for another 2 weeks, and 2 weeks after that, until you feel you're approaching your goal.

But even if you're modifying the plan or moving into the maintenance phase, I want you to keep thinking of your workout and eating plans in 2-week blocks. As you've discovered, small increments are much more doable mentally than taking huge steps. I recommend keeping to the 2-week theme. Set small goals for yourself for the next 2 weeks, and then the 2 weeks after that, and so on. And if you hit another plateau or you need another jumpstart—or if you have a big event coming up that you want to prepare for, go back to your 2-Week Total Body Turnaround!

I've designed this maintenance program for normal, busy people. It's a 20- to 30-minute cardio workout, done 3 to 5 days a week, plus 2 strength-training workouts a week.

For the cardio workouts, pick an activity that you know that you like and that you will do. For many of us, that means walking. And if that's worked for you before, great! Just remember to keep your intensity levels at a point of slight breathlessness, or a "6 to 7" on a scale of 1 to 10, if you're going for a solid 30-minute power walk. And don't forget to do your intervals. Try to do at least 2 cardio interval days a week, where you're alternating bursts of intensity with recovery. Use the interval workouts on the plan or try different levels of intensity to recovery. But keep in mind you have to really push those intensity bursts to get results, so power walk up the hills, climb stairs, or take it up to a jog if you can. You can even do what's called speed play, where you walk as fast as you can to a lamppost on the next block, or toward the next stop sign.

Keep the idea of "Motivation Monday" in mind: Remember you have 52 opportunities every year to make fitness count, so try to always do at least one of your workouts on a Monday. It will make you feel like you are starting the week off right. Then either double up your fitness and strength one day so you have a free "active" day the next, or just do them back-to-back over the course of the week.

WHAT OUR TEST PANELISTS TOLD US

"Here's what I loved about this plan: It wasn't a 'Get a perfect body in 2 weeks' diet or an 'Exercise your way to a beach body in 14 days' fitness plan. It was like a toolbox for a total life makeover. It brought together the mental, physical, nutrition—everything you need to change not just your body, but your mind. And as a side effect: It changes your life. How can you go back when you have felt this good? You can't!"
—**Linda A., 40**

Your Sample 2-Week Maintenance Program

DAY	CARDIO	STRENGTH
1	30 min.	None.
2	20 min.	**Lower body.** Pick one of the lower-body workouts from the 2-Week Total Body Turnaround, mix and match, or add on some moves of your own. Add the make-it-harder variations if possible.
3	Active rest day	
4	20 min.	**Total body.** Pick one of the total-body workouts from the 2-Week Total Body Turnaround, mix and match, or add on some moves of your own. Add the make-it-harder variations if possible.
5	30 min.	None.
6	Active rest day	
7	Choice: Do the cardio or strength routine of your choosing, or do a combo day where you do a few minutes of cardio in the morning and some strength moves at night (or try the FAST Track Routine on starting page 361 to combine both in one efficient workout).	
8	30 min.	None.
9	20 min.	**Upper body.** Pick one of the upper-body workouts from the 2-Week Total Body Turnaround, mix and match, or add on some moves of your own. Add the make-it-harder variations if possible.
10	Active rest day	
11	20 min.	**Total body.** Pick one of the total-body workouts from the 2-Week Total Body Turnaround, mix and match, or add on some moves of your own. Add the make-it-harder variations if possible.
12	30 min.	None.
13	Active rest day	
14	Choice: Do the cardio or strength routine of your choosing, or do a combo day where you do a few minutes of cardio in the morning and some strength moves at night (or try the FAST Track Routine starting on page 361 to combine both in one efficient workout).	

Remember that these workout times are just my minimum recommendation. More is always better. Most of us have movement engineered out of our lives: We ride to work, sit at a desk, and shop online. We have remote controls for almost all electronics so we don't have to stand up to change the TV or radio. The more you move, the better you'll feel! So if you have more time, crank your cardio up to 45 minutes or an hour, or add an extra workout on your "recovery" day. It doesn't have to be a formal at-the-gym session: Take a swim with your kids, go skating at the rink, or get on your bicycle and run your errands. And remember to mix up your strength routines with new moves and challenges to keep your muscles from hitting a plateau.

So now you may be asking yourself, "Where do I go from here?" I created this program to be a makeover for you, inside and out. By reprogramming your mind, you've started to change your body. What results do you want to continue to achieve? Do you want to take inches off your body? Lose pounds? Improve your body image? Boost your energy, your productivity, and your relationships? Health is not just about looking good—it's about the whole person, and being the healthiest you can be. As Eleanor Roosevelt said, "In the long run, we shape our lives, and we shape ourselves. The process never ends until we die. And the choices we make are ultimately our responsibility." The 2-Week Total Body Turnaround is about taking charge of your health—so keep going, you've earned it!

REAL TURNAROUND SUCCESS STORY
"I've reduced my insane stress levels."
STEPHANIE TEIG, 42

STEPHANIE'S NERVES WERE PUSHED to the breaking point. In the span of just a few months, she lost her grandmother, a cousin, some friends, and her ex-father-in-law. Then her father-in law committed suicide. Pile on two mortgages, chronic health concerns, a stressful job with a 40-mile commute each way, and four kids (8-year-old twins, an 11-year-old, and a 15-year-old), and it's no surprise the 42-year-old could barely find time to make a healthy meal, let alone exercise. She gained about 10 to 15 pounds and found herself in constant pain from her fibromyalgia, 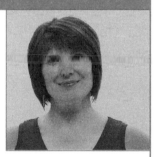 which she suffered since being in a bad car accident nearly 20 years ago. "I'd completely put myself on the back burner, and I was paying for it."

Almost immediately after starting the plan, she says, she felt her stress levels diminish. "I really took the time to focus on myself, and starting in the middle of the first week, my energy just kicked in. Both the cardio and strength workouts felt easier, so I could push myself harder." And her chronic pain began to diminish. After years of taking a low-dose muscle relaxant to help her sleep, she found herself able to cut back on the medication. Sleeping better at night helped as well. After a week, she says, her daughter, husband, and some co-workers were all commenting that they could see a difference. By the end of the 2 weeks, she'd lost nearly 4$\frac{1}{2}$ pounds and almost 9 inches.

"I wondered if the things I learned in the plan would become a habit once the 2 weeks were up, and to my surprise they really have," she says. "I'm not exercising quite as much, but I'm much more consistent than before. If I miss more than a couple of days of exercise, I find I'm really craving it."

Best of all, she says, she feels the change is permanent. "I feel like I'm back in control of my health. There's a long road ahead, but I'm excited to see what's around the next bend."

END NOTES

PART I

1. Audrey Cross, Patricia Peretz, Miguel Munoz-LaBoy, Ian Lapp, Donna Shelley, Allan Rosenfield, and Sidney Lerner, "Monday—A Social Framework to Enhance Health Promotion Efforts and Facilitate Sustainable Health Behavior Change," (White Paper, Columbia University Mailman School of Public Health), October 2006.

2. Suzanne C. Segerstrom, Shelley E. Taylor, Margaret E. Kemeny, and John L. Fahey, "Optimism Is Associated with Mood, Coping, and Immune Change in Response to Stress," *Journal of Personality and Social Psychology* 74, no. 6 (1998): 1646–55.

3. Faryle Nothwehr and Jingzhen Yang, "Goal Setting Frequency and the Use of Behavioral Strategies Related to Diet and Physical Activity," *Health Education Research* 22, no. 4 (August 2007): 532–38.

4. M. B. Zemel, J. Richards, A. Milstead, and P. Campbell, "Effects of Calcium and Dairy on Body Composition and Weight Loss in African-American Adults," *Obesity Research* 13, no. 7 (July 2005): 1218–25.

5. M. B. Zemel, W. Thompson, A. Milstead, K. Morris, and P. Campbell, "Calcium and Dairy Acceleration of Weight and Fat Loss during Energy Restriction in Obese Adults," *Obesity Research* 12, no. 4 (April 2004): 582–90.

6. J. O. Prochaska and W. F. Velicer, "The Transtheoretical Model of Health Behavior Change," *American Journal of Health Promotion* 12 (1997): 38–48.

7. Noël C. Barengo, Gang Hu, Timo A. Lakkaa, Heikki Pekkarinen, Aulikki Nissinen, and Jaakko Tuomilehto, "Low Physical Activity as a Predictor for Total and Cardiovascular Disease Mortality in Middle-Aged Men and Women in Finland," *European Heart Journal* 25, no. 24 (2004): 2204–221.

8. S. E. Sherman, R. B. D'Agostino, J. L. Cobb et al, "Physical Activity and Mortality in Women in the Framingham Heart Study," *American Heart Journal* 128, no. 5 (1994): 879–84.

9. Wayne Westcott, *Strength, Fitness, Physiological Principles and Training Techniques, 3rd edition.* William C. Brown, 1991, 74–75.

10. Wayne L. Westcott and Richard A. Winette, "Applying the ACSM Guidelines," *Fitness Management* (February 2006): 40–43.

11. Ibid.

12. P. C. Hilliard-Robertson, S. M. Schneider, S. L. Bishop, and M. E. Guilliams, "Strength Gains Following Different Combined Concentric and Eccentric Exercise Regimens," *Aviation, Space, and Environmental Medicine* 74, no. 4 (April 2003): 342–47.

13. T. Hortobágyi and P. DeVita, "Favorable Neuromuscular and Cardiovascular Responses to 7 Days of Exercise with an Eccentric Overload in Elderly Women," *Journals of Gerontology Series A: Biological Sciences and Medical Sciences* 55, no. 8 (August 2000): B401–10.

14. D. B. Hollander, R. R. Kraemer, M. W. Kilpatrick, Z. G. Ramadan, G. V. Reeves, M. Francois, E. P. Hebert, and J. L. Tryniecki, "Maximal Eccentric and Concentric Strength Discrepancies between Young Men and Women for Dynamic Resistance Exercise," *Journal of Strength and Conditioning Research* 21, no. 1 (February 2007): 34–40.

15. S. M. Nickols-Richardson, L. E. Miller, D. F. Wootten, W. K. Ramp, and W. G. Herbert, "Concentric and Eccentric Isokinetic Resistance Training Similarly Increases Muscular Strength, Fat-Free Soft Tissue Mass, and Specific Bone Mineral Measurements in Young Women," *Osteoporosis International* 18, no. 6 (June 2007): 789–96.

16. Timothy W. Puetz, Sara S. Flowers, and Patrick J. O'Connor, "A Randomized Controlled Trial

of the Effect of Aerobic Exercise Training on Feelings of Energy and Fatigue in Sedentary Young Adults with Persistent Fatigue," *Journal of Psychotherapy and Psychosomatics* 77, no. 3 (March 2008): 167–74.

17. W. L. Westcott, R. A. Winett, E. S. Anderson, J. R. Wojcik, R. L. Loud, E. Cleggett, and S. Glover, "Effects of Regular and Slow Speed Resistance Training on Muscle Strength," *Journal of Sports Medicine and Physical Fitness* 41, no. 2 (June 2001): 154–58.

18. B. A. Dolezal, J. A. Potteiger, D. J. Jacobsen, and S. H. Benedict, "Muscle Damage and Resting Metabolic Rate after Acute Resistance Exercise with an Eccentric Overload," *Medicine and Science in Sports and Exercise* 32, no. 7 (2000): 1202–7.

19. M.D. Schuenke, R. P. Mikat, and J. M. McBride, "Effect of an Acute Period of Resistance Exercise on Excess Post-Exercise Oxygen Consumption: Implications for Body Mass Management," *European Journal of Applied Physiology* 86, no. 5 (March 2002): 411–17.

20. "Exercise Walking Remains No. 1 as Fitness Activities Continue Participation Domination in 2007." April 2008. www.nsga.org.

21. Diabetes Prevention Program Research Group, "Reduction in the Incidence of Type 2 Diabetes with Lifestyle Intervention or Metformin," *New England Journal of Medicine* 346 (2002): 393–403.

22. Mark Hamer, Emmanual Stamatakis, and Andrew Steptoe, "Dose Response Relationship between Physical Activity and Mental Health: The Scottish Health Survey," *British Journal of Sports Medicine* (April 10, 2008).

23. Holly R. Wyatt, Suzanne Phelan, Rena R. Wing, and James O. Hill, "Lessons from Patients Who Have Successfully Maintained Weight Loss," *Obesity Management* 1, no. 2 (April 1, 2005): 56–61.

24. K. Ohkawara, S. Tanaka, M. Miyachi, K. Ishikasa-Takata, and I. Tabata, "A Dose-Response Relation between Aerobic Exercise and Visceral Fat Reduction: Systemic Review of

Clinical Trials," *International Journal of Obesity* 31 (2007): 1786–97.

25. J. L. Talanian, S. D. Galloway, G. J. Heigenhauser, A. Bonen, and L. L. Spriet, "Two Weeks of High-Intensity Aerobic Interval Training Increases the Capacity for Fat Oxidation during Exercise in Women," *Journal of Applied Physiology* 102, no. 4 (April 2007): 1439–47.

26. E. G. Trapp, D. J. Chisholm, J. Freund, and S. H. Boutcher, "The Effects of High-Intensity Intermittent Exercise Training on Fat Loss and Fasting Insulin Levels of Young Women," *International Journal of Obesity* 32 (2008): 684–91.

27. K. A. Burgomaster, S. C. Hughes, G. J. Heigenhauser, S. N. Bradwell, and M. J. Gibala, "Six Sessions of Sprint Interval Training Increases Muscle Oxidative Potential and Cycle Endurance Capacity in Humans," *Journal of Applied Physiology* 98, no. 6 (June 2005): 1985–90.

28. Anne McTiernan, Charles Kooperberg, Emily White, Sara Wilcox, Ralph Coates, Lucile L. Adams-Campbell, Nancy Woods, and Judith Ockene, "Recreational Physical Activity and the Risk of Breast Cancer in Postmenopausal Women," *Journal of American Medical Association* 290 (September 10, 2003): 1331–36.

29. JoAnn E. Manson, MD, DrPH; Frank B. Hu, MD, PhD; Janet W. Rich-Edwards, ScD; Graham A. Colditz, MD, DrPH; Meir J. Stampfer, MD, DrPH; Walter C. Willett, MD, DrPH; Frank E. Speizer, MD; and Charles H. Hennekens, MD, DrPH. "A Prospective Study of Walking as Compared with Vigorous Exercise in the Prevention of Coronary Heart Disease in Women." 341, no. 9 (August 26, 1999):650–58.

30. Mark Rakobowchuk, Sophie Tanguay, Kirsten A. Burgomaster, Krista R. Howarth, Martin J. Gibala, and Maureen J. MacDonald, "Sprint Interval and Traditional Endurance Training Induce Similar Improvements in Peripheral Arterial Stiffness and Flow-Mediated Dilation in Healthy Humans," *American Journal of Physiology:*

Regulatory, Integrative & Comparative Physiology 295 (July 2008): R236–42.

31. C. A. Vella and L. Kravitz, "Exercise After burn: A Research Update," *IDEA Fitness Journal* 1, no. 5 (2004): 42–47.

32. L. Kravitz, "Fat Facts," *IDEA Fitness Journal* 4, no. 8 (2007): 23–25.

33. John M. Jakicic, Kristine Clark, Ellen Coleman, Joseph E. Donnelly, John Foreyt, Edward Melanson, Jeff Volek and Stella L. Volpe. "ACSM Position Stand on the Appropriate Intervention Strategies for Weight Loss and Prevention of Weight Regain for Adults," *Medicine and Science in Sports and Exercise* 33, no. 12 (2001): 2145–56.

34. P. E. Alcaraz, J. Sánchez-Lorente, and A. J. Blazevich, "Physical Performance and Cardiovascular Responses to an Acute Bout of Heavy Resistance Circuit Training versus Traditional Strength Training," *Journal of Strength and Conditioning Research* 22, no. 3 (May 2008): 667–71.

35. M. Argevaren, G. Aufdemkampe, H.J. Verhaar, A. Aleman, L. Vanhees, "Physical activity and enhanced fitness to improve cognitive function in older people without known cognitive impairment." Cochrane Database Syst Rev. 2008 April 16, (2): CD005381.

36. N. Hamlyn, D. G. Behm, and W. B. Young, "Trunk Muscle Activation during Dynamic Weight-Training Exercises and Isometric Instability Activities," *Journal of Strength and Conditioning Research* 21, no. 4 (November 2007): 1108–12.

37. J. W. Bellew, P. C. Fenter, B. Chelette, R. Moore, and D. Loreno, "Effects of a Short-Term Dynamic Balance Training Program in Healthy Older Women," *Journal of Geriatric Physical Therapy* 28, no. 1 (2005): 4–8, 27.

38. M. J. Drummond, P. R. Vehrs, G. B. Schaaljeand, and A. C. Parcell, "Aerobic and Resistance Exercise Sequence Affects Excess Postexercise Oxygen Consumption," *Journal of Strength and Conditioning Research* 19, no. 2 (May 2005): 332–37.

39. Malachy P. McHugh, Declan A. J. Connolly, Roger G. Eston, Ian J. Kremenic, Stephen J. Nicholas, and Gilbert W. Gleim, "The Role of Passive Muscle Stiffness in Symptoms of Exercise-Induced Muscle Damage," *American Journal of Sports Medicine* 27 (September 1999): 594–99.

40. Christin Heidemann, Matthias B. Schulze, Oscar H. Franco, Rob M. van Dam, Christos S. Mantzoros, and Frank B. Hu, "Dietary Patterns and Risk of Mortality from Cardiovascular Disease, Cancer, and All Causes in a Prospective Cohort of Women," *Circulation* 118 (July 2008): 230–37.

41. Carol S. Johnston, "Strategies for Healthy Weight Loss: From Vitamin C to the Glycemic Response," *Journal of the American College of Nutrition* 24, no. 3 (2005): 158–65.

PART II

1. A. R. Skov, S. Toubro, B. Ronn, L. Holm, and A. Astrup, "Randomized Trial on Protein vs Carbohydrate in Ad Libitumfat Reduced Diet for the Treatment of Obesity," *International Journal of Obesity and Related Metabolic Disorders* 23 (1999): 528–36.

2. Douglas Paddon-Jones, Eric Westman, Richard D. Mattes, Robert R. Wolfe, Arne Astrup, and Margriet Westerterp-Plantenga, "Protein, Weight Management, and Satiety," *American Journal of Clinical Nutrition* 87, supplement (2008): 1558S–61S.

3. L. J. Appel, T. J. Moore, E. Obarzanek, et al., "A Clinical Trial of the Effects of Dietary Patterns on Blood Pressure. DASH Collaborative Research Group," *New England Journal of Medicine* 336, no. 16 (April 17, 1997): 1117–24.

4. "Osteoporosis: Fast Facts," National Osteoporosis Foundation, www.nof.org/osteoporosis/diseasefacts.htm (accessed October 31, 2008).

5. M.B. Zemel, W. Thompason, A. Milstead, K. Morris, and P. Campbell, "Calcium and Dairy Acceleration of Weight and Fat Loss during Energy Restriction in Obese Adults," *Obesity Research* 12 (2004): 582–90.

6. James A. Levine, Lorraine M. Lanningham-Foster, Shelly K. McCrady, Alisa C. Krizan, Leslie R. Olson, Paul H. Kane, Michael D. Jensen, and Matthew M. Clark, "Interindividual Variation in Posture Allocation: Possible Role in Human Obesity," *Science* 307, no. 5709 (January 28, 2005): 584–86.

7. Darcy L. Johannsen, Gregory J. Welk, Rick L. Sharp, and Paul J. Flakoll, "Differences in Daily Energy Expenditure in Lean and Obese Women: The Role of Posture Allocation," *Obesity* 16 (December 18, 2007): 34–39.

8. Lauren A Greene. "The Real Life Way to Lose," *Prevention* 60, no. 6 (June 2008): 133–36.

9. C. S. Johnston, P. D. Swan, and C. Corte, "Substrate Utilization and Work Efficiency during Submaximal Exercise in Vitamin C Depleted-Repleted Adults," *International Journal for Vitamin and Nutrition Research* 69 (1999): 41–44.

10. H. R. Wyatt, O. K. Grunwald, C. L. Mosca, M. L. Klem, R. R. Wing, and J. O. Hill, "Long-Term Weight Loss and Breakfast in Subjects in the National Weight Control Registry," *Obesity Research* 10, no. 2 (2002): 78–82.

11. J. S. Vander Wal, A. Gupta, P. Khosla, and N. V. Dhurandhar, "Egg Breakfast Enhances Weight Loss," *International Journal of Obesity* 32, no. 10 (October 2008): 1545-51.

12. J. S. Vander Wal, J. M. Marth, P. Khosla, K. L. Jen, and N. V. Dhurandhar, "Short-Term Effect of Eggs on Satiety in Overweight and Obese Subjects," *Journal of the American College of Nutrition* 24, no. 6 (December 2005): 510–15.

13. M. A, Wien, J. M. Sabaté, D. N. Iklé, S. E. Cole, and F. R. Kandeel, "Almonds *vs* Complex Carbohydrates in a Weight Reduction Program," *International Journal of Obesity* 27 (2003): 1365–72.

14. J. A. de La Paniagua, I. Romero, A. Vidal-Puig, J. M. Latre, E. Sanchez, P. Perez-Martinez, J. Lopez-Miranda, and F. Perez-Jimenez, "Monounsaturated Fat-Rich Diet Prevents Central Body Fat Distribution and Decreases Postprandial Adiponectin Expression Induced by a Carbohydrate-Rich Diet in Insulin-Resistant Subjects," *Diabetes Care* 30, no. 7 (July 1, 2007): 1717–23.

15. R. López Ledesma, A. C. Frati Munari, B. C. Hernández Domínguez, S. Cervantes Montalvo, M. H. Hernández Luna, C. Juárez, S. Morán Lira, "Monounsaturated Fatty Acid (Avocado) Rich Diet for Mild Hypercholesterolemia," *Archives of Medical Research* 27, no. 4 (Winter 1996): 519–23.

16. M. Conceição de Oliveira, R. Sichieri, and Moura A. Sanchez, "Weight Loss Associated with a Daily Intake of Three Apples or Three Pears among Overweight Women," *Nutrition* 19, no. 3 (March 2003): 253–56.

17. Julie Flood, "Apple Consumption and Calorie Control" (study presented at the Obesity Society annual meeting, New Orleans, Louisiana, October 23, 2007).

18. V. Nguyen, J. Brosnahan, A. Summers, R. Alvarado, D. Knapp, T. Angeopoulous, and J. Ripp, "Oatmeal as Part of a Healthy Weight-Loss Program" (study presented at the North American Association for the Study of Obesity, October 23, 2006).

19. C. M. Alper and R. D. Mattes, "Effects of Chronic Peanut Consumption on Energy Balance and Hedonics," *International Journal of Obesity* 26, no. 8 (August 2002): 1129–37.

20. C. R. Richardson, T. L. Newton, J. J. Abraham, A. Sen, M. Jimbo, and A. M. Swartz, "A Meta-Analysis of Pedometer-Based Walking Interventions and Weight Loss," *Annals of Family Medicine* 6, no. 1 (January-February 2008): 69–77.

21. S. A. Clemes, N. Matchett, and S. L. Wane, "Reactivity: An Issue for Short-Term Pedometer Studies?," *British Journal of Sports Medicine* 42, no. 1 (2008): 68–70.

22. J. Porcari, "Do You Do 10K a Day?," *ACE Fitness Matters* 12, no. 4 (July/August 2006): 9–12.

23. K. Zahour and J. Porcari, "Casual Day Equals Boosted Calorie Burn," *ACE Fitness Matters* 10, no. 4: 7–9.

24. Sid Kirchheimer, "Coffee: The New Health Food?," WebMd, http://men.webmd.com/features/coffee-new-health-food (accessed October 20, 2008).

25. Eduardo Salazar-Martinez, Walter C. Willett, Alberto Ascherio, JoAnn E. Manson, Michael F. Leitzmann, Meir J. Stampfer, and Frank B. Hu, "Coffee Consumption and Risk for Type 2 Diabetes Mellitus," *Annals of Internal Medicine* 140, no. 1 (January 6, 2004): 1–8.

26. K. J. Lee, M. Inoue, T. Otani, M. Iwasaki, S. Sasazuki, and S. Tsugane, JPHC Study Group, "Coffee Consumption and Risk of Colorectal Cancer in a Population-Based Prospective Cohort of Japanese Men and Women," *International Journal of Cancer* 121, no. 6 (September 15, 2007): 1312–18.

27. B. Sökmen, L. E. Armstrong, W. J. Kraemer, D. J. Casa, J. C. Dias, D. A. Judelson, and C. M. Maresh, "Caffeine Use in Sports: Considerations for the Athlete," *Journal of Strength and Conditioning Research* 22, no. 3 (May 2008): 978–86.

28. S. C. Segerstrom and L. Solberg Nes, "Heart Rate Variability Reflects Self-Regulatory Strength, Effort, and Fatigue," *Psychological Science* 18, no. 3 (2007): 275–81.

29. S. R. Bray, et al., "Effects of Self-Regulatory Strength Depletion on Muscular Performance and EMG Activation," *Psychophysiology* 45 (2008): 337–43.

30. John L. Ivy, Harold W. Goforth Jr., Bruce M. Damon, Thomas R. McCauley, Edward C. Parsons, and Thomas B. Price, "Early Postexercise Muscle Glycogen Recovery Is Enhanced with a Carbohydrate-Protein Supplement," *Journal of Applied Physiology* 93, no. 4 (October 2002): 1337–44.

31. V. S. Pereira Panza, E. Wazlawik, G. R. Schutz, L. Comin, K. C. Hecht, and E. L. da Silva, "Consumption of Green Tea Favorably Affects Oxidative Stress Markers in Weight-Trained Men," *Nutrition* 24, no. 5 (May 2008): 433–42.

32. Andrew Steptoe, E. Leigh Gibson, Raisa Vounonvirta, Emily D. Williams, Mark Hamer, Jane A. Rycroft, Jorge D. Erusalimsky, and Jane Wardle, "The Effects of Tea on Psychophysiological Stress Responsivity and Post-Stress Recovery: A Randomised Double-Blind Trial," *Psychopharmacology* 190, no. 1 (January 2007): 81–89.

PART III

1. Henning Boecker, Till Sprenger, Mary E. Spilker, Gjermund Henriksen, Marcus Koppenhoefer, Klaus J. Wagner, Michael Valet, Achim Berthele, and Thomas R. Tolle, "The Runner's High: Opioidergic Mechanisms in the Human Brain," *Cerebral Cortex* (February 21, 2008).

2. S. Ahmaidi, P. Granier, Z. Taoutaou, J. Mercier, H. Dubouchaud, and C. Prefaut, "Effects of Active Recovery on Plasma Lactate and Anaerobic Power Following Repeated Intensive Exercise," *Medicine and Science in Sports and Exercise* 28, no. 4 (April 1996): 450–56.

3. J. R. Karp, J. D. Johnston, S. Tecklenburg, T. D. Mickleborough, A. D. Fly, and J. M. Stager, "Chocolate Milk as a Post-Exercise Recovery Aid," *International Journal of Sport Nutrition and Exercise Metabolism* 16, no. 1 (February 2006): 78–91.

4. L. A. Frey Law, S. Evans, J. Knudtson, S. Nus, K. Scholl, and K. A. Sluka, "Massage Reduces Pain Perception and Hyperalgesia in Experimental Muscle Pain: A Randomized, Controlled Trial," *Journal of Pain* 9, no. 8 (August 2008): 714–21.

5. Zainal Zainuddin, Mike Newton, Paul Sacco, and Kazunori Nosaka, "Effects of Massage on Delayed-Onset Muscle Soreness, Swelling, and Recovery of Muscle Function," *Journal of Athletic Training* 40, no. 3 (July-September 2005): 174–80.

6. C. Carroll and T. Trappe, "Ibuprofen or Acetaminophen in Long-Term Resistance Training Increases Muscle Mass/Strength" (paper presented at the Experimental Biology

Conference, Federation of American Societies for Experimental Biology, San Diego, CA, 2008).

7. J. P. Chaput, J. P. Després, C. Bouchard, and A. Tremblay, "The Association between Sleep Duration and Weight Gain in Adults: A 6-Year Prospective Study from the Quebec Family Study," *Sleep* 31, no. 4 (April 1, 2008): 517–23.

8. American Academy of Sleep Medicine, "Extra Sleep Improves Athletic Performance," *ScienceDaily* (June 10, 2008), http://www. sciencedaily.com/releases/2008/06/08060907 1106.htm (accessed October 9, 2008).

9. Veronica Araya, "Aerobic Exercise Increases a Blood Protein That May Suppress Appetite" (paper presented at the Endocrine Society's 90th annual meeting, San Francisco, CA, June 17, 2008), http://www.endo-society.org/ media/ENDO-08/research/Aerobic-exercise-increases-a-blood-protein.cfm (accessed October 30, 2008).

10. S. D. Simpson and C. I. Karageorghis, "The Effects of Synchronous Music on 400-m Sprint Performance," *Journal of Sports Science* 24, no. 10 (October 2006): 1095–102.

11. Jo M. Welch, Katherine A. Kellner, Nina C. Laroche, Matthew J. MacCormick, Kathleen F. MacLean, and James A. Hemeon, "Motivational Music During Resistance Training Improves Strength Endurance" (paper presented at the American College of Sports Medicine annual conference, Indianapolis, IN, May 2008).

12. Jack F. Hollis, Christina M. Gullion, Victor J. Stevens, Phillip J. Brantley, Lawrence J. Appel, et al., "Weight Loss during the Intensive Intervention Phase of the Weight-Loss Maintenance Trial," *American Journal of Preventive Medicine* 35, no. 2 (August 2008): 118–26.

13. E. Wayne Askew, "Is Eight Enough? U Researcher Says Drink Up and Tells Why" (University of Utah University Health Care Media Center, Salt Lake City, UT, January 14, 2003). http://healthcare.utah.edu/publicaffairs/ news/archive/2003/news_74.html

14. Carol Johnston, "Strategies for Healthy Weight Loss: From Vitamin C to the Glycemic Response," *Journal of the American College of Nutrition* 24, no. 3 (2005): 158–65.

15. S. E. Swithers and T. L. Davidson, "A Role for Sweet Taste: Calorie Predictive Relations in Energy Regulation by Rats," *Behavioral Neuroscience* 122, no. 1 (February 2008): 161–73.

16. M. T. Timlin, M. A. Pereira, M. Story, and D. Neumark-Sztainer, "Breakfast Eating and Weight Change in a 5-Year Prospective Analysis of Adolescents: Project EAT (Eating Among Teens)," *Pediatrics* 121, no. 3 (March 2008): e638–45.

17. Marion M. Hetherington and Emma Boyland, "Short-Term Effects of Chewing Gum on Snack Intake and Appetite," *Appetite* 48, no. 3 (May 2007): 397–401.

18. C. H. Gilhooly, S. K. Das, J. K. Golden, M. A. McCrory, G. E. Dallal, E. Saltzman, F. M. Kramer, and S. B. Roberts, "Food Cravings and Energy Regulation: The Characteristics of Craved Foods and Their Relationship with Eating Behaviors and Weight Change during 6 Months of Dietary Energy Restriction," *International Journal of Obesity* 31 (June 26, 2007): 1849–58.

INDEX

Underscored page references indicate boxed text. **Boldface** references indicate photographs.

Chris Freytag, a fitness professional and mother of three teenagers, understands firsthand the challenges of balancing healthy habits with the demands of a busy life. A contributing editor at *Prevention Magazine* and author of *Shortcuts to Big Weight Loss,* Chris is also the founder of Motivating Bodies, Inc., a fitness coaching program. She has hosted many Prevention Fitness Systems' DVDs, is on the board of directors for the American Council on Exercise, teaches classes part-time at Life-Time Fitness, and is frequently featured in many magazines, newspapers, and TV shows. She lives in Minnesota with her husband and children.

ABOUT THE AUTHORS

Alyssa Shaffer is an award-winning writer and editor, specializing in health, fitness, and nutrition. She is a contributing editor to *Prevention* and the former fitness director of *Fitness* magazine. She also contributes to *Runner's World, Woman's Day, Parents,* and numerous other magazines and newspapers and is the author of *The A-List Workout.* Alyssa lives in New York City with her husband, Scott, and their twins, Nolan and Layla.

Jumpstart weight loss and maximize fat burn
with this tested 14-day program!

Do you want to see quick results that will really last? Then PREVENTION has the breakthrough DVD set you've been hoping for!

Each of these revolutionary workout DVDs is broken into ultra-efficient 15-minute segments, so you can shape up and trim down in just a few minutes a day. Choose your favorite segment for busy days, or use both DVDs together for a super-effective total body workout!

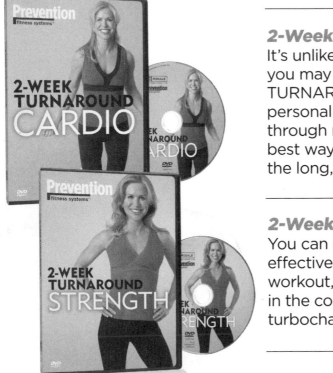

2-Week Turnaround: Strength—
It's unlike any strength-training routine you may have tried before. 2-WEEK TURNAROUND author and certified personal trainer Chris Freytag combed through research to determine the very best way to burn more calories and shape the long, lean muscles you crave!

2-Week Turnaround: Cardio—
You can enjoy one of the easiest, most effective workouts ever! With this DVD workout, you can blast fat and slim down in the comfort of your own home and turbocharge your weight loss!

See for yourself ... try it at home and step into a slim, new you in minutes a day!

Visit pvtwoweekturnaround.com/TR and order your set today!

201280001